The Rhetoric of Midwifery

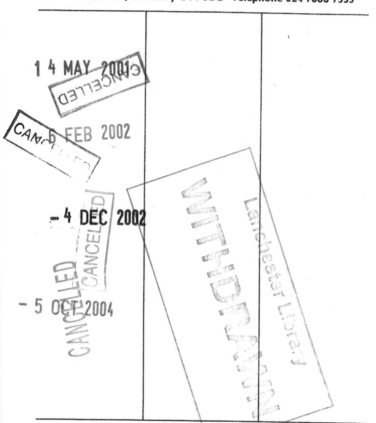

The Rhetoric of Midwifery

GENDER, KNOWLEDGE, AND POWER

MARY M. LAY

Rutgers University Press
New Brunswick, New Jersey, and London

Coventry University

Library of Congress Cataloging-in-Publication Data

Lay, Mary M.
    The rhetoric of midwifery : gender, knowledge, and power / Mary M. Lay.
      p. cm.
    Includes bibliographical references and index.
    ISBN 0-8135-2778-3 (cloth : alk. paper). — ISBN 0-8135-2779-1 (pbk. : alk. paper)
    1. Midwifery—Minnesota. 2. Midwives—Legal status, laws, etc.—Minnesota. 3. Midwifery—Political aspects—Minnesota. I. Title.
    RG950.L39   2000
    618.2′0233—dc21   199-43562
                                             CIP

British Cataloging-in-Publication data for this book is available from the British Library

Manufactured in the United States of America

To my parents

CONTENTS

PREFACE

Michel Foucault challenged scholars to investigate the local centers of the knowledge/discourse/power relationship, and, at first glance, this case study of the efforts of Minnesota traditional or direct-entry midwives to become licensed seemed an ideal way to meet that challenge. However, the study turned out to be much more than that. Between 1991 and 1995 the Minnesota Department of Health and Board of Medical Practice held public hearings to discuss the status of direct-entry midwives, who were practicing underground or a-legally in the state. Sitting across the table from each other for the first time were established physicians of obstetrics and gynecology, nurses and nurse-midwives who headed such organizations as Minnesota Nurses' Association and the regional chapter of the American College of Nurse-Midwives, malpractice lawyers, and direct-entry midwives. Although those midwives who belonged to the state midwifery Guild had been politically active, others were stepping into public view for the first time. Immediately, it became clear that this was a rare opportunity to study medical and midwifery practices in conflict, the use of discourse to maintain professional jurisdictions, the exclusive claim to scientific knowledge and discourse by dominant professions, and the cultural status granted to women's experience and knowledge of their bodies.

Certainly many fine books on midwives have been published in the last few decades. Many take a historical approach, some are based on interviews and life stories of practicing midwives, and some trace the legal battles of past and current midwives. This book is the first, I believe, to offer a rhetorical study of midwifery, to understand the arguments used to celebrate or suppress this centuries-old practice. Thus, the texts and public testimony originating within the Minnesota hearings provide the basis to understand the ideologies and value systems of midwifery and medical practice and why the two systems constantly seem in conflict. However, to place these texts and testimony in a broader context, I also looked back at the history of midwifery to capture the echoes from the past that resonated in the Minnesota hearings. I also relied on a source increasingly used by modern scholars: the Internet. Midwives across the United States and across the world share their feelings and protocols through computer mediated communication. They may still rely on natural remedies: herbs and the touch of their own hands to help mothers birth, but they depend on the computer keyboard to share birth stories with their sisters in other locations.

Finally, I hope that this book will not only offer its readers new understanding of how the hegemonic medical profession maintains its jurisdiction claims and how midwifery practice currently responds to those claims, but also insight into the role that discourse or language plays throughout these interactions. Scholars and students of rhetoric, women's studies, speech communication, history, women's health and medicine, public policy, medical ethics and humanities, and sociology should find the book of interest. I also hope that activists of alternative medicine and midwifery will learn much from the story of how the Minnesota midwives sought public and professional recognition.

This study would not have been possible without the warm and generous welcome I received from the Minnesota home birth community. The Minnesota midwives and their home birth clients invited me into their homes and to their meetings and helped me understand the philosophy and values of their special community. I also appreciate the support I received from the Minnesota Board of Medical Practice and Department of Health. These agencies provided me with audio tapes and the rule writing drafts from each public hearing and welcomed my presence at each meeting. I also want to thank my research assistants: Margaret Connelly assembled materials and transcribed tapes in the early stage of the study, Lise Hansen helped me compile secondary sources, and Amy Koerber located historical documents and read through the final drafts of the book. The reviewers and editors of the *Quarterly Journal of Speech*, and my co-writers of this early piece, showed me how to clarify my analysis. Charles Bazerman introduced me to the valuable work done on the professions by Andrew Abbott, Alan Gross encouraged me throughout the writing and publication process, Elizabeth Tebeaux introduced me to the work of Elizabeth Cellier, Laura Gurak advised me on issues of intellectual property but allowed me to make my own decisions, Bruce Henderson reminded me to tell a good story, and other friends and family encouraged me every step along the way. Jack Selzer and Deborah Kuhn McGregor gave excellent suggestions on earlier versions of the book. I presented various portions of this study at the Speech Communication Association in Chicago in October 1992, the Center on Women and Public Policy at the University of Minnesota in May 1993, the Conference on College Composition and Communication in Nashville in March 1994 and in Phoenix in March 1997, and the Gender, Women, and Science Conference in Minneapolis in May 1995. Finally, Robbie Davis-Floyd was generous in sharing information about the complex challenges that direct-entry midwives face at this time in their history, and, in some cases, Robbie provided me with the very language I needed to refine this book. Finally I thank David Myers, Brigitte Goldstein, and the staff at Rutgers University Press.

The Rhetoric of Midwifery

CHAPTER 1

The Current Debate over Direct-Entry Midwifery in the United States

I came to birth having been born at home. I had certain expectations that birth was a nonmedical event, due to my upbringing. I was born somewhere else; I was not born into this culture. And so, my first exposure to American medical health care came with the birth of my first child. Although medically speaking, the birth had a good outcome, emotionally speaking the birth to me was really disastrous and traumatic. I had no intention of becoming a midwife. I am entirely self-taught, self-trained, self-everything. It was the early 70s, and there were certain assumptions of the time, given the subculture that I lived in. The subculture that I lived in said that there were really no problems with birth, except those caused by the medical establishment.

*W*ith these words, in early November 1991, a traditional or direct-entry midwife, whom I call Rita Ortiz,[1] began her testimony before the Midwifery Study Advisory Group, a group charged with recommending to the Minnesota Department of Health and Board of Medical Practice whether direct-entry midwives should be regulated by the state. Direct-entry midwives enter directly into midwifery education and practice, rather than through the discipline of nursing, the route followed by their sister nurse-midwives. Rita Ortiz's testimony followed that of Rachel Waters, a pathologist at the University of Minnesota, who had just presented a statistical analysis of risks in pregnancy. For Waters's presentation, the room was darkened to accommodate the overhead projector that displayed her many graphs and charts. Out of a random sampling of five thousand hospital births from May 1988 to 1989 in Minnesota, her Minnesota Obstetrics Management Initiative or MOMI project identified and ranked twenty-five thousand risk factors in pregnancy, risk factors best managed in a hospital setting by health care professionals, according to Waters. By contrast, Ortiz, speaking with a slight accent, sat at the table, surrounded by physicians, nurses, nurse-midwives, direct-entry midwives, home birth parents, medical malpractice lawyers, and birth educators, and described her personal journey to midwifery.

At the time that Ortiz explained how she came to become a midwife, the Minnesota Board of Medical Practice had been charged by the state legislature for decades with licensing direct-entry midwives, but the board had never developed the required licensing examination. Therefore, on the day Ortiz gave her testimony, all of Minnesota's direct-entry midwives were practicing without a license in a sort of a-legal status. Tales of poor home birth outcomes, passed on by physicians, had recently reached the board in the Twin Cities and had become the catalyst for renewed scrutiny of the midwives. At the same time, the board and the Department of Health were not sure just how many planned home births actually occurred in the state, as midwives did not sign birth certificates, and, if a mother or infant had to be transported to the hospital, the midwife usually identified herself as a sister or friend to avoid scrutiny by the hospital or state. The two state agencies wanted these statistics.

Several members of the Minnesota Midwives' Guild actually welcomed this open discussion of their practices. They hoped the discussion might bring legal sanction for them to administer drugs, such as pitocin for postpartum hemorrhages, and to perform certain procedures at home, such as emergency episiotomies and suturing of first- and second-degree perineal tears (see appendix B for definitions of these and other birth terms). These measures would enable midwives to respond to emergencies at home; administering pitocin could stop sudden bleeding by encouraging the uterus to recover from labor, and an episiotomy or incision in the perineal tissue would allow the midwife to deliver a distressed baby quickly. If the midwives had permission to suture a slight tear the mother might experience as the baby passed from her body, they could avoid transporting the mother to the hospital. However, other direct-entry midwives in Minnesota—particularly those practicing in the religious communities where faith encouraged home births and home schools—feared any state interference and were not interested in incorporating these pharmaceuticals and specialized skills into their home birth practices.

Moreover, Minnesota's direct-entry midwives were aware of the controversies that emerged during other states' debates about the legal status of midwifery. During the period of the Minnesota public hearings (1991–1995), some states not only licensed direct-entry midwives but also set up schools of midwifery. For example, Florida's governor, Lawton Chiles, proclaimed October 10–14, 1994, Licensed Midwife Week, as he set the goal of having half the state's babies born with midwives in attendance. By the summer of 1996, Florida began graduating students from five direct-entry midwifery programs. By contrast, on December 13, 1995, midwife Roberta Devers-Scott was subjected to an undercover investigation in which employees of the New York State Education Department posed as potential clients to gather information about her practice. In New York, the only midwives who can be licensed are those who complete a program in midwifery whose admission requirements include a nursing degree and which leads to a baccalaureate degree. Therefore, direct-entry midwife Devers-Scott was arrested and charged with the felony of practicing midwifery without a license. In other states, such as Minnesota, direct-entry midwives were allowed to practice within a gray area of the law, ignored as long as they didn't step over certain nebulous boundaries.

Thus, as Ortiz described her personal journey to midwifery before the Midwifery Study Advisory Group, another story began, one that lasted for another seven years. This first advisory group made its recommendations to the state agencies in Minnesota to make midwifery more visible and to encourage cooperative agreements between midwives and medical care providers. Sympathetic legislators wrote bills that would have enacted their recommendations, but the bills were considered too controversial to bring before the state house and senate for debate. Because of its statutory obligation to license direct-entry midwives, the Board of Medical Practice convened a second advisory group, the Licensing Rule Writing Group, to write licensing laws but, after eighteen months, declared that the process had failed.

In the spring of 1997, the Board of Medical Practice set up a third task force, consisting of the current copresidents of the Minnesota Midwives' Guild, a consumer representative to the guild, a certified nurse-midwife, an obstetrician, a family practice physician, a lobbyist from the Minnesota Medical Association, a lobbyist from the Minnesota Nurses Association, a representative from the Minnesota Nursing Board, an attorney from the Minnesota Department of Health, and an attorney from the Minnesota Board of Medical Practice. Rather than conducting public testimony, this smaller and select group was charged with reaching consensus on what proved to be the most controversial part of licensing rules—scope of practice for direct-entry midwifery. However, in early 1998 the Minnesota board decided that the group did not meet their goal (Dixon, "Regional Reports—January 1998" 8). Had this process been successful, the Minnesota Midwives' Guild would still have faced some hurdles. The guild would have to had to write a bill on midwives' legal status to be presented to the 1998 legislature and to raise the money and "personpower" to lobby for the bill (Dixon, "Regional Reports—July 1997" 6). The collapse of this third task force meant that the Board of Medical Practice would most likely go to the legislature sometime in the future and ask that its statutory obligation to license direct-entry midwives be removed, making it possible to charge Minnesota direct-entry midwives with practicing medicine, nursing, or nurse-midwifery without a license. The Minnesota Midwives' Guild then became the Minnesota Council of Certified Professional Midwives, acknowledging members' status within their own international professional organization. However, in the fall of 1998, they were faced with the Board of Medical Practice's criminal investigation of one of Minnesota's direct-entry midwives (Dixon, "Regional Reports—September 1998" 9). At the time I write these words then, direct-entry midwives in Minnesota are still practicing within that a-legal, "gray" area—not legal, as they continue to practice without a license, and not illegal, as the state provides no way for them to become licensed.

The Minnesota Debates

To understand how the debates concerned the fate of direct-entry midwifery in Minnesota and to understand the national context for these public hearings, one must know the individuals and organizations as well as their relationships with each other. Initially, those participating in such debates could be cast into particular roles, given certain social and professional status, distinguished by their education and professional affiliations. However, during the Minnesota hearings these participants stepped out of these roles in order to try on others, or they were granted varying degrees of credibility, depending on the success of their arguments during the hearings.

The Direct-Entry Midwife

In the simplest terms, the direct-entry (also called the lay, empirical, independent, or traditional) midwife enters into a relationship with parents who plan to birth at home or at a birth clinic managed and staffed by direct-entry midwives. By one estimate, there are 2,000 to 3,000 direct-entry midwives currently practicing in the United States who attend between 11,500 and 12,500 births at home or in free-standing birth clinics per year (Sonnenstuhl; Davis-Floyd, "Development"; Rooks 9). During the time of the Minnesota hearings (1991–1995), seventeen states licensed, registered, or certified direct-entry midwives: Alaska, Arkansas, Arizona, California, Colorado, Delaware, Florida, Louisiana, Montana, New Hampshire, New Mexico, Oregon, Rhode Island, South Carolina, Texas, Washington, and Wyoming. In eleven states, direct-entry midwives were legal through judicial interpretation or statutory inference, and, in seven states, they were not legally defined but were not specifically prohibited from practice. In six states, direct-entry midwives were legal by statute but licensure was not available, and, in the remaining nine states, they were prohibited through statutory restriction or judicial interpretation.

Direct-entry midwives are primarily distinguished from nurse-midwives in that they generally do not have nursing degrees. Although, in the past, direct-entry midwives such as Rita Ortiz relied primarily on self-education and apprenticeship, today most direct-entry midwives combine apprenticeship with some university education or attendance at formal direct-entry schools such as the Seattle Midwifery School (Davis-Floyd, "Birth of a Dream"). However, the issue of apprenticeship is still seen by many midwives as the essential distinction between direct-entry midwives and nurse-midwives, because the apprenticeship confirms "connective and embodied experiential learning" and a "deep trust in women and in birth" (Davis-Floyd, "Development" 2). Apprenticeships involve observing and assisting practicing midwives who attend births; watching them as they deal with all stages of pregnancy, labor, and delivery; helping them deal with emergencies; and "talking endlessly with them about every detail of their care" (Davis-Floyd, "Birth of a Dream" 4). Judith Rooks summarizes the direct-entry midwifery community as follows:

> The direct-entry midwifery community retains a strong commitment to education through apprenticeship; a preference for experiential learning; belief in the validity of intuition and intuitive knowledge; confidence in private, tuition-based midwifery schools that are free-standing and under the control of midwives; and a general distrust of universities . . . they are psychologically and politically bonded by their common history, by out-of-hospital births as their mode of practice, by opposition to typical medical

obstetric care, and by the dichotomy between CNMs [certified nurse-mid-wives] and all other midwives. (229)

Direct-entry midwives focus on the normalcy of birth, on each woman as an individual within the unique context of her family and her life. As Rooks describes this philosophy, "The midwife strives to support the woman in ways that empower her to achieve her goals and hopes for her pregnancy, birth and baby, and for her role as mother. Midwives believe that women's bodies are well designed for birth and try to protect, support, and avoid interfering with the normal processes of labor, de-livery, and the reuniting of the mother and newborn after their separation of birth" (2). Direct-entry midwives view nurse-midwives, given their required nursing train-ing within nursing, as taught to be subordinate to physicians from whom they take orders and upon whom they rely in difficult cases. During lengthy interviews with direct-entry midwives, Davis-Floyd found that they tend to see nurse-midwives as more likely to accept a "medicalized, technological approach to birth that often cre-ates pathology" and that produces midwives who are afraid of birth ("Birth of a Dream" 4–5). Finally, whereas nurse-midwives might handle treatment of minor illnesses over a client's life span, direct-entry midwives focus exclusively on the independent care of normal birth and on management of complications, such as breech births, postpartum hemorrhage, and multiple births that, they believe, do not require technological interventions but in many cases can be handled successfully at home.

Much as Rita Ortiz defined herself in her November 1991 testimony during the Minnesota hearings, direct-entry midwives contrast themselves to those birth attendants with more professional status and medical background. Moreover, direct-entry midwives are legally defined as different than nurses, nurse-midwives, and physicians. For example, Arkansas' legal definition of "lay midwife" distinguishes her from others: "Any person other than a physician or certified nurse midwife who shall manage care during the pregnancy of any woman or of her newborn during the antepartum, intrapartum, or postpartum periods . . ." (Arkansas Department of Health 6). States such as Florida extend this distinction between direct-entry midwives and other medical care providers by emphasizing the degree of parental responsibility in deciding to birth with the aid of a direct-entry midwife: " 'Midwifery' " means the practice of supervising the conduct of a normal labor and childbirth, with the in-formed consent of the parent; the practice of advising the parents as to the progress of the childbirth; and the practice of rendering prenatal and postnatal care" (Florida Health Care Administration 2). Other states such as Alaska recognize not just the social and emotional aspects of midwifery care but also specify when a direct-entry midwife must consult with the medical community—when she must relinquish her independence:

> The "practice of midwifery" means providing necessary supervision, health care, and education to women during pregnancy, labor, and the postpartum period, conducting deliveries on the midwife's own responsibility, and pro-viding immediate postpartum care of the new born; "practice of midwifery" includes preventative measures, the identification of physical, social and

emotional needs of the newborn and the women, and *arranging for consultation, referral, and continued involvement when the care required extends beyond the abilities of the midwife, and the execution of emergency
measures in the absence of medical assistance . . .*

(Alaska Department of Commerce, 8, emphasis added)

Thus, the direct-entry midwife is legally defined in contrast to other health care
providers. Moreover, parents are informed about the risks and responsibilities of
choosing home birth, and, when a direct-entry midwife is required to interact with
the medical community, she finds herself in a subordinate position.

At the time of the Minnesota hearings, many direct-entry midwives belonged
to the Minnesota Midwives' Guild, a self-governing, peer-review group, which recognized three categories of birth attendants: Apprentice Midwife, Certified Traditional Midwife, and Senior Certified Traditional Midwife. Classification and
certification were based on the guild's requirements for number of births observed
and assisted, demonstrated ability to follow the guild's *Standards of Care and Certification Guide*, and, in the last two categories, a passing score on the North American Registry of Midwives exam. The guild was founded in 1988 and many of the
founding members, such as Rita Ortiz, came from Genesis, a midwives' group
formed in 1975, by "women who spontaneously evolved from being mothers to being midwives to fill the void left by the retirement of Minnesota's last licensed midwife, Ebba Kirschbaum" (Minnesota Midwives' Guild, *Standards of Care, 1st ed.*
3). The guild had about forty members at the time of the Minnesota hearings—although fewer were practicing at any one time—and the guild had as a lobbyist,
Mary Emerson, president of the International Cesarean Awareness Network/
Cesarean Prevention Movement of Southwest Minnesota, who actively participated
in the hearings. Those direct-entry midwives in Minnesota who chose not to belong
to the guild were often members of religious fellowships or ethnic communities
such as the large Southeast Asian community in the Twin Cities, or sought greater
freedom of practice outside the guild-dominated midwifery community.

Many direct-entry midwives in Minnesota and throughout the United States
also belong to the Midwives' Alliance of North America (MANA), founded in 1982
to "build cooperation among midwives and to promote midwifery as a standard of
health care for women and their families" (*MANA News*). MANA welcomes all
midwives, certified or not, and holds an annual conference. In October 1994 MANA
revised its Core Competencies to include a definition of the direct-entry midwife that
recognized such aspects as the midwife's autonomy, the normalcy of birth and the
uniqueness of each pregnancy, and the empowerment possible in birth:

> C. Midwives work as autonomous practitioners, collaborating with other
> health and social service providers when necessary . . .
> E. Midwives understand that female physiology and childbearing are
> normal processes, and work to optimize the well-being of mothers and their
> developing babies as the foundation of caregiving . . .
> H. Midwives recognize the empowerment inherent in the childbearing

experience and strive to support women to make informed decisions and take responsibility for their own well-being . . .
L. Midwives understand that the parameters of "normal" vary widely and recognize that each pregnancy and birth is unique.

(MANA Core Competencies 1994, 31)

MANA established the North American Registry of Midwives, which became a separate but affiliated organization. NARM began certifying midwives, called Certified Professional Midwives (CPMs), in 1994. The NARM exam is based on the Core Competencies established by MANA and on the results of a survey of 800 practicing home birth midwives (one-third of whom were certified nurse-midwives) made to determine what these practicing midwives felt were essential for entry-level practice in out-of-hospital settings. Later iterations of the exam (Forms C and D) added a skills component to the written portion of the exam and were psychometrically validated. MANA and NARM hoped to reach midwives practicing in the United States who, before CPM certification, were "hindered" in their interactions with other health professionals and in their dealings with "agencies such as governments and insurance companies" ("Setting the Standards" 17). Thus, one goal of the NARM exam was to professionalize direct-entry midwives. During the Minnesota hearings, the NARM exam was discussed as a potential exam for Minnesota licensing, as NARM and MANA were lobbying for similar results in at least twenty other states (Davis-Floyd, "Development" 4).

At the urging of direct-entry midwifery and home birth representatives who were inspired by the MANA Core Competencies, the August 30, 1994 draft of the Minnesota licensing rules defined the direct-entry midwife as "an autonomous health care professional who provides primary health care services during pregnancy, birth and the postpartum period for women and new borns" (Minnesota Board of Medical Practice, "Proposed Rules" 3). (See appendix C for a brief chronology of the hearings and the drafts produced.) This definition stressed the direct-entry midwife's independence from the medical community. Regardless of her individual background, goals, and values—the personal name and face she may take on in this story—the direct-entry midwife's emphasis on independence and her professional organization's certification options place her in potential legal conflict with other health care providers.

The Certified Nurse-Midwife

A certified nurse-midwife (CNM) is a registered nurse who has completed an university-affiliated educational program approved by the American College of Nurse-Midwives (ACNM), passed a national certification exam, and met the other criteria of ACNM. Nurse-midwives may complete a one-year certificate program or a two-year master's degree program in nursing, public health, or midwifery (Sonnenstuhl). The CNM works in collaboration with or under the supervision of a physician and aids in births that occur in hospital settings or in birth clinics and, in a few states, at home. Participating in the Minnesota conversations was the president of the Twin Cities Chapter of the American College of Nurse Midwives, a group that represents 80 percent of the certified nurse-midwives in Minnesota. During the 1990s in Minnesota, only one CNM attended home births.

Toward the end of the Minnesota conversations in 1995, a new accreditation offered by ACNM placed this professional organization of nurse-midwives in an uneasy relationship with direct-entry midwives. In an effort to "move their profession away from its embeddedness in nursing and toward greater independence and autonomy," ACNM's Division of Accreditation expanded its scope to include midwifery education and certification for non-nurse birth attendants (Davis-Floyd, "Development" 1). In a press release, the ACNM stressed the formal education and professional standing that it could offer non-nurse midwives: Graduates of its accredited basic midwifery educational programs "will possess no less than a baccalaureate degree from an institution for higher learning recognized by the U.S. Department of Education, and, upon successfully passing the national certification examination administered by the ACNM Certification Council, Inc. (ACC), will receive the professional designation of Certified Midwife (CM)" ("Women's Health Care Initiative" 1). This move on the part of the ACNM was predicted to "infuriate" those members who held nursing "dear" and to "thrill" those who wanted to be freed of supervision of nursing boards and to be regulated instead by midwifery boards (Davis-Floyd, "Development" 6).

However, this move proved problematic for direct-entry midwives who might be regulated by the same midwifery boards. The MANA president warned her members in the association's July 1995 newsletter that the ACNM intended to inform the states in which direct-entry midwives were licensed or were a-legal that ACNM leaders were "the only ones to set the standard for midwifery" (Barnes 3). While the route to MANA's certified professional midwife included the self-training that Rita Ortiz experienced and the apprenticeship possibilities that the Minnesota Midwives' Guild acknowledged, the ACNM's Certified Midwifery program stressed formal educational routes. ACNM's Division of Accreditation would recognize only midwifery schools with university affiliation and whose teachers were CNMs. Schools such as the Seattle Midwifery School, accredited by MANA's accrediting body, the Midwifery Education Accreditation Council (MEAC), would not be recognized by the ACNM's Division of Accreditation (Davis-Floyd, "Development" 3).

Decisions in some states reflected this conflict. In Georgia, nurse-midwives objected to NARM-certified midwives being called certified professional midwives in proposed legislation "on the ground that it will confuse the public" ("Regional Reports: Georgia" 6). In Vermont, the ACNM offered a position statement on direct-entry midwifery legislation: "The educational requirements are clearly unacceptable to ensure the health of mothers and babies in Vermont . . . We cannot compromise on the requirement of professional midwifery training being within an accredited educational program" ("Regional Reports: Vermont" 4). The conflict between direct-entry midwives and nurse-midwives over certification focused on the educational routes to midwifery.

NARM's certified professional midwife versus ACNM's certified midwife—the slight difference in the titles was not the only confusing issue. At the time that the Minnesota public hearings took place, ACNM and MANA seemed to work to cooperate with each other as both initially endorsed two different paths to certified midwifery—one based on nursing and one on direct entry with "equivalent midwifery skills" (Barnes, November 1994, 3). But by July 1995, the associations appeared so much in conflict that the president of MANA began a fundraising campaign to support MANA's "official certification route for direct entry or independent midwives" (Barnes, July 1995, 11). Communications sent out over computer listservs by ACNM members stressed how the nurse-midwifery model ensured quality of care:

> In the USA, Certified Nurse Midwives are growing and flourishing, numbering over 4000. They are making inroads in many ways, bringing midwifery care into the hospitals, providing care for low income families and becoming a respected provider and part of the team of providers in medical school programs, training residents in normal birthing. Usually, CNMs work in a collaborative or co-management relationship with physicians. This implies teamwork and promotes continuity of care.   (Sonnenstuhl)

With the arrest of direct-entry midwife Roberta Devers-Scott, MANA representatives believed that New York state was being used as a test case by ACNM and sympathetic legislators to create a single profession of midwifery (Schlinger 24).

Originally the New York Midwifery Practice Act seemed designed to increase midwifery care and to provide more medical backup for direct-entry midwives. Before the Act was passed, only CNMs were recognized and only under an obscure clause in the Sanitation Code (Davis-Floyd, "Birth of a Dream" 2–3). New York CNMs who actively support the new law envisioned a "new kind of professional midwife" who would be

> a graduate of one of numerous new programs they would design . . . [and] would graduate with the same skills as CNMs, but without having her life derailed by lengthy passage through nursing training, much of which is viewed as irrelevant to nursing. She would be likely to have more independence of thought and spirit than those who had been socialized into a nursing model, she would be more likely to work in freestanding birth centers and/or to attend home births, and she would be a pioneer who would help to reconstitute midwifery as an autonomous profession. . . . (2–3)

However, final revisions of the Act turned unlicensed midwifery from a misdemeanor into a felony and made it impossible for non-ACNM-certified direct-entry midwives to become licensed. To date, only one ACNM-accredited, university-based, direct-entry program has been recognized—in New York—and it accepts only a handful of direct-entry students per year; a lack of funding has curtailed the opening of other such programs (Davis-Floyd, "Development" 7).

When the Minnesota public hearings began, certified nurse-midwives at the table and behind the scenes kept in close contact with their ACNM colleagues, and both the nurse-midwives and the direct-entry midwives were well aware of the battles being fought in other states.

The Registered Nurse

A registered nurse graduates from an accredited, baccalaureate program or school of nursing and works under the supervision of a physician or other health care professional. Two professional nurses' organizations sent representatives to the Minnesota midwifery advisory groups: The Minnesota Board of Nursing sent its executive director and the Minnesota Nurses' Association sent a lobbyist. The formal and informal affiliations between nurses and nurse-midwives are strong. The Board of Nursing licenses the nurse-midwives as nurses, and the Minnesota Nurses' Association invites nurse-midwives into its membership. In fact, the lobbyist from the Minnesota Nurses' Association attended fewer of the public hearings but "took her lead" from the president of the Twin Cities Chapter of the ACNM.[2]

Again, the distinction between the certified nurse-midwives, registered nurses, and the direct-entry midwives is critical in some states where direct-entry midwives can be legally charged with practicing nursing or nurse-midwifery without a license. For example, in the fall of 1994 the Maryland Board of Nursing brought charges against Pennsylvania direct-entry midwife Judi Mentzer for practicing nursing without a license. Mentzer, who was certified by the Pennsylvania Midwives Association (comparable to the Minnesota Midwives' Guild), attended home births in both Pennsylvania and Maryland ("Regional Reports: Maryland"). The usual penalty for such charges: a fine and an injunction from further midwifery practice.

The Physician

Physicians graduate from medical school and are licensed by the state Board of Medical Practice and sit on its committees. Medical education and physicians' expertise constitute authoritative knowledge about birth in much of U.S. culture. As summarized by Judith Rooks, this authoritative knowledge promotes certain assumptions about the role of the physician in monitoring pregnancy:

> The main focus of medical education, training, knowledge, skills, and roles is pathology—the diagnosis and treatment of disease and trauma. . . . The physician's unique and awesome role lies in his or her ability to diagnose and treat disease, especially the use of medications and surgery. . . . Closer examination of *Williams Obstetrics* shows that its chapters on normal pregnancy focus primarily on the anatomy and physiology of the female reproductive system and the development of the embryo and fetus *at the level of the body's organs and the cells.* (126, original emphasis)

This view of medical authoritative knowledge critiques the focus on pathology that reinforces the impression that a woman's body is imperfect and that medicine can "improve on nature," that every pregnant woman and her infant are at risk, and the "you cannot assume that any birth is normal until it is over" (Rooks 127). The criteria that constitute *normal* for the physician, then, are much narrower than those assumed by the midwife. Risk assessment—such as that used in Rachel Waters's Minnesota Obstetrics Management Initiative or MOMI project as presented to the Minnesota Midwifery Study Advisory Group—relies on "tools that assign risk points to an extensive list of conditions that are statistically associated with higher-than-average perinatal mortality and formalized risk assessment processes that assign a risk score to women based on the sum of the points assigned to all of their high-risk factors" (Rooks 280). A direct-entry midwife might accept a pregnant woman whom a physician considered high risk, if the midwife were experienced in managing the condition and the client trusted her body and her midwife. Finally, monitoring devices used in hospital births, which even physicians now suspect might overdiagnose conditions, have expanded the proportion of pregnancies deemed "abnormal" or "pathological" so that, in the view of many midwives, "the distinction between risk factors and actual pathology has been lost, and women with high-risk factors are treated as though they have actual complications" (Rooks 448–449).

One of the more active participants in the Minnesota story was the Minnesota section chair of the American College of Obstetrics and Gynecology and president-elect of the Minnesota Ob/Gyn Society. This physician saw her role in the Minnesota conversations, particularly the licensing rule writing process, as "not only representing the physician community, but also as a resource to the traditional midwife as to what I thought might pass the Board of Medical Practice review from a medical standpoint."[3] Although she had her own opinions, her suggestions and responses were often framed in terms of how her colleagues would react.

Behind the scenes, the Minnesota Medical Association reviewed and commented on drafts of the licensing rules and communicated its reactions to the Board of Medical Practice staff. For example, the Minnesota Medical Association requested that the terms "autonomous" and "primary care services" be stricken from the definition of a direct-entry midwife in the licensing rules draft (Minnesota Medical Association). Again, Rachel Waters's MOMI project was considered a potential source of standards during the licensing process by the Board of Medical Practice.

Minnesota's as well as other states' agencies and legislatures struggle with what is "medical" and what is "natural" or "normal" about birthing procedures, terms that again distinguish between the practice of physicians and the practice of direct-entry midwives. In some states, this attempt to establish distinct jurisdictions has led to some awkward relations among birth care providers. For example, in Wyoming during the time of the Minnesota midwifery hearings, although direct-entry midwives could attend home births, they could not give prenatal or postnatal care, care considered by the Wyoming attorney general as diagnostic and therefore medical. Wyoming direct-entry midwives who offered prenatal and postnatal care were subject to prosecution for practicing medicine without a license (Becker et al., Wyoming Board of Medicine).

The State

In the Minnesota conversations, three groups represented the state: the Department of Health, the Board of Medical Practice, and the Legislature. The Health Occupations Program of the Department of Health made a commitment to the Board of Medical Practice to "study and make recommendations about the need to regulate traditional midwifery and how best to protect those individuals who decide to have homebirth" and formed the first advisory group (Marschall). This advisory group, before which Rita Ortiz testified in November 1991, produced a report that the commissioner of health endorsed with some uneasiness:

> I have a concern that the recommendations are insufficient to adequately protect the public from harm caused by untrained or incompetent home-birth attendants. We cannot abide practices and activity that result in serious, irreparable harm to women and infants. However, there are also limits to the control and regulation that government can exercise and effectively implement. Therefore, the recommendations in this report strike a balance, and I support them.   (Marschall np)

These recommendations included creating a Midwifery Advisory Council that would work with the Department of Health to develop a consumer education brochure for prospective parents considering home birth (Minnesota Department of Health, *Regulation* xiii).

In March 1993, Minnesota State Senators Sandra Pappas and Carol Flynn and House Representative Kay Brown wrote companion bills that were ruled "too controversial" to bring to the floor for full discussion. These bills would have repealed the requirement that the Board of Medical Practice provide a licensing route for direct-entry midwives and would have created an office of midwifery practice in the Department of Health in line with the first advisory group's recommendations. This office would

> investigate complaints and take and enforce disciplinary actions against all midwives for violations or prohibited conduct, as defined in section 148.498. The office shall also serve as a clearinghouse on midwifery services through the dissemination of objective information to consumers and through the development and performance of public education activities, including outreach, regarding the provision of midwifery services and midwives who provide these services.   (Minnesota State Senate 3)

Throughout all the Minnesota discussions, the Department of Health, the Legislature, and the Board of Medical Practice emphasized their obligation to "protect" Minnesota citizens from unsafe practices and practitioners. This obligation is echoed throughout the regulatory documents in other states. For example, in its purpose statement, Arkansas's "Regulations Governing Lay Midwife Practice" refers to the General Assembly's directive to the Arkansas Board of Health to "regulate and ultimately protect the health of the public" (Arkansas Department of Health 5). Similarly, Florida's Agency for Health Care Administration in the Division of Medical Quality Assurance states: "The Legislature finds that the interests of public health require the regulation of the practice of midwifery in this state for the purpose of protecting the health and welfare of mothers and infants" (1). The state agencies and legislatures, in essence, place their citizens under surveillance to protect them from unwise decisions and unsafe practices and call upon scientific and medical advisors to help them identify these practices.

The Minnesota Board of Medical Practice assigned a staff member to assist in writing the licensing rules and regulations for direct-entry midwifery. That staff member suggested procedures for creating the drafts, provided boilerplate language from the rules and regulations for other practices, explained the conventions of the genre and often the justification for the limits they placed on practices, and served as an informal co-chair during several hearings. This staff member held a nursing degree and was a lawyer. The director of the Board of Medical Practice attended the first of the licensing rule writing hearings to explain the process by which licensing rules and regulations were approved, and chaired the last hearings in which the board suspended the licensing rule writing effort. Finally, a representative from the Department of Health drafted the recommendations that emerged from the first Minnesota hearings, during which the general topic of regulation was debated.

Other than those representatives from the Board of Medical Practice and the Department of Health, it is much more difficult to put a face on members of the state agencies that were charged with considering the legal status of direct-entry midwifery. However, the relationship between the Minnesota Medical Association and the Board of Medical Practice is obvious. For example, in September 1996, the Public Policy Committee of the board reported on two of several new initiatives for discussion, one on infant circumcision and one on physician sexual misconduct. The Minnesota Medical Association was invited to send representatives to each working group (Minnesota Board Minutes). In November 1996, board membership consisted of sixteen members, ten of whom were physicians; one dentist and one lawyer served among the sixteen. In fact, Rachel Waters served as vice president of the board. The Board of Medical Practice, on the basis of membership alone, appeared to be very much a physicians' group.

The Home Birth Client

Another important player in the Minnesota debates was the home birth client, the citizen whom states feel obligated to protect. In a survey of home birth parents throughout the United States, Rooks found that they were usually white, married, and had had other children, either at home or in the hospital. They were a mixture of

> traditional, conservative, home-oriented women; college-educated, middle-class professionals and intellectuals; "New Agers"; members of certain religious groups; women who live in rural areas; women who need inexpensive care because they are not covered by any third-party health payment plan; "survivalists" and other people who are trying to live apart from the mainstream of American society; and Mexican women who want to give birth in the United States. (152)

In general, home birth clients strongly believe that birth is a natural and safe process and seek control of the birth environment. A few home birth clients want no men present during their deliveries or fear hospitals and physicians. In some states, one-third to one-half of home birth parents belong to religious groups that consider birth a spiritual event. Finally, the highest proportion of direct-entry, attended home births take place in the West or the Southwest (Rooks 152).

However, in the Minnesota hearings, neat divisions based on roles fell apart when the home birth parents spoke. Most direct-entry midwives were home birth parents. Uncomfortable questions arose during the hearings: Should a midwife speak in the hearings for those using or those offering midwifery services? If a midwife herself elected to give birth at home during a high-risk pregnancy, should she be protected from herself? If direct-entry midwives were regulated, would home birth parents lose some freedom to choose the degree of technology they would invite into their homes?

A few home birth parents who were not midwives did participate in the Minnesota conversations and contributed to the draft of the licensing rules. However, the roles became even murkier when one outspoken home birth parent revealed her medical profession: chiropractor. Finally, several of the home birth parents came from the religious fellowships in the Twin Cities where home births and home schools are a matter of faith or spiritual calling. At the June 15, 1995 Minnesota public hearing, two of these home birth parents spoke against pursuing regulation: "If you regulate the midwives, you will regulate the parents." From their point of view, the freedom of the home birth parents to choose where to birth conflicted with any regulation of direct-entry midwifery, even if that regulation might protect the direct-entry midwife from prosecution for "practicing" medicine, nursing, or nurse-midwifery without a license.

The Silent

Silent in the Minnesota story were those who sought anonymity or avoided intrusion into their cultural practices. For example, although the opinions of Southeast Asian and Native American midwives would have been welcome in the advisory groups, these midwives either chose not to attend the public hearings or were impossible for the Board of Health and Board of Medical Practice to identify. Often the "midwife" at a home birth in the Southeast Asian or Native American cultures in Minnesota is a mother, mother-in-law, grandmother, aunt, or sister who does not receive payment for her services. The majority of midwives within these cultures would not seek the protection of state agencies or follow their regulations. The Board of Medical Practice recognized this preference, and perhaps the impossibility of regulating these groups, in the March 10, 1995, draft of the licensing rules: "Midwifery services" did not include "gratuitous services provided by family members or services provided pursuant to the requirements or tenets of any established religion."

The Minnesota licensing drafts were not exceptional in excluding certain midwives from scrutiny. For example, the state of Washington's definition of midwifery practice notes that "[n]othing shall be construed in this chapter to prohibit gratuitous services" and that the regulations were not meant to "interfere with the practice of religion" (Washington 1). Therefore, although these absent midwives were considered in the Minnesota public hearings, they did not speak for themselves.

The Importance of the Minnesota Story

Why, then, is the story of the Minnesota hearings important if it had no result, if it led to no change, but simply left the state's direct-entry midwives to practice in a legal limbo? Why is the process of writing licensing rules for Minnesota's direct-entry midwives worthy of study if the process failed to reach its goal? Set within the centuries-old history of midwifery in the United States and other countries, the story is representative of the conflict between medical and state institutions and women's birth knowledge and craft. However, the substance of this story also offers opportunity for new understanding of this conflict and for the relationships within the professions among power, knowledge, gender, and discourse. The Minnesota midwives believe their own knowledge to be authoritative about birth, just as the medical community considers its knowledge to be authoritative. The medical knowledge system carries the authority of experts recognized by state agencies and by culture as a whole, while the knowledge system of the midwives is socially invisible and, in the opinion of many midwives and their supporters, legally oppressed. Within the hearings these two knowledge systems clashed, and the challenge of the midwives was to present their own body of knowledge in a way that would establish professional and social legitimacy, different in many ways from medical knowledge but valid in its own right.

In an important way, then, the Minnesota midwifery hearings demonstrate how the medical community uses discourse to establish its authoritative knowledge about birth and maintain its authority in opposition to other knowledge systems. Specifically, the testimony given at the Minnesota hearings illustrates the uneasy relationship between the hegemonic, technologically based knowledge systems of modern medicine and the marginalized, experientially based knowledge systems of midwifery. Anthropologist Brigitte Jordan has described how knowledge systems compete and gain a power basis; for example, she points out, "[F]or any particular domain several knowledge systems exist, some of which, by consensus, come to carry more weight than others, either because they explain the state of the world better for the purposes at hand (efficacy) or because they are associated with a stronger power base (structural superiority), and usually both" (56). The power of authoritative knowledge, therefore, is "not that it is correct but that it counts" (58). Authoritative knowledge is what participants in any situation consider important and according to which they make decisions and account for their actions. Through this legitimacy and official status, what members of a community consider authoritative knowledge determines accepted discourse about a subject.

At the time of the Minnesota hearing, both communities—the medical community and the midwifery community—had established what they considered authoritative knowledge about birth. These knowledge systems are not complete dichotomies, as midwives use and rely on scientific knowledge and medical tools when appropriate to their practices, just as physicians learn through personal experience. Moreover, scientific studies confirm that medical procedures cause iatrogenic harm and support the midwives' claims to be safe birth attendants. However, the ways the medical community and the midwifery community created their authoritative knowledge, how they established their credibility, what they considered as evidence to support their knowledge, and what educational routes they believed gave one access to their knowledge systems were at times very different. The challenge for the Minnesota direct-entry midwife who wanted professional status through licensing was to identify commonalities between the midwifery and medical knowledge systems while maintaining autonomy and ideological distinction.

Studying these conversations about midwifery and the competing knowledge systems of midwifery and medicine, then, reveals how a community uses discourse—or the written and spoken words that create and reflect the values and goals of a community—to maintain the authority of its knowledge system in a larger social setting, and how knowledge systems that originate in women's experiential knowledge may be devalued and silenced. As Carroll Smith-Rosenberg urges us to ask not what society tells us about gender but what gender tells us about society (19), this study increases our understanding of how women become knowers or the agents of knowledge within their own communities and within the larger society.[4] Because at least this portion of the story does have a definite ending, and the content of the story is reflected in words captured on tape, paper, and even the computer screen, the story enables us to study intersections of gender and power through actual discourse, a "local center" of a power-knowledge relationship, as defined by French philosopher Michel Foucault (*Sexuality* 52). Each community engaged in the Minnesota hearings about midwifery claimed to know the "truth" about birth and women's bodies, and that truth was expressed in definitions, knowledge claims, descriptions of personal experience, and interpretations of statistics. Moreover, because such truths are enshrined in law—laws that may empower or silence certain citizens—citizens may be placed under surveillance and their legal claim to scientific, medical, or technological tools controlled. An examination of the Minnesota midwifery hearings spotlights key intersections of the medical profession and women's rights and of the relationship between power and gender.

Looking again at Ortiz's testimony reveals some of this story's essential features—the clash between medical and midwifery knowledge—when Ortiz referred to the values and assumptions of cultures in conflict. An immigrant from Cuba and influenced by the Santa Cruz birth movement in the 1970s, Ortiz believed that birth was a natural, normal event and that medical intervention caused more problems than it solved. She came to midwifery through an intense personal experience, after she birthed her first child in a hospital. In her testimony, she contrasted the definition of a good outcome, determined by the medical "facts" or "logic," with her feelings and emotions. To become a midwife, Ortiz underwent self-training and apprenticeship, rather than engaging in formal education. Her next words describe her initial experience as a midwife:

> The first birth that I ever attended was in Rochester, Minnesota. It was cold; it was this time of year; there was a blizzard outside. The equipment that was taken to this birth was a pair of sewing scissors with orange handles, which were sterilized over boiling water with two chopsticks, and a pair of

white shoelaces which I obtained at Robert's Shoes on Chicago and Lake on my way out of town.

The woman that I would attend this birth with would later become an obstetrician, and she's now on staff on the Mayo Clinic. So we took divergent paths. The birth went very well. The woman had intended to have the birth by herself. So we came, so to speak, as "gravy." She had asked us to attend the birth and said that we were *it*. There was no one else in Minnesota at the time attending [home] birth.

This birth was definitely not "medical," as symbolized by the equipment Ortiz and her companion took to cut and tie the umbilical cord. The mother decided on the setting for her birth, the people who would witness it, and the degree to which they would assist her. It was the mother's birth experience; she owned it, and, as Ortiz said, the midwives were "gravy." Finally, Ortiz reminded her audience that obstetricians in Minnesota do not attend home births. Her companion at this birth now belongs to a different culture, a culture that Ortiz and her sister midwives will have to persuade of the legitimacy of midwifery and the value of their experiential knowledge about birth.

Because Rita Ortiz's characterization of her own entrance into the home birth community became formal testimony in a public hearing—her words were recorded, available for transcription and analysis—she offers a name and face to direct-entry midwifery at the end of the twentieth century. Along with many others who testified in the fall of 1991, she went on to contribute to the draft of licensing rules that the Board of Medical Practice eventually rejected in the second stage of the process. Ortiz, then, was part of the discourse community of home birth and of the communities of two advisory groups set up by the state agencies. In these contexts, such communities consist of people with a common goal, who interact by offering information and providing feedback. Community members create and use forms and systems of communication to provide and promote information inside and outside their community. Such communities share a language or vocabulary and often through communication create what they consider knowledge (see Swales, *Genre Analysis* 24–27). In an essential way then, discourse opens this story, marks its progress, and contributes to its ending. Moreover, the competing meanings of the story are contained within words: those words recorded during testimony; those appearing in the first advisory group's recommendations; those contained in the Minnesota statutes and the documents from the Minnesota Midwives' Guild; those written for the proposed legislation; those spoken behind the scenes of the public hearings that swayed the final outcome; and those causing irresolvable conflict in the process of drafting licensing rules. Moreover, these words are echoed in other state laws and in the discussions among midwives around the world who publish their thoughts in newsletters and magazines, discuss issues at conferences, and take advantage of modern technology to participate in computer listservs and create World Wide Web home pages (for a fuller description of methodology and these sources, see appendix A).

Therefore, this book begins with Rita Ortiz telling her story to the Minnesota

Midwifery Study Advisory Group and traces the testimony and arguments that took place within the Minnesota hearings and subsequent public debates over a four-year period (1991–1995). This study uses rhetorical theory to analyze the current testimony and debate as well as the historical conversations about midwifery and, in doing so, extends our understanding about the relationships among knowledge, discourse, gender, and power. Primarily, the study confirms how, through discourse, professional jurisdictions are maintained by culturally accepted appropriation of scientific discourse and claims to exclusive authority over scientific knowledge and how, again through discourse, competing bids for professional standing are combated by those monopolies. This study also casts new light on the role gender plays in the establishment of and the competition between the professions. In particular, the study demonstrates that women's experiential knowledge may be rejected as a potential basis for establishing a profession and for gaining legal sanction to perform certain procedures and make use of particular tools considered to be under the purview of scientific knowledge. Within this exploration of professional competition, the study focuses on how genres, or forms of communication, particularly licensing rules and regulations created by state agencies to recognize practitioners and to standardize their professions, may silence certain practitioners or negate practices and knowledge systems of particular discourse communities.

To understand the relationship of knowledge, gender, power, and discourse within such professional competition, this study looks at various rhetorical moves, decisions, and concepts: the rhetorical status negotiated throughout the Minnesota hearings by key speakers; the collaborative writing processes used in the second set of Minnesota hearings to grant equal voice to all participants regardless of professional status; the distinctions that key speakers made between themselves and those with less status, the "other" within a discourse community, and pervasive tendencies to define the normal in relation to the abnormal; the evidence used to establish and promote knowledge systems; and the boundary-spanning techniques used to question and expand what the medical community and much of society consider authoritative knowledge about birth. Finally, then, the testimony of Rita Ortiz, Rachel Waters, and others about birth and the place of midwifery in the birthing process affords the opportunity to extend our understanding about the nature of authoritative knowledge, the connection between professional standing and claims to exclusive authority over scientific procedures and technological tools, and the rhetorical means of persuasion and resistance a gendered group developed in attempting to find a place for their knowledge system and practices.

To follow the flow of discourse about direct-entry midwifery, much of this book is organized chronologically around the Minnesota public hearings about direct-entry midwifery. The second chapter provides a theoretical framework for appreciating the significance of those hearings. Chapter 2 gives a brief summary of current theories of interprofession competition, power and gender relations, genres, public discourse and public space, and social constructions of the body that help us understand the Minnesota hearings. Here I also explain my methodology in gathering data and the special challenge of using Internet research to inform my study. Because we must also appreciate how the Minnesota hearings reflect centuries of arguments about midwifery, the third chapter describes four periods in the history of midwifery in which recurring concerns emerged such as the ownership of knowledge about birth; the appropriate role of science and technology in birth; the conflict between status and autonomy during professionalization; and alternative settings and degrees of intervention in birth. I analyze the arguments within early midwifery texts, including Jane Sharp's *Midwives Book*, Elizabeth Cellier's 1687 proposal for an independent midwifery association, and Elizabeth Nihell's 1760 *Treatise on the Art of Midwifery*. I explain the impact of the invention of the obstetrical forceps and the debate at the end of the eighteenth century in the United States over the good or harm done by physicians who continued to use the forceps. I review the ninety-year debate over licensing of midwives in Britain and then delve into the debate over whether to educate and license or eliminate direct-entry midwives at the beginning of the twentieth century in the United States. Finally, I identify the philosophy and language of the home birth movement of the 1960s and 1970s in the United States.

The fourth chapter of the book tells the story of the first stage of the Minnesota debates, when the Midwifery Study Advisory Group wrote its recommendations for the Board of Health and the Board of Medical Practice—the recommendations that were reflected in the Pappas-Flynn-Brown bills. This chapter focuses on the key testimonies of Rachel Waters, Rita Ortiz, and other Minnesota Midwives' Guild representatives, and that of two non-guild midwives, to illustrate how the guild midwives established early rhetorical status by specifically pointing to the existence of an "other" midwife, one who could be shown to deserve lower social and rhetorical status. In focusing on an image of the undeserving other midwife, the guild persuaded the advisory group to empower those more seemingly responsible and knowledgeable midwives through the resulting report and its recommendations.

Chapters 5 and 6 analyze the development of the five drafts of the proposed midwifery licensing rules and regulations in Minnesota. These chapters discuss the direct-entry midwives' attempts to balance the benefits of professionalization, such as increased visibility, against potential disadvantages, such as decreased autonomy. Here I describe the genre conventions of licensing rules, in Minnesota and across the United States, and analyze the resistance of the direct-entry midwives to these conventions. Part of this analysis focuses on the collaborative processes chosen by the group and how the handling of conflict affected whose voices were represented in the emerging licensing rules. The chapters then analyze the jurisdictional battles between competing systems of authoritative knowledge—the medical knowledge of the culturally recognized experts and the experiential knowledge developed and highly valued within the midwifery community. Chapter 6 explores the appropriation of science by the medical community to justify its insistence on the authority of its ways of knowing and to defend its jurisdictional boundaries and how this defense contributed to the failure of the midwifery rule writing process. The final chapter of the book focuses on how the Minnesota debates inform our understanding of women's sense of self and body in relation to embodied and experiential knowledge.

CHAPTER 2

Rhetorical Analysis and the Midwifery Debates

꧁ॐ꧂

*The female body that is an effect of the construction of
identity/authority of obstetricians in nineteenth-century medical
discourse is a hybrid creature formed through the articulations among
social practices, the development of new knowledge, and changing
patterns of power and authority. In this sense, the female body
functions as a border case; it is at once defined as part of a natural
order and as an intensely fascinating and yet threatening object of
cultural control. Its excessiveness strains the cultural authority of
medical knowledge. As such it is a site of potential transgression
against the boundaries of social order, at once constituted within the
dominant discourses of science and medicine but threatening to the
epistemological certainty of that discourse.*
(Anne Balsamo, 27–28)

*R*hetorical analysis provides the essential
means of interpreting the Minnesota midwifery story. We might consider rhetorical analysis, quite simply, as "the study of how people persuade" (McCloskey 29), or, as defined by Aristotle, "the faculty of observing in any given case the available means of persuasion" (153). This study then examines the persuasive strategies that key spokespeople in rhetorical analysis, called rhetors, used throughout the Minnesota hearings to present and defend their views of the midwifery and medical knowledge systems. In the broadest sense, then, rhetorical study focuses on "how people use language and other symbols to realize human goals and carry out human activities" (Bazerman, Shaping Written Knowledge 6). Language or discourse creates and negotiates knowledge, standardizes and modifies practice, and urges or suppresses action. Although rhetorical analysis assumes that every speaker or writer—every rhetor—can select from common persuasive devices, such as metaphor, analogy, enthymeme, and definition,[1] a rhetor's field, experience, expertise, purpose, audience, and situation determine which devices most persuade others. Therefore, this study goes beyond tracing specific language choice in key testimony; it focuses on how the various arguments framed by the midwives, nurse-midwives, home birth parents, physicians, and nurses involved in the hearings reflect their values and the degree of authority their knowledge carries.

Those choices not only reflect and often reinforce the thoughts and values of the individual rhetor—and his or her community and culture—but they also lead to concrete action and create abstract knowledge. Through language or discourse, knowledge and actions are negotiated within a community, sustained or modified when new experiences or theories are realized, and become authoritative when the community decides to recommend or establish a certain tool, procedure, or theory.

Often the most interesting and enlightening rhetorical studies focus on a community in conflict, coming internally from its own members or externally from a competing community. During that conflict, knowledge and values are often articulated publicly, statements are certified as "fact" or "truth" by the community, and the community may actively consider, absorb, or reject competing knowledge. During these times of conflict, rhetorical scholars can understand what the community believes is truth, what constitutes its authoritative knowledge about important subjects, and what evidence the community uses to sustain or alter its knowledge. Rhetorical scholars can also examine what status and power competing knowledge systems may have in broader society if the conflict is aired publicly. The Minnesota midwifery hearings afford just such an opportunity.

These studies are possible because, in the words of John Nelson, Allan Megill, and Donald McCloskey, specialists or members of discourse communities are "creatures of rhetoric," and all fields are defined by special "textures of rhetoric" (4–5). The rhetors who testified before the Midwifery Advisory Study Group in the fall of 1991, who participated in the efforts to write licensing rules in Minnesota, who created the *Standards of Care and Certification Guide* of the Minnesota Midwives' Guild, who debated the licensing laws in other states, who contribute to the Midwives' Alliance of North America newsletter, who participate in computer listservs on midwifery, and so on, are such creatures of rhetoric. These rhetors brought to the public hearings on midwifery the accepted rhetorical strategies and vocabulary of their communities. For example, on the one hand, direct-entry midwives, such as Rita Ortiz, who was introduced in the first chapter of this book, offered birth stories as evidence, and a speaker's credibility was established not only by the number and outcome of births attended but also by her own mothering experience—her embodied knowledge. On the other hand, physicians, such as Rachel Waters who headed up the MOMI project described in the first chapter, relied on their professional training and formal quantitative research studies to establish acceptance for their views about safe birth. Moreover, the advisory and licensing writing groups constituted their own communities, in which certain rhetorical devices became more persuasive than others. For example, in the Minnesota midwifery hearings, those direct-entry midwives who linked their proposals to the common good, to the protection of mothers and infants, were often granted more authority to define effective midwifery practice.

Finally, such discourse communities are not static: The goal of the Minnesota midwifery hearings was to achieve a consensus among representatives from competing communities about how to regulate direct-entry midwifery. In making these decisions, the participants were given a chance to negotiate knowledge about birth, regardless of what their own communities identified as authoritative knowledge at the time. As Dorothy Winsor comments on the nature of such situations, "a common vision of reality is also a rhetorical achievement because knowledge of the world is not something that is once achieved and then forever remains the same" (*Writing* 6).[2] The hearing participants were asked to achieve a common vision of birth—the definitions of normal and abnormal birth and the procedures to make both safe—or a type of reality that, in this case, would be legitimized through professional status for direct-entry midwives and through official documents such as licensing rules and regulations. Because knowledge does not exist separate from its knowers but instead is continually socially constructed, this study asks how, in a particular discourse community such as the Minnesota hearings, one gets to be a knower, an expert whose judgment and knowledge count. It also asks how rhetors who seem less powerful than their opposition negotiate the common reality, the knowledge systems, within any particular discourse community they join or argue against. In particular, this study traces the rhetorical moves that the direct-entry midwives make within the midwifery hearings to question the medical authoritative knowledge about birth and to defend an alternative knowledge system. Finally, the study attempts to explain why these rhetorical strategies ultimately failed.

Theories of the Body

Among the many specific theories that inform this rhetorical study of the Minnesota midwifery hearings are those on the body—its materiality and its social and discursive construction. The statement that opens this chapter, from Anne Balsamo's *Technologies of the Gendered Body*, exemplifies how complex our thinking about the body has become. The female body not only is *a material and physical entity,* one defined, examined, diagnosed, and treated by bioscience, but it also is *socially constructed* by medical and other knowledge systems. Our bodies exist—but they also seem to take on a certain nature because we talk about them, measure them, imagine them, in ways determined by our social and cultural values. At one time, we believed that our bodies were constituted of the four humors—blood, phlegm, choler, and black bile—and whichever humor predominated an individual determined that person's health. Later, we imagined our bodies as well-run machines, but machines open to invasion by germs if exposed to unclean environments. Now, as discussed later in this section, we often consider our bodies to be flexible and agile systems, producing antibodies to combat invasion by germs and sustain health. Women's bodies, in particular—how they are described and defined through language—seem to reflect gender values and hierarchies within various moments of our cultural history. For example, Aristotle believed that the genitals of human females and apes were the same, supporting his view that women were directly linked to these primates. On the other hand, male apes' genitals were too "doglike" to be similar to that of the human male, supporting his belief that the human male was the most advanced of all creatures (Schiebinger 89). This social and discursive formation of the body, then, often creates a picture of the "normal" body that may view women's bodies as less capable than men's or that may negate women's varied experiences. These values and hierarchies often compete with individual women's embodied and experiential knowledge. For example, in the late nineteenth century, physicians concerned with abortion practices among midwives and homeopaths began to standardize the viability of fetal life according to specific stages of pregnancy. However, women themselves determined this defining moment in their pregnancy by when, as individuals, they first felt quickening or fetal movement; only then did they feel obligated to bring the pregnancy to term (Reagan 8–9). Today, pregnant women often identify the first time at which they began to fully sense their babies as that moment when their physicians or technicians share with them an ultrasound image. Bodies, then, as noted by Elizabeth Grosz, are "not only inscribed, marked, engraved, by social pressures external to them but are the products, the direct effects, of the very social constitution of nature itself" (*x*). Throughout social history, women have been variously identified in terms of their relationship to the body. For example, in mind/body, culture/nature dualisms, women have been "cast into the role of the body" or the caretaker of the body (Bordo 5–6). Their bodies have been defined in negative terms, as impure, chaotic, uncontrollable, seductive. This body has been, to use the words of Susan Bordo, "mediated by language: by metaphors (for instance, microbes as 'invading,' egg as 'waiting' for sperm) and semantical grids (such as binary oppositions as male/female, inner/outer) that organize and animate our perception and experience. We thus have no direct, innocent, or unconstructed knowledge of our bodies; rather, we are always reading our bodies according to various interpretive schemes" (288–289).

Moreover, with increasing use of new reproductive technologies, bodies take on the nature of cyborg or cybernetic organisms, according to such scholars as Donna Haraway, hybrids of machine and organism that change "what counts as women's experience in the late twentieth century" (147). Haraway sees this blurring of boundaries as potentially positive, in that cultural assignments of masculinity and femininity become less discrete, and "[n]ature and culture are reworked; the one can no longer be the resource for appropriation or incorporation by the other" (151). To others, this reconceptualization of the body makes it the site for struggles for new meanings, an "ideological tug-of-war between competing systems of meaning" (Balsamo 5), the focal point for power struggles (Bordo 17). Within the Minnesota midwifery hearings, the struggle over the definitions and boundaries of such concepts as "normal" and "safe" reflects the competing aspects of medical and midwifery knowledge systems. Whoever gets to define the body—and what makes it safe and normal—claims a great deal of authority and power to determine standards of practice among medical and alternative caregivers.

Today, because of social and discursive perceptions of the body, the pregnant woman and the baby are often conceived as separate entities and may end up as competitors, a further alienation of women from their bodies. In fact, Bordo speculates that because the pregnant woman is defined by "her biological, purely mechanical roles in preserving the life of another," her own claims to subjectivity, "her valuations, choices, consciousness are expendable" (79). For example, when faced with a persistent breech baby—one not turning head down in the womb—she might be urged to schedule a cesarean rather than being given information on how she or her caregiver might successfully turn the baby. Through new reproductive technologies, the fetus is increasingly seen as a person—a separate body from its mother—an autonomous patient confirmed in its ultrasound image. Such perceptions and models of the body, therefore, impact not only how physicians might view pregnancy but also how the mother herself might experience labor and birth. No longer relying on quickening to confirm her baby's existence, she learns to distrust her own body's progress through pregnancy and instead to trust the expert who interprets and presents her with the first image of her baby. She might also perceive her body as fragmented—as a womb, a breast, a limb, monitored by a machine—instead of as an integrated whole.

Alternative caregivers, such as direct-entry midwives, also must reconcile their practices with the discursive definitions and perceptions of the body posed by hegemonic medical knowledge systems—or else find a means to resist. In a similar study, Emily Martin traced changing models of the body's immune system from the 1940s to the present. Early images of the immune system involved a body defending itself against an invasion of germs, entering through any openings within the body, coming from an unclean environment. The body was a machine, whose parts could break down to invite invasion or would break down upon invasion (*Flexible* 26–29). Now the body's immune system is considered part of an active complex series of systems, producing new antibodies to preserve health and meet each new challenge. The healthy body is flexible, agile, adroit, and innovative. Such new perceptions of the flexible body would seem to provide space for alternative therapies, and, in fact, Martin speculates that such alternative practitioners as acupuncturists share with biomedicine at least this perception of the flexible immune system (83–84). Indeed, the direct-entry midwives engaged in the Minnesota hearings often suggested that they shared with physicians certain standards of cleanliness—for example, they used gloves during deliveries and were attentive to the mother's nutritional habits.

However, despite these commonalities, mothers' and midwives' birth stories suggest persistent conflicts between the ways they view their bodies and the ways their bodies might be viewed within biomedical systems. For example, a Belgian midwife found that her own body's reaction to a standard medical procedure went counter to the norm:

> Two years ago my first baby was born. . . . It was a pretty hard delivery that ended with a cesarean. The gynecologist used catgut for my wound. In my hospital, they always use this kind of wire and there never was a problem. But after several weeks, I was loosing little pieces of that catgut. My body didn't accept this "foreign body." Nevertheless my cesarean healed and after almost two years the problem seemed dissolved. After the delivery of my 2nd baby . . . , I had lots of pain at my seam of the cesarean. The doctor decided to operate. It was the catgut. . . . After two years the catgut was almost new! Now they used another wire for the wound (Vicryl). Let's hope that my body reacts well.   (listserv communication, August 5, 1996) [3]

This midwife and mother experienced what standard medical practice determined she should not—pain and undissolved stitches from a previous cesarean. Her body, challenged by a "foreign" body, reacted in what she and her physician considered an abnormal way. According to her interpretation, despite the fact that the hospital now preferred Vicryl for stitching, it wasn't that the catgut failed to dissolve after her surgery—her body failed to dissolve the catgut. Additionally, because of this earlier failure, she lost faith in her system's ability to handle future invasion.

Frequently defined as caretakers of the body, and especially the reproductive system, women and their midwives are often caught up in the complexities of the body. Are our bodies material objects that can be felt by us and teach us how best to manage our own care and needs? Are these material entities that can be described, measured, and treated effectively by our caregivers? Or are our bodies defined by cultural experts to such an extent that we fail to know and trust them and so experience them according to some primary hegemonic norm? Who knows and owns our bodies during pregnancy and birth—biomedical experts, mothers, midwives? Are babies part of their mothers' bodies before birth, or are they separate citizens and patients with their own rights and needs? The Minnesota midwifery hearings inspire these questions and more as the hearings demonstrate the ideological struggles between competing knowledge systems about the body.

Interprofessional Competition: Social, Rhetorical, and Professional Status

Because the purpose of the Minnesota midwifery hearings was to determine the legal status of direct-entry midwifery, this study also follows how the rhetorical, social, and professional status of the key rhetors shifted during the hearings to enable rhetors to argue effectively for certain definitions of midwifery legal status. In particular, the study recognizes any increase in a rhetor's status within the hearings that helped the rhetor affirm or renegotiate her group's professional status and marks the loss of status that silenced a rhetor or negated her remarks. Finally, the study identifies why the Minnesota Board of Medical Practice decided to suspend the hearings and leave the midwives without legal sanction to practice and what rhetorical strategies the board's spokespersons used to persuade all participants that such suspension was necessary. Although this analysis focuses on specific Minnesota hearings held between 1991 and 1995, the rhetors who came to the hearings already had a certain degree of social and professional status. To understand the role that interprofessional competition played within the hearings, it is important to recognize that status and how it might be achieved.

We afford individuals and groups social status based on their age, gender, profession, education, experience, income, and other demographic characteristics. We often rank the importance of what they say or grant them rhetorical ethos according to this social status and their conduct during a particular event or activity (Logue and Miller 25). In the broadest sense, ethos is reflected in a rhetor's social status and conduct, and a rhetor's status and conduct contribute to her credibility or authority. Moreover, a rhetor's ethos reflects upon the communities to which she belongs, and her choices and successes impact the status of that group. Finally, a rhetor "enacts" her community, represents to her audience the goals and knowledge systems of her community in unique ways—she characterizes her community in ways that may be distinct from other members of that community, and her choices to do so might be based on what she considers a persuasive move in a certain situation (Miller and Halloran 121). In the Minnesota hearings, it is important to realize that in general,society has conferred on members of the medical profession high social status. Their ethos is well established by their education and culturally assigned expertise as long as their professional conduct is not questioned. By one estimate only one-half of one percent of babies born in Minnesota in the early 1990s were born at home (Illg). In 1994, in the entire United States, only about 17,600 home births were attended by direct-entry midwives (Rooks 227). Thus, Rachel Waters, whose testimony preceded Rita Ortiz's in the first discussions about direct-entry midwifery, would be granted high social status because of her occupation and professional credentials. This social status would carry over into the opening discussions of the Minnesota hearings. In turn, Ortiz, although she was a founder of the Minnesota Midwives' Guild and was well-respected among the home birth community, was practically invisible in a society whose majority did not even realize that home birth was an option and that direct-entry midwives still practiced. Rhetors, such as Ortiz and Waters, came to the hearings with differing social status, which initially affected their personal ethos before the group involved in the hearings. They also enacted their own discourse communities in distinct ways at the hearings.

These enactments and the persuasive devices chosen by such rhetors as Waters and Ortiz contributed to the rhetorical status that rhetors might achieve during the course of the hearings. Rhetorical status is not static; it might change in an instant, given the reception a statement receives, the perceived conduct of a rhetor, or the rhetorical move of another rhetor (Logue and Miller 22). The heart of this study lies in these changes in rhetorical status. Shifts in rhetorical status within specific contexts such as the Minnesota hearings empower or silence individuals and their discourse communities during conflict. In essence, the task of the direct-entry midwives in the public hearings was to establish a credible and sustained rhetorical status that, for those midwives who desired licensing, meant a state-sanctioned professional status. Moreover, only high rhetorical status during the hearings would enable the direct-entry midwives to affect the licensing rule genre in a way that would accommodate their alternative knowledge about birth.

If the heart of this study rests in tracing these shifts in rhetorical status, the importance of the study lies in what new understanding the study brings to how, through discourse, professions maintain their status and have impact on competing knowledge systems, in particular the knowledge that women and their midwives bring to birth. Many of the direct-entry midwives involved in the Minnesota hearings realized that state-sanctioned professional status would enable them to expand their practice through advertising, to apply for third-party insurance reimbursement and malpractice insurance, to obtain and carry drugs, to encourage open medical backup and transfer of care, and to set up and help govern their own educational programs. Many of the midwives had professional status within their national organizations, such as the Midwives' Alliance of North America, and had just obtained or were pursuing the title of certified professional midwife through the North American Registry of Midwives. However, they still needed state-sanctioned professional status to legally carry out certain procedures and use certain tools at home.

The professional status of the medical profession has been well documented in studies such as Paul Starr's Pulitzer Prizewinning book, *The Social Transformation of American Medicine*. According to Starr, that status of the medical profession is pervasive within our society:

> The dominance of the medical profession, however, goes considerably beyond this rational foundation. Its authority spills over its clinical boundaries into arenas of moral and political action for which medical judgment is only partially relevant and often incompletely equipped. Moreover, the profession has been able to turn its authority into social privilege, economic power, and political influence. (5)

With that professional status, medical experts have considerable voice in conversations about birth; their authoritative knowledge about birth hinges on the expertise they have achieved socially, economically, and politically. By contrast, the history of midwifery in the United States reveals a general failure to professionalize. For example, in a study of the practices of Wisconsin midwives in the early part of the twentieth century, Charlotte Borst found that midwifery organizations and schools failed to promote the professionalism of midwifery (30–34). In fact, Starr directly contrasts midwifery with the powerful knowledge systems of professional medicine:

> Feminists claimed that as patients, as nurses, and in other roles in health care, they were denied the right to participate in medical decisions by paternalistic doctors who refused to share information or take their intelligence seriously. They objected that much of what passed for scientific knowledge was sexist prejudice and that male physicians had deliberately excluded women from competence by keeping them out of medical schools and suppressing alternative practitioners such as midwives. (391)

Thus, at the beginning of the midwifery hearings, medical practitioners had the state-sanctioned professional status that acknowledged their authoritative knowledge about birth. They were licensed professionals who populated the Board of Medical Practice and who were generally able to monitor their own professional practices. By contrast, direct-entry midwives lacked any state-sanctioned professional status in Minnesota and had to seek that status by breaching the jurisdictional barriers erected by those practitioners whom much of society had placed in charge of birth. In order to do so, the midwives had to gain legitimacy for their own knowledge.

Professional status is achieved when specific jurisdictional boundaries are drawn to distinguish one practice from others, and when these boundaries are accepted by society, by other professions, and by agencies able to grant legal sanction.

These boundaries are often distinguished by the specific knowledge systems that a profession develops or claims, and these knowledge systems may be disputed when a competing practice requests professional status or advances alternative knowledge systems. Thus, these knowledge claims are usually exclusive and carry with them a powerful social, economic, and political voice and status. For example, Andrew Abbott, who has done a study of professional systems, describes these jurisdictional boundaries in their social contexts:

> In claiming jurisdiction, a profession asks society to recognize its cognitive structure through exclusive rights; jurisdiction has not only a culture, but also a social structure. These claimed rights may include absolute monopoly of practice and of public payments, rights of self-discipline and of unconstrained employment, control of professional training, of recruitment, and of licensing, to mention only a few. (34, 59)

A profession's ability to establish and sustain its jurisdiction in the twentieth century has, in part, depended on prestigious academic knowledge and on exclusive claim to aspects of science and technology. That claim grants the profession the authority to monitor its own practice and to select those practitioners it wants to recognize and recruit (Andrew Abbott 53–54).

The expert scientific and technical knowledge that a profession claims within its jurisdictional boundaries makes the client dependent on the sanctioned professional to interpret aspects of that scientific and technological world. Medicine occupies a special position in terms of that dependency. According to Starr, medical professionals interpret personal, physical conditions for their clients by using their scientific expertise:

> Even among the sciences, medicine occupies a special position. Its practitioners come into direct and intimate contact with people in their daily lives; they are present at the critical transitional moments of existence. They serve as intermediaries between science and private experience, interpreting personal troubles in the abstract language of scientific knowledge. (4)

The client asks the medical practitioner to interpret physical symptoms, to diagnose personal ailments, and to administer treatment according to scientific abstractions. Although certainly physicians consider the patient's specific case, their professional status relies on their ability to bring scientific learning to that case. As Emily Martin describes this relationship in her study of reproductive metaphors, this dependency has the potential to demean women: "Medical culture has a powerful system of socialization which exacts conformity as the price of participation. It is also a cultural system whose ideas and practices pervade popular culture and in which, therefore, we all participate to some degree" (*Woman* 13).

To gain professional status, the direct-entry midwives would have to claim a jurisdiction that clarified and legally acknowledged their relationship to scientific knowledge and medical tools and procedures. Also, the midwives would have to find an exclusive jurisdictional niche within the system of professions that administered to birthing mothers and their infants. The knowledge system of direct-entry midwifery is established in part through direct experience with birth, almost always first experienced when midwives themselves become mothers. This experience is conveyed through birth stories, passed on within apprenticeships, and, although made abstract through standards of practice, safeguards the mother's and the midwife's right and responsibility to base decisions on the particular physical and emotional situation. However, while maintaining these distinct ways of knowing about birth, the Minnesota direct-entry midwives sought through professional status the legal right to carry drugs, to perform episiotomies, and to suture perineal tears—techniques that many found compatible with birth stories, apprenticeships, and individual choice of birth attendant and setting.

Power and Gender

Moreover, this study relies on current understanding of the role of discourse in maintaining and challenging professional jurisdictions by considering the *gendered* practice of midwifery. Most studies of professional systems have not focused on gender as a component in establishing and defending jurisdictional boundaries or on resistance to legitimizing women's experiential knowledge through professional status. Rita Ortiz's journey to midwifery began with her own experience with birth, an embodied experience that, despite the good medical outcome, she interpreted to be disastrous and traumatic. Moreover, her education as a midwife came primarily from attending the births of others, rather than learning anatomy and physiology in a formal setting. Therefore, this study extends our knowledge about how, through discourse, professional boundaries are maintained and challenged by offering a specific case study of the debate about the legitimacy of women's knowledge.

In contexts in which technology impacts health and safety, rhetorical scholars are just beginning to recognize how, as Beverly Sauer observes, "the conventions of public discourse sanction the exclusion of alternative voices and thus perpetuate [a] salient and silent power structure" and how "the notion of expertise excludes women's experiential knowledge" (65–66). In a study of the documents describing a mining accident, Sauer found that wives of miners knew from the amount of dust they washed out of their husbands' work clothes that the mines were unsafe, but this experiential knowledge had been disregarded. The Minnesota direct-entry midwives and their home birth clients challenge the categories of evidence generally accepted as authoritative by the hegemonic medical community. They identify themselves as women and as mothers and celebrate the experience that defines their attitudes toward birth and their sense of self.

The women who choose home births with direct-entry midwives comment that the experience empowers them as women, and that experience may convince them to become midwives themselves. As Gloria Olson, one direct-entry midwife involved in the Minnesota hearings, noted about her own home birth experience: "It was the most empowering, wonderful experience of my life. It was like I did it, I can do it, I woke up to my power as a woman. I just went on to have the rest of my kids at home."[4] (See appendix C for a list of the key rhetors in the Minnesota hearings.) The desire to regain a sense of personal power through birth is expressed by other midwives around the United States. For example, Clara, a direct-entry midwife practicing in another state, believed that the gendered nature of the home birth setting was what attracted women to the practice:

> Women choose homebirth for a variety of reasons, but for most of the women I attend the fact that I and my assistant are women, and that the only man present both during and after the birth is her husband is a big factor . . . In the hospital, the caregiver is expected to be an authority figure, and authority figures are traditionally male. . . . My ladies were all greatly relieved when I had a baby because finally I "understood what us women go through."   (listserv communication, July 13, 1996)

In a way, women such as Gloria Olson and Clara are attempting to regain female dominance in the birth room, a dominance that was lost when medical men gained authority through birthing tools and techniques such as the forceps and the drugs that induced twilight sleep. For example, in her study of childbirth from 1750 to 1950, Judith Leavitt stressed the centrality of gender in the birth room before medical men became involved in birth:

> Gender played an important part in the birthing experiences of American women above and beyond the domestic female context in which birth took place. It was a significant factor in the choice of birth attendant for those groups of Americans who worried about modesty and about the cost of delivery. For millennia women attended other women during labor and delivery because birth was women's private business. Women knew how to help because they had themselves experienced the pain and anguish of delivery. They knew how to comfort because they knew what women felt and needed at their times of travail. And they knew how to intervene because they had watched others manage labor and delivery. Furthermore, many birthing women could accept only other women witnessing the intimate physical details of birth. (108)

The history of midwifery testifies to the knowledge that women brought to and derived from the birth room (see chapter 3, "The Rhetorical History of Midwifery"). It is the perception of control over their own physical being and of physical and emotional empowerment that attracts women to birth at home. For these women, birth is not a health problem but a personally enhancing experience. As with Rita Ortiz's first client, the woman selects where and with whom she will birth, and the midwife's task is to respect and support those choices. Thus, women and their direct-entry midwives expect that birth at home will empower them as women— and to some extent overcome their social subjugation because of gender. To legitimize midwifery by granting professional status to midwives, then, would seem to recognize a knowledge system based on women's experiential and embodied knowledge.

When considering gender and power, it is essential to distinguish between a sense of personal power and the power granted or gained by a subject or a rhetor through public discourse. Women who birth at home express their increased personal power, but this study asks to what extent, through discourse, knowledge may be legitimized or negated by those with professional power. One of the most relevant but controversial theories of discourse and power has been proposed by philosopher Michel Foucault, who speculated that power is reflected in and distributed by discourse: "Indeed, it is in discourse that power and knowledge are joined together" (*Sexuality* 100). Rather than focusing on power as strictly a matter of social or professional status, Foucault asserted, in essence, that rhetorical status contributes to power:

> we must conceive of discourse as a series of discontinuous segments whose tactical function is neither uniform nor stable. To be more precise, we must not imagine a world of discourse divided between accepted discourse and excluded discourse, or between the dominant discourse and the dominated one; but as a multiplicity of discursive elements that can come into play in various strategies. *It is this distribution that we must reconstruct, with the things said and those concealed, the enunciations required and those forbidden* . . . (*Sexuality* 100, emphasis added)

When one group's terms and evidence are favored over another's, that group has the power to shape public discourse about particular issues. That power enables that group or discourse community to influence law and social and professional practices within our society. As Joan Scott observes, "[G]ender is a primary way of signifying relationships of power" (1069; see also Condit 7). Thus, the negotiation and distribution of power during the Minnesota hearings reflects the value assigned to women's knowledge.

For example, direct-entry midwives rely on their intuition to help their home birth clients through the birth process. By the same token, direct-entry midwives rely on their clients' intuitions to determine what help they might need. Thus, the Minnesota direct-entry midwives and their home birth clients rely on what Carole Browner and Nancy Press call "embodied knowledge" or the knowledge derived from a woman's perceptions of her body's natural processes throughout the course of pregnancy (113). In their study of women and their experiences during pregnancy, Browner and Press found that women accepted caregivers' recommendations when they were confirmed by embodied knowledge and rejected those that contradicted that knowledge. In other words, the women in the Browner and Press study considered their embodied knowledge to be authoritative. Robbie Davis-Floyd and Elizabeth Davis maintain that the physical, emotional, intellectual, and psychic connections direct-entry midwives achieve with their clients "quite regularly expose the contradictions that the voice of rationality proves, in the domain of birth, to be unable to exclude" (320). These connections successfully carry mothers through various stages of the birth for which the hegemonic medical system of knowledge would dictate intervention. Moreover, the connection that direct-entry midwives are able to achieve with their clients depends on how connected they are to their own thoughts and feelings, their own intuitive sense of self. Davis-Floyd and Davis suggest that the more familiar midwives are with biomedical diagnostic technologies, the less they trust this intuition (324, 327). However, although women might seek empowerment through home birth, the "evidence" of embodied knowledge and intuition is often pre-empted in public discussions about birth. As Davis-Floyd and Davis say, "The voice of reason is loud and aggressive; the harder task, as the midwives see it, is to identify and heed the truths spoken by the still, small, and culturally devalued inner voice" (330). This study, then, traces the rhetorical strategies used to counter the authoritative knowledge of that voice of reason and to propose the alternative authority of that intuitive inner voice and the embodied knowledge that voice represents for women.

Genres

Professions maintain their authoritative knowledge and their professional and social status through particular types or forms of communication or genres. Genres are rhetorical forms created in response to recurrent situations and "serve to stabilize experience and give it coherence and meaning" (Berkenkotter and Huckin 4).[5] The Minnesota hearings about direct-entry midwifery produced extensive drafts and documents of licensing rules and regulations, a genre created by state agencies and legislatures in cooperation with professional organizations to define and govern practices. The conventions of the genre of licensing rules and regulations are not neutral but instead assume a particular knowledge system linked to formal education, abstract standards, and hierarchical relationships among practitioners. The degree to which rhetors in the Minnesota hearings were able to increase or maintain their rhetorical status depended to some degree on how they could manipulate this genre. Conflict over medical and midwifery systems of knowledge became most obvious in the Minnesota hearings when participants discussed how to apply the conventions of the licensing genre to direct-entry midwifery.

Because the Minnesota hearings about direct-entry midwifery produced extensive drafts and documents, this study explores whose knowledge about birth is reflected in the carefully chosen words and meticulously crafted phrases in these documents. At the time of the hearings (1991–1995), direct-entry midwifery was legally defined in the state of Minnesota. Therefore, the Minnesota Board of Medical Practice was charged with administering the licensing rules created in hearings and to enforce the scope and limitations designated by the definition of midwifery practice created within the hearings and recorded in the licensing rules. These definitions set boundaries and limits and distinguished between acceptable and unacceptable practices. The debates and the negotiations over midwifery that took place in the public hearings reflected various meanings of birth, safety, risk, rights, and informed consent, held by nurses, doctors, nurse-midwives, home birth parents, direct-entry midwives, lawyers, and government agency staff members. The meanings that individuals and groups assigned to these concepts were diverse and often conflicting. However, in the midwifery hearings, participants were asked to collaboratively select words and phrases—often expressed in definitions—that would become laws and rules. These laws and rules would set up the scope of practice for the midwives and would list the contraindications for home birth and the limits that could not be crossed without prosecution and penalty.[6] The scope of practice for direct-entry midwives and the contraindications for home birth expressed in licensing rules could expand or limit the current practice; could reflect the values and knowledge system of the medical community, those of the home birth community, or a compromise position; and could encourage the majority of midwives to seek licensing or to force them to go further underground.

In tracing the negotiations among hearing participants over certain key words and phrases, this study analyzes to what extent the genre of state statutes and licensing rules perpetuate medical knowledge about birth or can accommodate midwifery knowledge. The participants in the Minnesota hearings reacted to the conventions of the licensing rules and regulations, discussed how to modify these conventions to accommodate midwifery knowledge, and, at times, resisted the aspects of medical knowledge that the conventions represented. Because a genre is a rhetorical response to a recurrent situation, it represents a community's ideology and norms. Therefore, examining the conversations and debates about midwifery reveals assumptions underlying medical authoritative knowledge about birth. For example, the licensing rules that regulate the professions were developed to identify those practitioners whom the state recognizes as having appropriate education and training, to protect the public from unsafe practices and practitioners, to legally define the scope of practice and contraindications for care that the profession and the state agree upon, and to set up mechanisms to curtail or abolish the practices of those practitioners who violate the professional standards. As genres, licensing rules serve a rhetorical purpose: They are used by government agencies to regulate the professions and to establish state-sanctioned authoritative knowledge within a practice. However, because genres are dynamic, serve certain purposes, support actions, and respond to situations, the Minnesota debates over the conventions of the licensing rules and regulations illuminate how, through discourse, a profession may refute competing knowledge systems.

The conventions of a genre may limit or silence members of a discourse community, such as the discourse community formed by the diverse participants in the Minnesota hearings, and may also maintain the professional and social status of a community such as the medical profession. As Lloyd Bitzer points out, "The situations recur and, because we experience situations and the rhetorical responses to them, a form of discourse is not only established but comes to have a power of its own—the tradition itself tends to function as a constraint upon any new response in the form" (13). Genres contribute to the construction of the "other," the silenced, suppressed, or oppressed; genres affect power, status, and resources.[7] Thus, this study describes how the licensing rule genre reflects the power relations between the Minnesota midwifery and medical communities in the Minnesota hearings. The study focuses on such forms and content of the licensing rule genre to explore the extent to which, in this situation, authoritative knowledge about birth, as offered by the state and its medical experts, was maintained. Also, the study analyzes how the form and content of the genre itself became part of the argument to exclude opposing knowledge systems about birth, and how it was challenged by the direct-entry midwives.

Public Discourse and the Public Sphere

Finally, it is important to recognize that the discourse analyzed within much of this book took place within the public sphere, a forum in which rhetorical scholars, such as Celeste Condit, contend that "material realities [can be] expressed and ideas materialized" (3). Thus, public discourse not only is productive but also can ideally accommodate the voices of many discourse communities: Ideas can be generated, public vocabularies created, and social conditions articulated through discussions in the public sphere. For example, as rhetorical scholar Thomas Goodnight suggests, argument within the public sphere pertains to probable knowledge where the "full worth of a policy is always yet to be seen," a place in which participants may collaboratively construct a future (214). The midwifery hearings, then, afford their participants an opportunity to negotiate authoritative knowledge about birth, to reconsider what constitutes evidence and truth about birth, not only within midwifery or medicine but also potentially within the broader society. However, according to rhetorical theory, certain arguments are more effective in the public sphere than others. For example, arguments that appeal to the public good—to health, safety, and general welfare—are recognized as legitimate within the public sphere. To contribute to probable or emerging knowledge about birth, rhetors might couch their arguments in the "good reasons" most acceptable within the public sphere (Condit 6). For example, the Minnesota midwifery advisory groups were charged by the state with protecting the public from harm, and those rhetors who allied themselves with this goal were most successful in persuading their listeners that their knowledge systems were legitimate.

Keeping the argument about birth within the public sphere seemed advantageous to those direct-entry midwives who sought professional recognition for their knowledge about birth and who were willing to offer good reasons acceptable in the public sphere to support their knowledge system. However, other rhetors, particularly those within the medical community, argue to keep the conversation about birth within the technical sphere, a forum in which medical and scientific experts construct authoritative knowledge. Arguments in the technical sphere are restricted to the argument practice of professional communities and depend on "considerable expertise" and evidence presented through the conventions of scholarly argument to "advance a special kind of knowledge" (Goodnight 220, 217). Participants in the Minnesota hearings representing the medical community might prefer to keep the debate over safe birth practices within the technical sphere, where arguments would be best supported by health care professionals' expert knowledge and the scientific methodology of such studies as Rachel Waters's MOMI project. On the other hand, many of the Minnesota rhetors speaking for direct-entry midwifery seemed to sense that, within the public sphere, their voices needed to be heard; only in the public sphere could they gain professional status necessary for licensing and for legal access to the scientific and technological tools they felt they needed, and so they worked to develop persuasive strategies that would best articulate their views about birth. Thus, within the hearings, rhetors often attempted to shift the conversation back to the technical sphere or to maintain public discourse, and used arguments more appropriate to one sphere than the other. Such shifts—and the persuasive strategies that support them—often reveal certain aspects of conflicting knowledge systems of discourse communities and signal important turns in the Minnesota hearings.

Finally, although many of the direct-entry midwives involved in the hearings argued to sustain public discourse about birth, others argued that decisions involving birth were best made in the private sphere. They were content with the general invisibility of their practices and refused any state-imposed limits on their midwifery knowledge about birth. In the private sphere, knowledge claims require more informal and even anecdotal evidence (Goodnight 220). Thus, in the private sphere, the decision to home birth would be negotiated between each midwife and parent and would be based on such differing aspects as health history, personality, and religious faith, with few abstract standards limiting practice. Such decisions would not be subject to the logic and abstractions of the technical sphere or the open debate of the public sphere. This impulse to keep the conversation about birth within the private sphere divided the Minnesota direct-entry midwifery community. After all, asserted some midwives, their own knowledge about birth was developed within that sphere in which evidence was expressed in personal birth stories rather than statistics and medical case histories. For example, Rita Ortiz described in her initial testimony how such a decision to birth at home might be made in the private sphere:

> The first phone call sets off a course of events that will help that woman either have her baby at home or not have her baby at home. I try to assess her motivation for wanting to stay home. . . . I ask her about her world view, how self-sufficient she is, how does she view safety and security, what are her fears surrounding birth, life, and death, and why is she choosing to ask me of all people . . . [Does she] see herself as being weak or strong, ambivalent or straightforward, in an unstable and conflicting relationship or a stable family life, . . . ? [What are her] feelings of womanhood, superiority or inferiority to other women, . . . ? [Does she] see herself as a sex-object, reject the major aspects of being a woman? [8]

The rhetorical challenge facing the Minnesota direct-entry midwives who sought state-sanctioned professional status also involved arguing that the public discourse about midwifery must embrace the very personal nature of birth. The personal nature of birth included the rights of the home birth parents and midwives to decide that birth must be a private rather than medical event. At the same time, the direct-entry midwifery community split over whether arguing for a public conversation about birth would negate the very knowledge system that originated in private decisions and values and in personal experience.

This rhetorical analysis of the Minnesota midwifery hearings, then, is enhanced by our current theories of how bodily images are discursively constructed within communities and cultures. The study also relies on our knowledge of interprofessional competition and the status or credibility granted to and established by rhetors with different social, professional, and rhetorical status. Tracing how and why this status changes during the hearings provides a picture of medical and midwifery ideologies. It would be impossible to discuss past and current midwifery practice without acknowledging the relationships between gender and power. These relationships are maintained or resisted through discourse, and in this study the licensing rules and regulations genre provides one focus of that discourse. Finally, because the Minnesota debates took place within the public sphere—in hearings open to the public—we can see the challenge faced by women seeking to have their very personal experiential and embodied knowledge about birth publicly and legally sanctioned.

Methodology

This book results from a qualitative case study of the Minnesota midwifery hearings, a study in which ethnographic means of data collection were used. Rather than writing a primer on rhetorical theory and using the hearings as an example, my purpose is to use rhetorical theory to understand the midwifery hearings and then, whenever possible, to comment on or extend theory based on what I learned from the hearings. Therefore, in the majority of the chapters that follow I present chronologically the progression of the hearings, the arguments posed, and the documents produced. However, in presenting various stages and aspects of the hearings, I identify which theories and rhetorical tools seem best to illuminate a particular argument or document and to identify what we might learn from an in-depth look at that argument or document. These later chapters, then, return to and expand upon many of the issues about knowledge, gender, power, and discourse introduced in earlier sections of this chapter.

Although, in appendix A, I offer a more personal reflection on my methodology, list my data sources, and describe the midwifery listserv that I used to contextualize the Minnesota hearings, here I comment on how my initial research questions necessarily changed over the five years during which I collected data and the challenge of using Internet research to contextualize the Minnesota hearings. My study began with one question that remained important throughout the five years: What were the commonalties and differences between the two systems of medical and midwifery knowledge about birth, and how were these features articulated publicly by representatives from the medical community and from the midwifery or home birth community? The essential nature of this question became clear during the first hearing I observed, in which both Rachel Waters and Rita Ortiz testified. For example, Waters used statistical analysis to support her community's authoritative knowledge about birth while Ortiz relied on her personal experiences with her own and others' births. However, at the end of this hearing, it was clear that because one knowledge system had been accepted within our broader culture more than the other, I needed to add a second question: What rhetorical strategies would Rita Ortiz and her sister midwives use to convince their listeners that their midwifery knowledge was a legitimate way of knowing about birth in order to gain rhetorical and, eventually, professional status? At the end of the first round of hearings, which took place between October 1991 and May 1992, I concluded that Ortiz and the Minnesota Midwives' Guild representatives at the hearings had used boundary-spanning techniques to legitimize their knowledge system and had benefited from the depiction and presence of an "other" midwife whose knowledge about birth might be interpreted through religious dictates and therefore would contrast unfavorably with guild practices. Although a faction of the Minnesota home birth community had been silenced by such rhetorical strategies, the guild midwives who sought greater legal recognition of their practices gained increased visibility and approval. Although they still could not legally carry certain drugs or perform particular procedures, they could sign birth certificates and contribute to a brochure distributed by the Department of Health that described their services.

When I learned that another set of hearings was to take place, one in which licensing rules and regulations were to be produced, I wanted to study the collaborative process used by the participants. I intended to record field notes and to study the drafts produced. I imagined that my primary contribution would be another study of workplace composition practices. However, although the collaborative process chosen by the hearing participants was intended to grant all an equal voice, I saw once again that the issue of competing knowledge systems would taint the collaborative process. For example, many direct-entry midwives participating in the hearings found that conventions of the licensing rules and regulations would not accommodate their knowledge about birth but instead would place them under the supervision of the medical community. Therefore, I needed to ask another related question as I observed this second round of hearings: How did the established profession of medicine use the particular genre of licensing rules and regulations to maintain its jurisdictional boundaries in the face of competing knowledge systems? To answer this question, I studied the features of the genre and observed which features seemed to accommodate and which seemed to negate midwifery knowledge systems. The hearing participants clearly identified these features in their discussions.

Finally, when the Board of Medical Practice suspended the hearings in August of 1994, I needed to know why. Although a qualitative study seldom allows the researcher to assign cause, it seemed to me that some aspect of the conflict had taken on additional importance and led to the breakdown of the process. My notes and subsequent face-to-face consultations with key rhetors from the hearings confirmed that the midwives' bid for legal sanction to carry drugs and diagnostic tools and to perform so-called medical procedures, and their assertion that their experiential knowledge and informal educational systems should allow them to do so, prompted medical representatives to lobby the board to suspend the hearings. At this same time, some midwives asserted that their knowledge should allow them to support at home pregnancies that medical expertise considered high risk, an assertion that divided the midwifery community and alienated the medical community by directly challenging medical authoritative knowledge about birth.

Although I have identified my research questions here in a somewhat traditional sense, I was quite aware throughout the five years I studied the midwifery community in Minnesota that this community was one not yet examined by rhetorical theory. Moreover, because the community was one of women, I wanted to capture the nature of women's experiential knowledge and the midwives' and home birth parents' sense of themselves as women as much as possible. Lurking on a midwifery listserv, joining MANA, and reading historical and contemporary midwifery publications allowed me to contextualize the Minnesota hearings and midwifery community. I deliberately focused on this hidden and almost invisible community, leaving similar infiltration of the more visible medical community to previous scholars. My aim was simple: to explore through my own disciplinary lens one of the abiding yet hidden worlds of women.

Also, I need to comment on my approach to the third chapter of this book. Although this chapter on the history of midwifery appears before those that analyze the modern debates over midwifery, it was written after the first version of that analysis. Knowing that I did not want to write yet another comprehensive history of midwifery—in particular, one that, given the main emphasis of this book, must be compressed into one section—I chose the following approach. First, I identified the issues that drove the 1990s debates. Next, I reread the overall history of traditional midwifery to see to what extent these issues appeared in what historians had identified as important arguments about midwifery in the past. Finally, I located the public and private texts in which these arguments were detailed; those texts provide the rhetorical sites described within this chapter. During this process, I tried to avoid generalizations that dismiss the context and history of the particular rhetorical sites, but at the same time I tried to prepare the reader for the issues that arose in the 1990s Minnesota debates. I am sure that, like me, the reader will be struck by the remarkable similarity between the issues that emerge, not only in the four periods that I cover, but also throughout the centuries of debates about midwifery.

Finally, I want to comment on the special challenges of doing Internet research to contextualize the Minnesota midwifery hearings. I lurked on the public midwifery listserv located at *midwife@fensende.com* to determine whether the issues raised in the hearings were currently being discussed by midwives elsewhere and whether practices such as attending breech babies at home, a skill that some of Minnesota's direct-entry midwives claimed, were common elsewhere. I did not study the specific nature of the exchanges in the listserv. However, I need to comment on how much credibility I could grant listserv messages and on issues of community, audience, and author's intent that impacted my consideration of listserv comments.

Scholars of Internet research methodology do not agree to what extent computer-mediated communication (CMC) creates communities. For example, James Costigan proposes that

> There is no existing parallel social construct, and in many ways, the Internet creates wholly new social constructs. The medium and its uses are creating communities that not only would not but could not have formed without the use of the Internet. The development and use of chat rooms, for example, has driven a language and community that is closely knit yet extremely diverse and dispersed. (*xix*)

Costigan also argues that, although CMC creates these new communities, they are immediate and fluid; although special languages are created to support the community, usually little effort is made to maintain community structure (*xxii*). Jan Fernback describes the catalyst for these CMC communities as a commonality of interests or locations, whose boundaries are continuously renegotiated and whose connectedness is enabled only by the medium of the Internet (204–206). Although CMC is "socially constructed space," these cybercommunities, notes Fernback, are characterized by "common value systems, norms, rules, and the sense of identity, commitment, and association that also characterize various physical communities and other communities of interest" (211). However, scholars such as Stephen Doheny-Farina disagree that the Internet and CMC create communities. Doheny-Farina contends that communities must be bound by physical place and by social and environmental factors: "You can't subscribe to a community as you subscribe to a discussion group on the net. It must be lived. It is entwined, contradictory, and involves all our senses" (37). On the other hand, Laura Gurak considers CMC communication as capable of forming a "new kind of public space," "an electronic and virtual place of such speed and simultaneity" that people with common values can use to discuss and take action on issues (8).

It is clear that the midwifery listserv participants believed that they had established a community based on common values and a common sense of commitment. Even though men and women share the list—a few male midwives and at least two male obstetricians participated in the listserv during the time I read postings—in general, the community consisted of female direct-entry and nurse-midwives, who frequently attest to their dependence on the listserv for emotional support after difficult births and for advice on their practices. The attitudes of the midwives toward their computer listserv are exemplified below in two threads—one in which participants define the listserv community and one in which they react to flaming.[9]

The midwifery listserv is "for discussion of midwifery issues"; however, Sabrina also maintains Lady's Hands, a "pagan birth list," and confusion about a message posted to midwife@fensende.com, which was meant for Lady's Hands, started one thread in which the purpose of the listserv was discussed. Lilly asked the midwife list, believing that she was really posting to Lady's Hands, whether any one had become "paranoid" about lurkers who were not "pagan friendly" (listserv communication, September 15, 1996). By the time Nancy spotted Lilly's error— "Lady's Hands is a pagan list to my understanding, but the midwife list is a conglomerate. . . . [I]f I am wrong, I would appreciate someone letting me know"(September 16, 1996)— the group had already begun to respond with their impressions of the purpose of the listserv:

> I don't believe we've discussed religious views enough for me to have any clue to what the others' viewpoints are in this area. The same would be true about sexual preferences. Actually, it is none of my business unless someone chooses to share this with me. I feel we are a tolerent group, with the same goal of healthy mom and baby.
> (Suzanne, listserv communication, September 15, 1996)

I may be overstepping myself here since I am new, but here goes. We're all professionals here, or at least aspiring to be, right? So, what does it matter if the sister midwife from whom we learn is Pagan, Christian, heterosexual, lesbian or otherwise? I am a Christian, however, I am not now "lurking" nor have I ever done so in search of anything more than the information that is so helpful in my study of our common craft. Please, no more flaming on the issue. There is too much that we can learn from each other for this kind of pettiness. We do a disservice to the women who have worked so hard to revive our sacred profession/calling by this kind of behavior.

> (Amy from Texas, listserv communication, September 16, 1996)

This is really too bad. I've never seen this list as anything other than midwives supporting midwives, regardless of religious beliefs. I appreciate all of you very much, and I don't really care who is lurking. Maybe they'll learn compassion from us. . . .

> (Grace, CNM—a Christian who loves goddess statues,
> listserv communication, 16 September 1996)

The person who brought this up and seemed so agitated by the "lurking" issue seems to have her/his own ax to grind and I thought that the sister from my sister state said it well. Midwifery is bigger than our minds can comprehend.

> (Tammy in Texas, listserv communication, September 17, 1996)

I appologise [sic] for my ignorance, but, have I missed something here? What are you all talking about ? This pagan /wigwam/christian. What the dif; are we or are we not MIDWIVES. That means "with women" and I don't see whether we are blue or black or polkadotted [sic] what difference it makes as long as we are true to our clients, ourselves and support our peers.   (April, listserv communication, September 17, 1996)

The listserv participants who engage in this thread stress the inclusive nature of the list and their dedication to their clients. Therefore, flaming is not acceptable on the list. Quite often a participant will preface or end her remarks with a comment such as "with all due respect, not a flame" (Betty, listserv communication, September 16, 1996). But, when one participant reacts to what she thinks was disapproval of oral sex, she flames, as shown in the second thread:

> HOW DARE YOU?!?!?!?! How can you claim, in the same post, to be "in love with the multiplicity of human experience," and chastise someone else for their supposed judgemental [sic] response to oral sex . . . and then imply that other's sexual activities . . . show evidence of "psychological pathologies" and give you "good cause" for referral?
>
> (Jackie—whose palms are sweating and hands are shaking from rage!
> listserv communication, September 7, 1996)

However, it becomes quite clear that, although Jackie's emotions are acceptable, her flaming is not:

Jackie—slow down and take a few deep breaths [sic]. Gotta say I think you have over-reacted on this one. . . . Not quite sure where all your rage and sweating palms are coming from, but personal attacks on other midwives really aren't appreciated in this forum. Remember, this is a list where we should try to hear and respond in a civil fashion. That is not to say we should not disagree, but I personally feel your post really goes beyond [what] I consider appropriate participation.

(listserv communication, September 7, 1996)

Thus, the midwifery listserv constituted a community in which the participants, for the most part, freely exchanged ideas, gave support, accepted difference, and discouraged any messages that silenced others.[10] The community supported its members as a way to improve their practices and help their clients, regardless of the specific protocols involved in those practices. The community existed in the minds of the listserv participants.

Once having accepted that the listserv functioned as a community in the minds of the participants, I had to decide to what extent I could accept the messages of the participants as reflective of actual practice and to what extent messages might have been modified to argue a point or create a persona. Scholars such as Sherry Turkle have proposed that on the Internet "players" become "authors not only of text but of themselves, constructing new selves through social interaction," and that these selves were "multiple, fluid, and constituted in interaction with machine connections . . . made and transformed by language" (*Life* 12). On the Internet, Turkle proposes that new personae are created, that participants "self-fashion and self-create," that "real-life selves" may learn lessons from "virtual selves," and that these newly created selves are similar to those that emerge during psychoanalysis, fragmented for some but for others self-transformed (180, 256, 260). Of course, participants engaging in face-to-face public discourse may assume a persona in order to be more persuasive; in fact, my rhetorical analysis of the Minnesota hearings depends on tracing which arguments key rhetors decide to present and which "face" of midwifery or medicine they assume in making those arguments. Moreover, the midwifery listserv participants themselves described their purpose in contributing to and maintaining their listserv: They were not playing games or joining chat rooms, but instead seeking and sharing information to improve their practices. Therefore, I assumed, even though midwives without Internet access could not participate in the midwifery listserv, that the long list of participants provided a wide range of comments on practice. I assumed that the majority of participants engaged in listserv conversations for professional development; trying on different personae was of secondary importance to them. Finally, unless credibility of a message was directly challenged by other listserv participants, I assumed that a message was truly reflective of practice. As Gurak states:

In online discourse, the ethical character of the speaker is often unchallenged; the sense of trust among some members of the Internet community is often based on a person's stated professional affiliations and subsequent contributions of life on the Internet. Individuals can be accepted as moral and credible even though the many recipients of an Internet message have never met the author or authors of the message and cannot be sure that authors are who they say they are. In addition, pseudonyms, for example can be used to mask the name of a speaker, so that often it is the ethos of the *texts,* not the character of the speaker, that does or does not convince others. (14–15)

Thus, although I acknowledge the complexities of Internet research, the midwifery listserv messages provided a way to contextualize the Minnesota hearings. These listserv messages, then, function much as the rules and regulations within other states, which provide a way to determine the commonality or uniqueness of the Minnesota debates. The listserv messages also contextualize my study of the rhetorical strategies used to defend or defeat midwifery in other centuries, as described in the next chapter.

CHAPTER 3

The Rhetorical History of Midwifery

❧❦❧

*I am well aware that many practitioners do not wait for these
conditions to arise but put on the forceps early in the labor, but I want
to make a plea for conservative action in this event. Give nature a
chance before interfering. The more experience gained the less and
less frequently do I find forceps necessary. Many a time Mother Nature
has come to reassert herself when it seemed that instrumental delivery
was inevitable.*
—*(Mosher 35)*

*Is labor a natural process? To this we may reply with another question:
If labor be the natural process which you assume, why is it necessary
to call in a physician at all? And we may also ask: Are human beings
to-day natural? Is not our whole life, in civilized countries, artificial?*
—*("Are Our Obstetrical Principles Unscientific" 155)*

$\mathcal{T}$he history of midwifery foreshadows many
of the issues that drive modern conversations about midwifery. Or, to reverse this
point of view, modern public debates about midwifery resonate with echoes from
the history of midwifery, particularly in its relationship to medicine and the state.
This is not surprising, in that direct-entry midwifery celebrates its connections with
past philosophies, because it adapts many of the practices and remedies of its earliest practitioners. Modern midwives still rely on touch and intuition before they
turn to drugs and invasive procedures. Also, state, church, and medical communities have long struggled to define the limits of midwifery practice in relation to
other practitioners, while the direct-entry midwives, attracted to professionalization, have continued to fear loss of autonomy. This chapter identifies and describes
those echoes within the spoken and written words of midwives, nurses, birthing
mothers, and physicians across four centuries. Such a review provides an additional
interpretive framework for the current debates over the licensing and professionalization of direct-entry midwifery. In particular, at four key historical periods, midwives and their supporters or opponents have debated the issue of who holds
authoritative knowledge about birth, including the appropriate role of science and
technology in the birth process, the need for intervention in the birth process, jurisdictional distinctions between medical and midwifery practice, and the differing

values of abstract scientific theory, principles of anatomy and physiology, and women's experiential knowledge.

For example, in the first quotation that opens this chapter, George Mosher observed in an 1892 issue of the *Journal of the American Medical Association* that mother nature would "reassert" herself before the forceps were needed to deliver a child, particularly given the birthing mother's fear that the physician was about to use instruments. Mosher cited a case in which the mother delivered her baby while Mosher was walking across the street to borrow forceps from a colleague. However, as seen in the second opening quotation, the editors of *JAMA* argued that labor and birth were no longer natural processes, if they had ever been; labor and birth were therefore best overseen and managed by a physician armed with the latest technology. Such questions about the normalcy of birth and appropriate intervention surface again in modern midwifery debates.

This chapter identifies themes within the history of midwifery, primarily in the United States and England, which reemerge within debates over modern direct-entry midwifery. Because there are already many fine general histories on midwifery[1] and because my study is a rhetorical one, I focus on four periods of relevant public debate over midwifery. This focus recalls the arguments and issues that arose in previous decades—even centuries—about midwives' knowledge, the relationship of their knowledge to science and technology, their professional status, and their ideology in relation to legal agencies and medical communities.

The first period I explore, some three centuries ago, saw the publication of early midwifery texts that argued for the relevance of women's experiential knowledge, including the first text written by a midwife, Jane Sharp's *The Midwives Book*. In 1671 Sharp attempted to teach midwives all they needed to know about the anatomy and physiology of their clients. In 1687, Elizabeth Cellier presented a proposal for an independent midwifery corporation to run a hospital and midwifery school in London. Finally, Elizabeth Nihell's 1760 *A Treatise on the Art of Midwifery* was a direct argument against encroaching on female midwives. The second period begins with the invention of the obstetrical forceps and other tools by the Chamberlen family of London in the early 1700s and highlights their insistence that female midwives not be permitted to possess or learn how to use these instruments. At the end of the nineteenth century in the United States, reproductive technology such as the forceps again became the focus of debate over the good or harm done by physicians who continued to use these instruments. The third historical period, in the 1920s, centers on the discussion about whether to educate and license or eliminate midwives in the United States. This period encompasses the public health movement and the Sheppard-Towner Act. In discussing this period, I also briefly review the earlier debate over licensing midwives in Britain, which involved a schism between nurses and midwives. Finally, I analyze the philosophy and language of the home birth movement of the 1960s and 1970s in the United States, which was initiated by the Santa Cruz Birth Center in California and The Farm in Tennessee. I also mark the subsequent arrests of midwives for practicing medicine without a license and for murder.

Knowledge and Practice of Early Midwives: A Woman's Touch

Although scholars have certainly documented women's involvement in, if not ownership of, birth from biblical times until the middle of the sixteenth century, few of these early midwives' words are available to us. As Jane Donegan notes, "As women, most midwives were socialized to view themselves as innately inferior beings, that is, beings whose sexual natures assigned them positions and roles subordinate to those held by men. One consequence was that literate women who could have left records were unlikely to consider their work worth reading" (20). References to early midwives are found primarily in male surgeons' and physicians' written cases; midwives' oaths and licensing requirements; accusations that midwives were engaged in witchcraft, abortion, or infanticide; and allusions to midwives in autobiographical texts (Donegan 20–21).[2]

Jane Sharp's The Midwives Book: Arguing for Education

Among the exceptions are the words of Jane Sharp, Elizabeth Cellier, and Elizabeth Nihell. Sharp's *The Midwives Book* (1671), was written to better educate midwives, as she expressed in her dedication:

> To the Midwives of England. Sisters. I have often sate down sad in the Consideration of the many Miseries Women endure in the Hands of unskilful Midwives; many professing the Art (without any skill in Anatomy, which is the Principal part effectually necessary for a Midwife) meerly for Lucres Sake. (1)

However, Sharp was well aware that she addressed another audience, one skeptical about the ability of midwives to learn anatomy and physiology and one advocating the exclusion of women from formal education:

> Some perhaps may think that then it is not proper for women to be of this profession, because they cannot attain so rarely to the knowledge of things as men may, who are bred up in Universities, Schools of learning, or serve their Apprentiships for that end and purpose, where Anatomy Lectures being frequently read, the situation of the parts both of men and women and other things of great consequence are often made plain to them. (2)

Sharp alluded to the Bible to emphasize that midwives had been responsible for birth throughout history, and she contended that, although women might not be suited to formal study because of their natures, their practical skills and experiential knowledge outweighed their lack of theoretical knowledge: "[T]hough nature be not alone sufficient to the perfection of it, yet farther knowledge may be gain'd by a long and dilligent practice, and be communicated to others of our own sex" (3).

Sharp's book appeared at a time when midwives had almost exclusive jurisdiction over normal birth throughout Europe. English midwives were not regulated until the middle of the sixteenth century, when early regulatory stipulations focused primarily on the midwife's character, her possible involvement in witchcraft and magic, and her responsibility to see that children were baptized in the Church of England or properly buried, and that paternity was correctly identified. Birth was considered a normal event, although in complicated deliveries the midwife was expected to call on a male surgeon who usually had little knowledge about birth and could only extract the child piecemeal to save the mother's life or perform a Cesarean section on the mother after her death to save the baby.[3] At the time Sharp was writing, only a few texts were geared to boosting the midwife's knowledge about birth, and these texts revealed Sharp's male contemporaries' narrow views of the midwife's practice.[4]

For example, John Maubray's 1724 *The Female Physician* focused on the general conduct of the midwife and recommended that with abnormal cases she take "immediate *Recourse* to the ablest *Practiser* in the ART, and freely submit her Thoughts to the discerning *Faculty* of the more Learned and Skilful" (quoted. in Cutter and Viets 13, emphasis in original). Edmund Chapman's 1730 *Treatise on the Improvement of Midwifery* omitted anatomical descriptions that might "raise and encourage *impure* Thoughts in the Reader's Mind, rather than to convey any real Instruction," a reflection of the modesty expected of the midwife and her clients (*xx*, original emphasis). Chapman, however, assumed that some midwives might attend problematic presentations but criticized the midwives' popular techniques for handling these, such as dipping the infant's hand in cold water so that the infant might withdraw it and emerge head first (113). Nicholas Culpeper's 1724 *A Directory of Midwives* also included instructions for how to turn a baby but did not include necessary anatomical information so that the midwife could visualize what she was attempting. And, *Dr. Chamberlains' Midwives Practice,* probably authored by Paul Chamberlen in 1665, noted that midwives needed to be educated primarily so that they could judge which cases they were capable of handling. Therefore, the midwives whom Jane Sharp addressed were expected to attend normal births, which to some midwives included problematic presentations such as breeches and twins; know when to call on a more learned midwife or a physician or surgeon; and maintain good conduct, religious laws, and modesty in attending births (see appendix B for a description of how a midwife might manage breech birth).

Within her text, Sharp carefully balances her acknowledgment of men's superior social place with her instructions to the midwives. The midwives must know anatomy so "that we may be able to help and give directions to such women as send for us in their extremities, and had we not some competent insight into the *Theory*, we could never know how to proceed to practice, that we may be able to give a handsome account of what we come for" (166). But first Sharp must describe the male anatomy "because it is commonly maintain'd, that the Masculine gender is more worthy than the Feminine"(4). She acknowledges, according to the medical beliefs of her day, that "Mens parts for Generation are compleat and appear outwardly by reason of heat, but womens are not so compleat, and are made within by reason of their small heat" (37). Then, drawing her anatomical theory from Hippocrates, Galen, and Aristotle, Sharp gives a thorough description of such anatomical parts as the womb, acknowledging not only the man's contribution to procreation but also the female's sexual pleasures:

> The Matrix or Womb hath two parts: the great hollow part within, and the neck that leads to it, and it is a member made by Nature for propagation of children. The substance of the concavity of it is sinewy, mingled with flesh, so that it is not very quick of feeling, it is covered with sinewy Coat that it may stretch in time of Copulation, and may give way when the Child is born; when it takes in the Seed from Man the whole concavity moves toward the Center, and embraceth it, and toucheth it with both its sides. The substance of the neck of it is musculous and gristly with some fat, and it hath one wrinkle upon another, and these cause pleasure in the time of Copulation; this part is very quick of feeling. (34–35)

Ultimately, however, Sharp stresses the difference between men and women, rather than the male's superiority: "Man in the act of procreation is the agent and tiller and sower of the Ground, Woman is the Patient or Ground to be tilled . . . [W]e women have no more cause to be angry, or be ashamed of what Nature hath given us than men have, we cannot be without ours no more than they can want theirs" (33). Therefore, within the text, readers find Sharp poking fun at assumptions of male superiority: Even though a woman's vagina should "fit" any size penis, Sharp says, "yet I have heard a *French* man complain sadly, that when he first married his Wife, it was no bigger nor wider than would fit his turn, but now it was grown as a Sack; Perhaps the fault was not the womans but his own, his weapon shrunk and was grown too little for the scabbard" (53).

Within the heart of her text, Sharp teaches her readers not only anatomy but also non-invasive diagnostic techniques and natural remedies. These techniques and remedies reflect her knowledge of herbs, for example, and the superstitions of the time. To tell whether the woman or her mate is barren, the midwife must "take some small quantity of Barley, or any other Corn that will soon grow, and soak part of it in the mans Urine, and part in the womans Urine, for a whole day and a night; then take the Corn out of both their Urines and lay them apart upon some floor, or in parts where it may dry, and in every morning water them both with their own Urine, and continue; that Corn that grows first is the most fruitful, and so is the person whose Urine was the cause of it . . ." (164). Although prayer is the only remedy for barrenness, Sharp does offer remedies for other conditions: "If the womb be too windy, eat ten Juniper berries every morning, if too moist, the woman must exersize, or sweat in a Stove. . . . " (176). For ulcerated wombs, she offers a remedy that seems extreme to modern eyes: "Take Oyl of worms, of Foxes, and of the Lillies of the Vallies, each alike, boyl a young blind Puppey in them so long that his flesh part from the bones. . . . " (195).[5] Finally, to alleviate pain, the laboring woman could sit in a warm bath (184), a remedy used by midwives today.

Regardless of how Sharp's remedies might amuse a modern reader, her midwives—as will their twentieth-century sisters—rely on herbs, touch, intuition, and the laboring mother's own instincts. All women "do not keep the same posture in their delivery" and so the midwife must allow them their choice, Sharp cautions (199). And, with her hands anointed with "Oyl of Lillies, and the Womans Secrets, or with Oyl of Almonds," the midwife can visualize the position of the child" (199) or aid in a normal delivery: "The woman must hold her breath in and strive to be delivered, and the Midwife must stroke down the birth from above the Navel easily with her hand, for that will, as I said before, make the Infant move downwards" (205).

Sharp assures her readers that a footling can be turned, not by instruments but by the midwife's hands:

> If the child come forth with both legs and feet first, and the Childs hands both lifted above the head, this is the worst for danger of the rest; she [the midwife] must strive to turn the Child, and if she cannot she must try to bring the hands down to the sides, and to keep the legs close that it may come forth, or else to bind the feet as they come out with some linnen Cloath, and tenderly to help delivery, but it will be hard to it. (201)

With the knowledge Sharp offers, a midwife can also deliver twins: "If they come one with his feet, the other with the head forward at the same time, she must receive that first which is most likely, and next the passage, and that which cometh with the feet first, if she can, receive last, taking heed that they do not hurt one the other" (203–204).

However, Sharp's confidence that, given their intuition and experience, her midwives could attend malpresented and multiple births was not shared by her male contemporaries (see appendix B for a glossary of birth terms). Hugh Chamberlen declared that midwives must call in the physician for a malpresentation or a baby who threatens not to emerge head first from the womb. And, William Giffard cautioned that midwives must send for help "when a Child comes Footling, and not to venture (unless they are very skilful) to bring it forwards" (quoted. in Donegan 39–40). Chapman warned that "Women-Midwives" who attempted to turn a child might encounter "many unforseen Difficulties" best handled by a physician (*xii*). As seen in subsequent chapters in this book, disagreement about whether midwives could handle malpresentations and twins reappears at a critical juncture in the Minnesota conversations about the scope of practice for direct-entry midwives.

Finally, Sharp cautions the midwife generally not to intervene in natural birth except in extreme cases. For example, she should not break the laboring mother's membranes to speed labor: "These waters make the parts slippery and the birth easie, if the child come presently with them, but if it stay longer till the parts grow dry it will be hard, therefore Midwives do ill to rend these skins open with their nails to make way for the water to come, nature will make it come forth only when she needs it and not before; but if the water break away long before the birth, it is safe to give medicaments to drive the birth after the water" (207).

The midwife would use instruments only if their remedies fail to deliver the mother of a child who has died in the womb. "That disease," Sharp says, "is beyond the power of medicine or ordinary Midwifery, then we must come to chigurgery" (191). Perhaps acknowledging those midwives who practiced far away from surgical help, rather than simply cautioning to send for the surgeon, Sharp includes exact instructions for the midwife: "fasten a hook to one eye of it [the head], or under the chin, or to the roof of the mouth, or upon one of the shoulders, which of these you find best, and then draw the Child out gently that you do the woman no hurt" (191–192).

Jane Sharp taught her midwives anatomy, shared her diagnostic techniques and remedies, and affirmed that the midwives' hands and herbs in combination with the natural birthing process were sufficient to handle most cases. Sharp also carefully positioned the female midwife, within a society that viewed females as naturally inferior to males, as the sole practitioner of birth, including some of the most challenging cases.

Elizabeth Cellier's Midwives' College: Asking for Self-Governance

Elizabeth Cellier proposed another scheme for training midwives and maintaining their place in birthing practices. In 1616, Peter Chamberlen, surgeon to the Queen, had proposed a midwives' corporation, which, rather than granting the midwives control, would have given him a monopoly on licensing and instructing the midwives and on attending their difficult cases. The College of Physicians opposed Chamberlen's plan and asserted instead that midwives were best regulated through a Bishop's license and examination by the College. A later attempt by Chamberlen's nephew to revive the midwives' corporation proposal also failed, and this time the midwives themselves accused the Chamberlens of wishing to benefit financially by restricting the midwives' education and abilities and thereby expanding the number of "abnormal" cases (Donnison 13–14). On one hand, Sharp's text increased the midwives' knowledge; on the other hand, if Cellier's Midwives' College had been approved, the College would have increased the midwives' professional standing but set strict limits on their jurisdictional boundaries. Similar to the Hôtel-Dieu in Paris, Cellier's lying-in hospital would incorporate all midwives in London, provide for their instruction, and offer a setting for their professional discussions.[6] Cellier's bid for self-governance for midwives in 1687 raised issues of jurisdiction and autonomy that reappear in modern debates over direct-entry midwifery.

Whereas Sharp balanced her need to improve the anatomical knowledge of her midwife readers with her acknowledgment of the lesser social position of women in general, Cellier's scheme would have expanded the midwives' professional position but would have necessarily limited their autonomy. Aware of the growing interest among male practitioners in the "business" of birth, Cellier began her argument with the warrant that the education midwives obtained at her Midwives' College would save the lives of women and children who had "in all Probability perished, for Want of due Skill and Care, in those Women who practise the Art of Midwifery" ("Scheme"1). Cellier reminded her readers that history identified many honored, educated, and self-directed midwives ("An Answer" 4). However, throughout her proposal, Cellier carefully defined how the midwives must interact with the medical community and the state. She promised that the midwives would confine their activities to midwifery and not engage in surgery and pharmacology, thereby avoiding jurisdictional competition ("An Answer" 4). The midwives would conduct their own peer review, but their formal education would be orchestrated by male practitioners:

That a Woman, sufficiently skilled in Writing and Accounts, be appointed
Secretary to the Governers and Company of Midwives to be present at all
Controversies about the Art of Midwifery, to register all the extraordinary
Accidents happening in the Practice, which all licensed Midwives are, from
time to time, to report to the Society. . . . That the principle Physician, or
Man-midwife, examine all extraordinary Accidents, and, once a Month at
least, read a publick Lecture to the whole Society of licensed Midwives,
who are all obligated to be present at it, if not employed in their Practice;
and he shall deliver a Copy of such Reading, to be entered into the Book
to be kept for that Purpose. . . . ("Scheme" 6)

The College, and the Royal Foundling Hospital it would support, could expand into
"twelve of the greatest Parishes" to establish more lying-in-hospitals to be governed
by matrons from the Corporation of Midwives," but the King and his representatives
would make the higher appointments in the College ("Scheme" 2–3). Achieving
this balance between the midwives' control and their obligation to interact with the
state and medical communities seems a deliberate rhetorical strategy on Cellier's
part. She wished to define limits and relationships rather than having others do so
for her. For example, she replied to hostile questions about her proposal: "Wherein
we desire you not to concern your selves, until we desire your Company, which we
will certainly do as often as we have occasion for your Advice in any thing *we do
not understand, or which doth not appertain to our Practice*" ("An Answer" 5).

Historians predict that if King James had favored Cellier's proposal, the College of Physicians would still have successfully opposed the Midwives' College
based on the same objections they raised about the Chamberlens's schemes (Donnison 19). As more men took up the practice of midwifery, attending routine cases
in direct competition with their female counterparts, female midwives were challenged to survive within this competitive arena. Male practitioners had several advantages: They had access to new birth technologies such as the forceps; the first
lying-in hospitals established in London provided medical men with clinical cases
for study; the family who could afford the more expensive male practitioner often
felt it had achieved a higher social and economic status; and the less powerful An-
glican Church granted fewer and fewer midwifery licenses to women (Donnison
22). Although male practitioners such as John Douglas thought men belonged in
the birthing room only in "abnormal cases" (quoted in Jex-Blake 22), others such
as Thomas Dawkes continued to narrow the limits of normalcy and midwives'
capabilities.

Elizabeth Nihell's Treatise: Arguing Against Birth Instruments
In reaction to this narrowing of midwifery practices, Sarah Stone published
her *Complete Practice of Midwifery* to help midwives handle difficult cases without calling in a male practitioner. Moreover, Elizabeth Nihell, who studied at the famous training hospital Hôtel-Dieu in Paris and lived with her surgeon-apothecary
husband in the Haymarket, argued in 1760 that interventions by instruments, brought

into the birthing room by male practitioners, were seldom necessary. Nihell's observations at the Hôtel-Dieu are summed up in such words as: "One [male practitioner], upon some most learnedly erroneous hypothesis, pulls and hauls the arm of an innocent infant yet living, so that he plucks it off; or repels it with such violence, that he breaks it: another unmercifully opens the infant's head, and takes the brain out: some bring the whole away piece-meal: operations often to be defended only by hard words and harder hearts" (10–11). Rather than accepting that female midwives were less useful during birth because they had no access to or training in the emerging technologies, Nihell argued that these technologies caused more damage than good, a charge often raised by twentieth-century direct-entry midwives and their home birth clients.

To make her case, Nihell takes the power to make decisions out of the hands of male practitioners. She assures her readers—mother and fathers alike—that they have the common sense and reason to make their own birthing decisions. This constituted an early type of informed consent: "Fashion, sillily fostering a preference of men to women in the practice of midwifery" along with "Fear" caused "errors and pernicious innovations" in birth (*ii, iii–iv*). Nihell attributes these errors directly to male midwives, who offend nature rather than assist her, and who rely on theories "which, when reduced to practice, are infinitely worse than any deficiency in some particular female-practitioners," theories which are "fit for nothing so much, as to prepare dreadful work for their instruments" (*v*). These male midwives are motivated, Nihell claims, by interest in obtaining an income through extending their jurisdictions, and her own purpose is to "undeceive the public," to "remove the prejudices that support male-midwifery," and to demonstrate the "destructiveness of instruments in the art of midwifery" (*vi, x–xi*).

Nihell sets up a series of objections to female midwives and then refutes these objections, often arguing directly with the words of such famous male practitioners as William Smellie. For example, to those who object to female midwives because the art of midwifery is a branch of the "art of physic" and "must have been originally in the hands of man, the inventor of all arts," Nihell responds that Eve had sufficient knowledge to deliver her children herself (14). To those who assert that a "good practitioner of midwifery" must understand anatomy, a science that is the "province of man," Nihell responds: "It is sufficient that a woman understands and knows the structure and mechanical disposition of the internal parts which more particularly distinguish her sex; that she can discern the container from the contents, what belongs to the mother from what belongs to the child, as well as what is foreign to both" (32–33). Experienced midwives have this knowledge; more knowledge is not necessary: "It is true, that these poor midwives do not understand anatomy enough to make a dissection; but I fancy that the ladies who want assistence in their lying-ins, are not very curious of having one that can dissect instead of delivering them" (33–34).

Although Nihell offers a range of objections and responses, she focuses on intervention and instruments. Nihell sums up the arguments of those who claim that technology has eliminated the need for the female midwife:

The different instruments which the men have invented in aid of, and supplement to the deficiency of nature, and of which they are frequently obligated to make use in different labors, ought not to be put into the hands of midwives: and were it but for this reason alone, they ought to be excluded from the practice of this art. As, why multiply attendants unnecessarily? A man-midwife, with his instruments which he ought always to have about him, is enough for every thing: whereas a midwife, if the case requires instruments, will be obligated to have recourse to a man: consequently double embarrassment, double expence. (35–36)

Nihell responds by contrasting the female midwife's more effective hands to the male midwife's brutal instruments:

The keen instruments bring an argument they imagine capable of banishing or exterminating all the midwives. The men, they say, enjoy alone the glorious privilege of using instruments, in order, as they pretend, to assist nature. But . . . where is the person that would prefer iron and steel to a hand of flesh, tender, soft, duly supple, dextrous, and trusting to its own feelings for what it is about: a hand that has no need of recourse to such an extremity as the use of instruments, always blind, dangerous, and especially for ever useless? (36–37)

Of the 900 births that Nihell attended, she never saw any occasion to use such instruments (46, 54). The experienced midwife "with less learning and more patience," "well acquainted with the power and custom of Nature" is less likely to injure mother or child (76). She will call for help when needed, but from the physician or surgeon, not from the male midwife, whose "shew must be made of doing something, *will* most probably determine him improperly, if not fatall, to random prescriptions . . ." (122–123, emphasis in original). The female midwife and the physician have mutual respect for their differing knowledge systems and approaches, Nihell asserts (126, 251).

As did Jane Sharp, Nihell defines the female midwife's sense of touch as her most useful technique, "the most nice and essential point of the art of midwifery" (311). To Sharp, the body is certainly material, and touching is an essential diagnostic tool as well as remedy: "When, by *touching,* I perceive, there is an obliquity of the uterus in the case, in the proper time, I desire the patient to lay on her back, and introducing my finger, endeavor to come at the orifice of the uterus. Upon getting hold of it, I support it so long as the labor-throw continues, and I take care the child should not engage itself too much" (347–348, emphasis in original). Male midwives do not possess the art of touching, as their hands are "naturally none of the softest, and perhaps callous with handling iron and steel instruments" (317). Therefore, Nihell argues, the female midwife belongs in the birthing room: "The infinitely important service of predisposing the passages, and of obviating difficulties, to be only ascertained by that faculty of touching, is palpably and peculiarly appropriated by Nature to the women only . . ."(318). Touching is natural to women, and touching imitates Nature, which "proceeds leisurely," whereas the forceps "goes too quick to work" (415). Nihell concludes:

> The art of midwifery then, in its management by women, carries with it, in the recommendation of order, modestly, propriety, ease, diminution of pain and danger, all the marks of the providential care of Nature. . . . Whereas the function of this art, officiated by men, has ever something barbarously uncouth, indecent, mean, nauseous, shockingly unmanly and out of character: and, above all, of lame or imperfect in it. (452–53)

Jane Sharp argued that midwives needed anatomical education, and Elizabeth Cellier contended that midwives needed professional recognition and self-governance; both writers saw possibilities for midwives improving their practices and positions. However, Elizabeth Nihell argued against a growing tide of male midwives who entered the birthing room with technology to which female midwives had no easy access—instruments that promised to free women and their infants from long labors and possible death but wrought their own brand of destruction. To survive, Nihell felt that the female midwives had to define their jurisdictional practices in contrast to these instruments.

Midwifery's Relationship to Science and Technology

Many historians believe that despite the efforts of Nihell and others, the invention and use of the forceps marked the end of female midwives' control over birth. For example, Donegan says: "It was the surgeons' possession of the forceps that enabled them to challenge directly the women midwives' traditional role as the attendants at all normal cases" (47). Donnison agrees: "[I]t was probably the introduction of the midwifery forceps, a development which occurred about 1720, which precipitated this rapid acceleration in what was already an existing trend" (21–22).[7] While many women feared the instruments, and both midwives and physicians warned of the damage they could cause, birthing mothers whose labors didn't progress normally welcomed the rapid delivery that the instruments often made possible. As Leavitt remarks: "If physicians used forceps too often, or if they intervened in the birth process too eagerly, it was because they were more persuaded by the faces of women in agony than by the cautions of their elders. The instrument provided one important differentiation between the skills of doctors and the skills of midwives, and doctors needed to remind their patients of this distinction" (48).

Intervention: Narrowing the Definition of the
Good Midwife and Normal Birth

The forceps were invented in 1598 and initially kept secret by the Chamberlen family of England; this enabled male members of the family to claim skills beyond the ken of their female counterparts. Later instructions for how to use the forceps, written by Benjamin Pugh in his 1754 *Treatise on Midwifery* and by William Smellie in his 1756 *Treatise on the Theory and Practice of Midwifery*, addressed only male midwives. One exception was Margaret Stephen who in 1790 taught female midwives in London the use of forceps (Wilson 202).

Before the invention of the forceps (as well as the fillet and vectis—see appendix B for a description of these instruments), the male practitioner called in to deal with a difficult birth could usually only deliver a dead child through craniotomy by hook and crotchet; female midwives usually attempted to turn the malpresented child with their hands or by repositioning the laboring mother (Wilson 49, 52, 54). The forceps, fillet, and vectis allowed the male practitioner to deliver a living child in some of the most difficult cases and so claim that his practices were superior to those of the female midwife.

However important these instruments, birth practices changed for a number of other reasons. For centuries, birth had been a female ritual that maintained the midwife's status among all classes. Wilson describes the ritual of birth within the community of women:

> What we must remember is that the traditional role of the midwife was embedded in the collective culture of women. It was the ceremony of childbirth that conferred authority on the midwife; the mother's personal choice extended only to the selection of *which* midwife, of those locally available would deliver her. What gave the ritual its immense power was collective female authority . . . Mothers, midwives and gossips were bound together by the same web of social bonds that constituted the collective culture of women in general. That culture was made possible by the range of experiences and activities shared by mothers of all social ranks. The basis of this sharing was the patriarchal order, that is, the laws and customs that conferred upon husbands property in the sexuality, the goods and the labour of their wives. Even the aristocratic wife was subsumed within this order; all women found themselves bound by it. Hence the fact that the relatively humble midwife could assert power over a mother who belonged to the ruling class. (185)

Initially women feared the male midwife, who broke into the circle with his immodest and seemingly violent instruments. To overcome this fear, the male midwife had to deliver living children—to save not just the mother but also the child.

New class distinctions also strengthened the male midwife's position. A new culture of ladies of leisure in the middle and upper classes began to distinguish itself from the lower classes. To this new class, the new male midwife symbolized a superior social status (Wilson 186–192). Childbirth was "no longer a collective event" but a solitary one, if at home, and a "medicalized" one, if in the lying-in hospital (Wilson 204, 206). Moreover, it was "unthinkable" to many to include midwives, or any women, in medical training (Wertz and Wertz 45).

As a result, the definitions of the good midwife and the normal or natural birth were changing. For example, William Giffard in his *Cases in Midwifery* defined the good midwife as the one who diagnosed by touching and then sent promptly for the male practitioner when needed; she was the one who recognized her subordination, could give a case history to the male practitioner, and then would step aside, returning only when called back to cut the umbilical cord (Giffard 89).[8] Sir Richard Manningham, who established the first lying-in infirmary in London, taught midwives how to manage normal births, and male practitioners to manage normal and abnormal births. To Manningham, birth "was implicitly guilty until proven innocent," and the good midwife summoned the male practitioner immediately upon sensing trouble, an attitude still expressed today by many physicians and reflected within many states' licensing rules and regulations on direct-entry midwifery (quoted in Cutter and Viets 15–16; see also Wilson 115).

This narrowing of the scope of practice of the midwife and the parameters of normal or natural birth was carried into the United States by those trained abroad. For example, William Shippen, educated in London and Edinburgh, lectured exclusively to male students on anatomy, natural and unnatural birth, and obstetrical instruments, with the expectation that physicians would intervene in the normal birth process. Leavitt remarks that "for those women who chose physicians instead of or in addition to midwives, birth became less a natural, immutable process and more an event that could be altered and influenced by a wide selection of interventions" (49).

The first midwifery manual written in the United States was Valentine Seaman's 1800 *The Midwives Monitor and Mother's Mirror*, in which he defined natural labors as those "where the head presented with no 'artificial assistance' necessary and with a duration of up to twenty-four hours . . . whereas 'complicated' labors were those accompanied by 'floodings,' 'convulsions,' or other unusual conditions" (80–81). The good midwife was to attend only natural labors and "to bolster her patient's morale during labor, to examine her to determine the degree of dilation achieved, to support the perineum at the moment of birth, to tie off the umbilical cord, and above all, to refrain from pulling on the cord in an effort to hasten the expulsion of the placenta" (90–99).

As male practitioners gained more experience with birth and with their instruments, they began to exclude twin births and malpresented babies from their definitions of normal birth. While most midwives left the delivery of the second twin up to natural processes, male practitioners believed that the second twin should be pulled from the birth canal immediately—and often by the feet. Wilson speculates that because the midwives attended more spontaneous deliveries of the first twin, they also saw normal delivery of the second twin. Male practitioners, often called in when the mother had difficulty delivering the first twin, needed to help the exhausted mother quickly deliver the second (163). Much the same thing happened with malpresentations. Male practitioners were called in when the midwife couldn't turn the child to the head or deliver by the feet; instruments such as the forceps provided the traction needed to turn the child to the feet "without depending on the natural powers" (Wilson 163). In promoting this form of podalic version, possible with the forceps, male practitioners reinforced the notion that such malpresentations were abnormal births and therefore beyond the female midwives' scope of practice.

Regardless of whether the invention and use of the forceps, fillet, and vectis directly caused or simply contributed to the decline of midwifery, by the end of the nineteenth century in Britain and in the United States, the female midwife had lost control of birth. Now an important part of her role was to know when to summon the male practitioner with his instruments, and she was told that, despite her knowledge about birth, many birth situations, including twins and malpresentations, were beyond her skills.

The Science and Technology of Birth: A Masculine Domain

These definitions and boundaries are affirmed in what appears to be the final debate about the forceps, a debate that took place within the pages of the *Journal of the American Medical Association* at the end of the nineteenth century. The debate raised a number of issues: the best type of forceps, the frequency of their use, the knowledge needed to use them effectively, and their safety. The debate also reflected many physicians' attitudes about the natural process of birth and about the knowledge and values of the women they treated and of female birth attendants who assisted the physicians. However, the debate surfaced within the medical community and became an argument among physicians, rather than an argument between midwives and male practitioners as it had been two centuries before.

Early in the debate, a group of practitioners expressed their belief in the natural birth process. Responding to the assertion that the forceps be used before the mother was fully dilated, they countered that the use of the forceps was "seldom indicated," regardless of the "modern idea" that the forceps was "an instrument with which it is practically impossible to injure either mother or fœtus" ("Complete Dilation" 239). For example, Dr. Hiram Corson offered his personal philosophy of birth: "I have considered labor a natural process, and that my duty consisted in awaiting the action of the patient's forces; not setting them aside and myself usurping the duties which the natural efforts would have performed without difficulty; but coming to my patient's aid only when her forces seemed inadequate to the performance of their duties" (138). George Mosher (see the first quote at the chapter opening) affirmed this belief in the natural process.

Corson's remarks sparked the most controversy when he claimed that physicians used the forceps so frequently "not because nature is inadequate to the work," but because the physician "wished to get away speedily" to handle as many patients as possible. Although the forceps might cause lacerations of the cervix and perineum, the practitioners earned "large renumerations" from repairing these tears (138). However, the *JAMA* editors responded to Corson by questioning how natural birth really was (see the second quote opening this chapter), as they called Corson's argument "not logically sequential" or "rhetorically connected" ("Are Our Obstetrical Principles Unscientific?" 155).

Other physicians continued to argue that the forceps and force were seldom needed if the physician relied on the natural birth process. For example, one female physician, E. S. Mead, notes that unskilled practitioners "put on a pair of forceps, and with great strong muscles that could lift probably two hundred pound dumbbells, they pull. They seem to think that the only thing to be done is to deliver the child; if they cut off its circulation or bruise the mother, that is a matter of minor importance . . ." (277). She commented that she was not a strong woman but strong enough to assert any force needed without supplementing that force with instruments: "It seems to me that it is a lack of anatomic knowledge that destroys so many and makes so many failures" (277).

As other physicians joined the debate about the degree to which the physician could rely on the natural birth process, their language reflected their depersonalization of the mother and her infant, their distrust of female birth attendants, and their affirmation of differing class attitudes toward birth. For example, Henry Fry, who considered labor "absolutely a physical act, accomplished according to a well-defined mechanism," argued that the laws "governing the passage of the *passenger*" must be understood by the physician, who should avoid brute force and remove the forceps if nature begins to take over (651–653, emphasis added). The physician's task was to analyze each situation and to be versed in several types of forceps: "*according to the circumstances of the case, always selecting that instrument which best enables him to apply the blades to the sides of the head*" (651, original emphasis).[9] Fry designed forceps for several situations, including transverse positions for which the forceps "curve adopted is the result of experimentation upon *fresh fœtal heads and articulated female pelves*" (654, emphasis added).

H. C. Coe proposed that the damage done by the forceps was justified, even when the mother was only partially dilated, if infant mortality was thereby reduced. Coe found the instruments particularly useful in his private practice, as "it was this class of patients, in whom the accoucheur was most frequently obligated to perform version, who were most anxious to have living children" (101). And, promoting his new version of the forceps, William Stewart cautioned that the forceps "should never be used simply to gratify nervous patients, interfering nurses or meddlesome women, nor to save time of a practitioner, busy or otherwise" (770). Finally, Mosher himself longed for "the Utopian age where we can trust our patient to the care of a conscientious, obedient, intelligent and discreet nurse upon whose judgment we can rely to conduct the case in the interim between the first examination and such time as the physician's skill is ultimately necessary. . . . But this will require an education vastly superior to that now possessed by the average nurse, and also of the patient, and more especially of her friends and over solicitous neighbors, as well" (33).

Although the physicians arguing within the pages of *JAMA* disagreed on the extent to which they could rely on the natural process of birth, they assumed that the decision of whether to use the forceps was theirs. They also assumed that neither the mother nor female birth attendants could be relied on to make informed decisions or to monitor births, and that, as physicians, they were the appropriate attendants of not only abnormal but also normal births. Thus, in the end, the invention of birthing instruments narrowed the role of the midwife and the definition of normal birth and further devalued midwives' knowledge.

The Question of Professionalization of Midwifery

Before discussing the debates about the place of midwifery and the definitions of public health that took place at the beginning of the twentieth century in the

United States, I offer a brief review of the status of midwives in Britain during roughly the same period. My purpose is not to identify parallel discussions in the two countries, as Britain took a very different course than did the United States. Instead, first I demonstrate the nature of British physicians' and nurses' opposition to midwifery regulation—and the compromises that British midwives made to win professional status. My purpose here is to illustrate the dilemma that arises with professionalization: Midwives gain higher status but lose autonomy. This is the same dilemma facing modern midwives. I point to the characteristics that the British midwifery legislation has in common with the licensing rules for modern direct-entry midwives. Then I illustrate, primarily through the arguments raised in professional journals and government reports, the warrants used either to call for the elimination of United States midwives, to extend the jurisdictional boundaries of the medical community, or to argue for the professionalization of midwifery. Within these debates, the definition of birth ranged from a normal process to a pathological condition, while questions were raised about whose authoritative knowledge about birth counted the most. Finally, I explain how these issues were complicated in the United States by the 1920 public health movement.

British Midwives Become State-Recognized Professionals: The Ninety-Year Debate

It took ninety years for the Midwives' Act to be passed in Britain. Several influences delayed its final passage until 1902. The British government was reluctant to become involved in what seemed an issue of free trade. Although medical practitioners agreed on the benefits conferred on women by better-educated midwives, many felt that women in general had no place in medicine and that midwives would disappear once clients could afford male practitioners. Although midwifery had strong leaders in its ranks, overall, many midwives were uneducated and illiterate—a difficult group to rally (in fact, it was impossible to even know how many midwives were practicing at any one time and who they all were). The midwives who worked for regulation had to garner the support of the male medical practitioners who believed that midwifery practices should be restricted and overseen by medical men. Finally, the newly organized British nurses opposed the midwives' bid for professional status (Donnison 117, 125, 176–177). However difficult its passage, the 1902 Midwives' Bill gave midwives a professional standing that they still maintain, to a great extent, in Britain today; it also involved a compromise that United States direct-entry midwives continue to debate.

The issue of regulating midwives resurfaced several times in Britain since the Chamberlens and Elizabeth Cellier came up with their alternative plans two centuries before. For example, in 1874, Dr. J. J. Aveling, who founded the Sheffield Hospital for Women, supported the registration of midwives in his *English Midwives: Their History and Prospects* and believed that midwives were capable of educating themselves while remaining independent of male practitioners. About the same time, the Female Medical Society suggested that midwives be admitted to the Medical Register with status equal to that of medical practitioners; a group of London midwives formed the Obstetrical Association of Midwives in support of this suggestion. The association's leader, Maria Firth, an ex-matron of the British Lying-in Hospital, believed, based on her experience, that midwives need not restrict themselves to attending only normal births.

In a counterproposal, the Obstetrical Society supported regulation of midwives by the General Medical Council but wished to place them in a subordinate position, both in terms of knowledge and practice, to medical practitioners and to expel those midwives who attended abnormal births without seeking medical assistance. Although no regulatory scheme was instigated as of that point, the Obstetrical Society's view of the registered midwife seemed persuasive to many for several reasons: Restrictions, such as the 1868 Pharmacy Act, already forbade the dispensing of drugs by anyone but chemists and druggists, so the midwives would benefit from having a professional relationship with these specialists; the medical profession considered it beneath its dignity to testify to the skills and practices of women as "medical advisors" rather than as subordinates; and the public as well as medical practitioners feared that too highly educated and independent midwives might demand a fee that many of their poorer, rural clients could not afford (Donnison 80–82, 88, 90). However, the registration and examination costs for midwives proved a problem. The number of midwives who sought regulation couldn't pay a fee that would adequately finance the registration process. If the government stepped in to subsidize the midwives, then the Obstetrical Society objected that its members would lose control of the registration process (Donnison 96).

In 1880, another midwives' society was founded by Louisa Hubbard; the Midwives' Aid or Trained Midwives' Registration Society worked for recruitment of educated women into the profession and for state recognition. This new society tried a new and eventually more successful tactic: It worked in cooperation with male medical practitioners, particularly obstetricians. The midwives in the society accepted that their practice would be confined to normal births and that they would be required to call for medical assistance in abnormal cases. The society recruited respectable middle-class women into its ranks, promoting midwifery as a "sphere of usefulness" that was natural for women (Donnison 100–102; see also *Pall Mall Gazette* 11). And in 1882, the society proposed another regulatory scheme with two important differences. First, midwives would be treated more harshly than doctors for professional misconduct. This decision acknowledged physicians' status and power in British society. Second, the society accepted the fact that not all midwives would seek licensing, so a compromise was struck that would split the more educated, probably urban midwife from her less educated, rural counterpart (Donnison 104). The bill received impressive backing, although even physician Sophia Jex-Blake warned the midwives that under the regulation they would be examined and governed by medical practitioners who might not be educated in midwifery themselves. Jex-Blake also warned that midwives could not sit on the Central Board in charge of regulation, and that all midwives would be forbidden from attending any condition defined as abnormal, regardless of their individual training, experience, and expertise (Donnison 105). Although this version of the bill also failed, the debates went on as the society took on the title of Midwives' Institute and continued with the task of educating its members. In cooperation with the society, the Workhouse Nursing Infirmary Association published *Nursing Notes*, in which the institute publicized its regulatory proposals, promoting many of the same compromises.

These moves by the Midwives' Institute were particularly important given the activities of Britain's nurses. By 1887, Bedford Fenwick helped found the British Nurses' Association to fight for the professional advancement and state registration of nurses, and the Nurses' Association used its own publication, *Nursing Record*, to promote nursing. Rather than waiting for the midwives to set the precedent for regulation and professional recognition of female practitioners, Fenwick urged the midwives to join the nurses in a common effort. However, the Midwives' Institute rejected Fenwick's invitation. The midwives were much closer to registration than the nurses, and, even given their realization that the regulation would lead to some subordination, the midwives thought their practice distinct in its degree of independence from medicine and in its close relationship with clients. To add to the tension between the midwives and the nurses, physicians thought the British Nurses' Association members should register as midwives or midwifery nurses because they saw little difference between the midwives' and nurses' practices. Over the next decade, Fenwick would do everything in her power to oppose the registration of midwives and to argue that it was the midwives who should have nursing training (Donnison 113, 115, 127).

When finally passed in 1902, the Midwives' Act placed the midwives in what Donnison has called a "uniquely disadvantaged position among the professions" (174):

> First, although conferring State registration of midwives, the Act subjected them to the local authority supervision otherwise associated with the local licensing of tradesmen. Second, although midwives, like other professions, were liable to erasure from the register for professional misconduct, this misconduct was in their case more widely, and more minutely, defined. Moreover, midwives also risked erasure if their *private* lives met with the disapproval of their disciplinary body. Lastly, in contrast with other professions, midwives were not to regulate themselves—indeed, a rival profession was to have a dominant voice in their government. (174–175, original emphasis)

The law itself opened with the admonition that no midwife could "imply that she is by law recognised as a medical practitioner" and therefore the midwife was distinguished by what she was not—she was the exception to the dominant birth practitioner ("British Midwifery Law" Section 1–5). Finally, those who believed that birth could not be defined as a natural process—or that problem-free births were the exception—greatly influenced the finer points of the Midwives' Act. The Central Midwives' Board, ruled by a medical majority, laid down a strict code of conduct for the midwife, her dress, her tools, her records, and the number of visits she must pay the mother, but, most important, the conditions that dictated when she should send for the doctor. Eventually, all new midwives had to take the board's examination and the period of required training stretched from three months to two years.

And, even in the mid–twentieth century, British midwives had to meet stricter requirements for their professional "conduct" than those required for other professions (Donnison 179, 181).

Thus, by 1902 British midwives had achieved a national professional status that direct-entry midwives throughout the United States still do not have. However, the British midwives also realized that with professionalization came compromise: The midwives would have more access to formal education and relationships with physicians, but they would have to accept medical practitioners' definitions of normal and natural births. Furthermore, the practice of midwifery would be sustained in Britain, but all midwives would have to follow the same protocols regardless of their individual knowledge and experience.

The Debate over Sustaining or Eliminating the U.S. Midwife

At about the same time, four groups were discussing the midwifery "problem" in the United States: (1) those seeking to abolish the midwife and legally prosecute those who continued to practice, such as the State Legislature in Massachusetts; (2) those arguing for eventual abolition of midwifery, but tolerance of the midwives until substitutes (usually physicians) could be trained; (3) those, such as New York City and State, arguing that regulation and education would ensure safe midwifery care such as that found in England; and (4) those (mostly southerners) who "felt that if, somehow, midwives could be made to wash their hands and to use silver nitrate drops for the babies' eyes" that was all that could be expected (Kobrin 353–354).

These groups expressed concern about infant and mother mortality in cases handled by uneducated midwives or poorly prepared physicians. They also worried that a potential double standard for obstetrical care would become the norm should the midwives continue to practice. They argued about whether midwifery care should be confined to so-called normal births and whose authoritative knowledge about birth would prevail. Those advocating the abolition or maintenance of midwifery spoke adamantly and publicly, in journals and government reports. Although these issues were not unique to the United States, the debate was complicated by the Sheppard-Towner Act and the 1920s public health movement.

As early as the 1820s, opponents to midwifery suggested that midwives were responsible for alarming numbers of deaths. For example, a report to the Medical Society of the County of New York stated that "the mortality among newly born children would be materially diminished if the practice of midwifery was more restricted to male attendants" (*Medical Repository*, quoted in Donegan 130). However, others suggested that poorly trained physicians were responsible for greater numbers of deaths, and that the solution was not to eliminate the midwives, but to better train both physicians and midwives (see, for example, Litoff, *American Midwives* 91).

By the turn of the twentieth century, the midwives of New York served as an interesting microcosm for the midwifery debates: To some they represented the very best in care; to others they symbolized all the reasons to eliminate the practice. For example, in 1907 Elisabeth Crowell, assistant secretary of the New York State branch of the Public Health League, reported on her investigations for the Public Health Committee of the Association of Neighborhood Workers. Crowell had interviewed 500 of the estimated 950 midwives handling 42 percent of the births in Manhattan. Crowell was greatly disturbed by the midwives' practices, addressing her concern primarily to medical practitioners:

> To the medical man the facts concerned with the methods of practice of these women will undoubtedly appeal with greatest force. Three-fifths of the total number visited stated frankly that they would undertake the care and treatment of abnormal cases. Many did not hesitate at the removal of an adherent placenta, others will perform version, and all of them will treat a *postpartum* hemorrhage, calling in a physician only when they find themselves entirely unable to cope with the situation at hand. Practically all of them claimed that they used antiseptics, which meant very little if the midwife was dirty, her bag filthy, and if she appeared generally ignorant and incompetent. (reprinted in Litoff, *Midwife Debate* 41–42)

Based on these findings and her discovery that some midwives performed abortions, administered drugs, and gave advice about other illnesses, Crowell suggested that by law the midwife be restricted to natural labor (Litoff, *Midwife Debate* 48). Midwives in New York were registered by the Board of Health, but Crowell believed that licensing of those midwives "only as can meet a high standard of education, training, experience and morals" would eliminate those whose practices were questionable. Crowell maintained that the current form of registration "does not guarantee that the midwife so registered is in the possession of even a modicum of intelligence, let alone any fitness, professional or otherwise" (Litoff, *Midwife Debate* 47).[10]

In contrast to Crowell's condemnation, S. Josephine Baker publicly supported New York's midwives. In a 1912 issue of the *American Journal of Obstetrics and the Diseases of Women and Children,* Baker used a warrant similar to Elizabeth Cellier's:

> The practice of midwifery dates back to the beginning of human life in this world . . . its history runs parallel with the history of the people, and its functions antedate any record we have of medicine as an applied science. To deny its right to exist as a calling is to take issue with the external verities of life. The only points upon which we may argue are the training required for its safe and lawful practice, and the essential fitness of those who follow this calling requisite for the safeguarding of the mother and child. (reprinted in Litoff, *Midwife Debate* 153)

Baker reminded her readers that Socrates's mother was a midwife and she asserted that Europe provided a model for how to treat midwives. She also suggested that mortality rates would drop if midwives' practices were clearly defined, a definite course of study at a registered midwifery school were required, midwifery licenses were issued and renewed yearly by local boards of health that continued to supervise midwives, and all midwives were instructed in how to manage normal labor and diagnose abnormal presentations and complications (166). Baker and others considered the Bellevue School of Midwifery a model for midwifery training (Rule 992).

However, those who advocated the elimination of the midwife questioned whether any birth was "normal"; at the very least, they wished to drastically narrow the definition of "normal." For example, James Huntington reminded the readers of the 1913 *Boston Medical and Surgical Journal:* "There is less and less talk of the '*normal* case' so frequently spoken of by those in favor of the midwife as a practitioner. The trained obstetrician knows that no case is normal until it is over. At any moment complications are liable to arise capable of taxing the skill of the obstetrician to the utmost" (quoted in Litoff, *Midwife Debate* 112; original emphasis). Joseph De Lee agreed in his 1915 *Transactions of the American Association for the Study and Prevention of Infant Mortality:* "Certainly, having babies is a natural process, and, in the intention of nature should be a normal function, yet there is no one here who can deny that it is a destructive one. We all know that even natural deliveries damage both mothers and babies often and much. If child-bearing is destructive, it is pathogenic, and if it is pathogenic it is pathologic" (reprinted in Litoff, *Midwife Debate* 104).

If few or no births were normal, then there was no need for the midwife. Her practice created a double standard of care that endangered the mother and infant. As De Lee put it: "Why should there be a double standard in obstetrics?" At the same time that standards were being raised in medical schools, "we are to try to educate, in a few months, an ignorant woman up to responsibilities of cases with mortalities which would stagger the best of surgeons" (103). Such a double standard only hurt the client, as Huntington said: "How can we with any justice suggest one class of service for the poor and ignorant and another for the well to do and educated? No other branch of medicine tolerates this dual standard—two classes of practitioners, one semi-trained and the other thoroughly educated" (115).

Moreover, if obstetrics were to be recognized as a profession, it had to generate, control, and maintain the authoritative knowledge about birth. The midwife, according to Huntington, contributed "nothing to the knowledge of obstetrics" (113). She could not learn proper birth management, said De Lee: "Obstetrics is a major science. It requires the highest kind of skill in addition to much knowledge to do even tolerable work. The high class of work and superior knowledge required of the infant welfare nurses, the child saving societies, public health movements, all throw into relief the impossibility of training the midwife for any good purpose" (108). Finally, the midwife threatened the ability of physicians to make a living. According to Huntington, writing with Arthur Emmons in 1912, these physicians would be "forced by law to respond to the call of the midwife in trouble" (Emmons and Huntington, reported in Litoff, *Midwife Debate* 123). To De Lee, Emmons, and Huntington, the midwife must be eliminated, and physicians should handle all childbirth, a dangerous condition requiring the knowledge that was solely within the purview of medical science.

However, among opponents and proponents of the midwife, some saw the possibility of different, rather than competing, care. For example, Abraham Jacobi, president of the American Medical Association in 1912, specified the midwife's scope of practice:

> As long as these cases are uncomplicated, the presence of a bright trained woman should be, and is, welcome. She must have learned to distinguish the position of the fetus, and know when to call a doctor; how to do, in his absence, a version of cases of emergency; how to attend the eyes; hemorrhages depending on incomplete uterine contraction or from injuries—one of which is tearing off of the placenta—and how to recognize eclampsia, inversion of the uterus, the presence of a mechanical obstacle like fibroma or a contracted pelvis. She must know how to deal with asphyxia. More than anything, she must have been taught to appreciate two things: first, how to keep absolutely clean—that means to disinfect herself and her hands; second—and therein lies a secret of success—not to leave the woman. (reprinted in Litoff, *Midwife Debate* 197)

The midwife was not to medicate, operate, or correct "as a rule, wrong fetal positions" (196). Moreover, Carolyn Van Blarcom in the *American Journal of Public Health* pointed out that the midwife "acts not only as a visiting nurse, but as general advisor and woman friend at a period which is fraught with much anxiety and terror. She frequently prepares the meals and gives aid in a variety of forms which an attending physician could not and would not attempt to offer" (reprinted in Litoff, *Midwife Debate* 173). The general public should be educated about the "wide differences" between the midwife and the physician:

> The midwife should not vie with the doctor, but rather should be a competent visiting nurse with midwife training, who would be permitted to conduct only normal deliveries, and be obligated to secure medical attention for her patients upon the appearance of carefully defined symptoms of abnormality or complication. Accordingly, the greatest value of her services would in giving intelligent nursing care to the mother and her infant during the twelve or fourteen days following delivery; advising the mother as to her own hygiene before and after labor and arming her with that most valuable and desirable possession, knowledge as to the care of her own infant. (174)

Even J. Clifton Edgar, writing in the *American Journal of Obstetrics and the Diseases of Women and Children* in 1916, cautioned readers that "any plan for the elimination of the midwife" must consider "the fact, that the midwife not merely delivers the woman, but often bathes the mother and baby, cares for the other children of the household, and frequently acts as housekeeper and cook as well" (reprinted in Litoff, *Midwife Debate* 132–133).

At this time, one of the most outspoken and influential opponents of midwifery joined the discussion. In 1913, Charles Ziegler published his "The Elimination of the Midwife" in *JAMA*. The medical community should be concentrating on raising the level of education and experience of the physician, Ziegler argued. No training of the midwife, even temporary or in rural locations, was wise: "My own feeling is that the great danger lies in the possibility of attempting to educate the midwife and in licensing her to practice midwifery, giving her thereby a legal status which later cannot perhaps be altered. If she once becomes a fixed element in our social and economic system, as she now is in the British Isles and on the Continent, we may never be able to get rid of her" (32).

Ziegler saw no possibility that the midwife could coexist with the physician: "The fact is, as I shall attempt to point out, that we can get along very nicely without the midwife, whereas all are agreed that the physician is indispensable. It thus seems that the sensible thing to do is to train the physician until he is capable of doing good obstetrics, and then make it financially possible for him to do it, by eliminating the midwife and giving him such other support as may be necessary" (32–33). Obstetrics was an "important branch of medicine," Ziegler said, that required knowledge of physiology and pathology as well as general medicine. He agreed with others that not only was the midwife incapable of learning this knowledge, but she also contributed nothing to the subject (33).

The Sheppard-Towner Act and the Public Health Movement Encounter the Forces of the AMA

These debates were complicated by the public health movement in the United States in the 1920s. The movement focused on the education of mothers but had potential for positive impact on the status of midwifery. The Sheppard-Towner Act of 1921 initially provided funding for educational and public services, but then was subsequently challenged and overturned. The Act was one part of this public health movement and has been called "enfranchised women's first public act" (Wertz and Wertz 209). The Act was designed to improve women's knowledge of prenatal and obstetrical care and to provide community resources for that care. Public health agencies in each state would spend 1.48 million dollars in the first year and 1.24 million dollars in the second on these efforts. Fourteen of the states decided that licensing, supervising, and instructing midwives would be their priority. Other states set up infant welfare centers, trained public health nurses, supported home visits by nurses, and created prenatal clinics. By 1929 when the act was overturned, infant mortality had dropped from seventy-five in one thousand to sixty-four (Wertz and Wertz 209–210).[11] However, although the Sheppard-Towner Act demonstrated how much of the public could be helped by preventive medicine, the American Medical Association lobbied against it—and contributed to its repeal in 1929 (Litoff, *American Midwives* 99).

The Sheppard-Towner Act assumed that physicians offered remedial medical services rather than preventive health care. Although inspired by the New York City Bureau of Child Hygiene, the act focused on rural areas and small towns, where midwives were sometimes the primary caregivers. Public health nurses were charged with upgrading the midwives' skills. The repeal of the act exemplified the American Medical Association's growing political strength and further placed medical doctors at the forefront of care for pregnant women. With the act's repeal, the supervision of pregnancy was deemed more than previously within the physician's jurisdiction and the pathology of birth became the prevailing norm. At the same time, nurses and midwives lost independent authority. Within the Children's Bureaus physicians began to set the standards for prenatal care.

In Minnesota, the newly created Division of Child Hygiene financed a survey of midwives in the state in 1924. The survey revealed that out of 166 midwives identified, 118 were licensed by the state. The survey predicted that the number of midwives would continue declining, noting that the St. Paul school, in which many had taken their training, no longer existed. Alarming to the physicians who read the survey was the assertion that the "great majority" of midwives in the state failed to "show a proper understanding of the meaning of aspesis, or of the conduct of a normal delivery," which included "particularly those who apparently had no proper conception of their limitations in the presence of obstetrical complications" or "who failed to show a basis upon which they would be able to recognize such complications" (Hartley and Boynton 443). Physicians discussing the survey recommended that "we should not lessen our efforts to bring about the desired result of getting the number of women delivered by midwives down to zero" (Hartley and Boynton 445).

The opposition to professionalizing direct-entry midwives in the United States centered around several issues:

- the alarming mortality rates among mothers and their infants;
- the possibility of a double standard of obstetrical care even if midwives were regulated;
- the tendency to define birth as a pathology rather than a normal process;
- reports that midwives continued to care for so-called complicated pregnancies, including malpresentations; and
- the question of whose authoritative knowledge about birth counted.

Those who argued for the elimination of midwives backed their arguments with stories about uneducated and unsanitary midwives who attempted to deliver infants in jeopardy. They defined obstetrics as a medical science and birth as a dangerous condition, and they believed that only physicians had authoritative knowledge about how the condition could best be handled. They also contended that physicians should not be required to examine or back up "semi-trained" caregivers. Those who defended midwifery saw history and tradition as essential warrants, believed that European midwifery regulation could serve as a model, and reminded their opponents that midwifery practice could be different and yet useful. These defenders used the Sheppard-Towner Act to educate midwives, public health nurses, and their clients. The Act demonstrated that preventive, rather than remedial care, could raise the survival rates of infants and their mothers. The repeal of the Sheppard-Towner Act struck a blow to the independence as well as the professionalization of midwives. They continued to practice in both urban and rural settings, but, unlike British midwives, failed to be accorded consistent legal treatment. Some states were willing to regulate and educate them; other states ignored their existence; still others took steps to eliminate their involvement in birth as physicians and hospitals took control of birth.[12]

The 1970s Natural and Home Birth Movement: Women Reclaim Birth

For the next few decades, midwives faded into the background. They served primarily in rural communities, as medical care providers continued to develop the specialty of obstetrics and gynecology. In the 1970s, small but significant groups of women began to reclaim birth after decades in which birth almost always took place in a hospital and the cesarean section rate grew, when mothers were regularly shaved, given enemas, urged to take a variety of pain-killing drugs, placed in "twi-light sleep," administered pitocin when their labors "failed to progress," and sub-jected to episiotomies regardless of their baby's condition or position. These women wanted birth to be more natural, and they wanted to make the decisions about their birth settings, their support systems, and the degree of medical intervention in their births. They were convinced that hospital births were more dangerous.[13] Many women and their families helped create alternative communes and birth centers; others decided to birth at home. Associations were founded such as the National Association of Parents and Professionals for Safe Alternatives in Childbirth and the Midwives' Alliance of North America; periodicals were published such as *Birth, Mothering*, and *The Practicing Midwife;* and books appeared such as Suzanne Arms' *Immaculate Deception*, Raven Lang's *Birth Book*, the Boston Women's Health Book Collective's *Our Bodies, Ourselves*, and Ina May Gaskin's *Spiritual Midwifery*. The women's health movement encouraged women to be informed and confident about their bodies. Although birth outside the hospital cost less, the majority of those who chose home births in the 1970s were not poor and were not rural; they wished to have more spiritual, more natural births, and the appropriate attendant was the midwife (Hazell).

Some physicians joined and even led the movement. Earlier, alternative birth and labor advice was offered by Grantly Dick-Read, the British doctor who in the 1930s attributed labor pain to fear and lack of knowledge; Dick-Read's advice crossed the Atlantic in the 1940s and caught on in the 1950s. Fernand Lamaze, who started educating mothers in the 1950s, became popular in the 1960s and 1970s as he helped mothers take a more active role in birth. Robert Bradley, a Denver physi-cian, taught breathing techniques and encouraged fathers to enter the delivery room and mothers to go home as quickly as possible; he advocated these measures in the 1950s but they were adopted by the women's health movement of the 1970s. Fam-ily birthing centers inside hospitals were created to meet the needs of this emerg-ing consumer movement. But the majority of physicians were convinced that birth outside the hospital was unsafe. For example, the former director of the American College of Obstetricians and Gynecologists called home birth "in utero child abuse" (quoted in DeVries 53). Also, physicians knew that they would lose their malprac-tice insurance and hospital privileges if they participated in home births.

In this section, I focus on the warrants and ideologies for midwifery practice, birth centers, and home birth as offered by two groups: the Santa Cruz Birth Center in California and the Farm in Tennessee. I also identify a new form of informational and persuasive narrative that took root in these communities—the birth story. Finally, I raise the legal issues that confounded direct-entry midwives and their clients in California in the 1970s and the early 1980s. This review provides an important transition into the 1990s public hearings on direct-entry midwifery, as many of the voices heard in the rest of this book, such as Rita Ortiz's, gained their education and experience and developed their birth ideologies during this turbulent time.

The Santa Cruz Birth Center

The philosophy of the Santa Cruz Birth Center reflects the feelings not only of the women's health movement but also of the Vietnam War protesters. Raven Lang, the Center's primary creator and spokesperson, quoted both Bobby Seale and Jerry Rubin as she framed the Center's history and philosophy in her *Birth Book*. The AMA and "the ruling class" contributed to women's oppression, according to Lang. She summarized the social and political climate as follows:

> If home birth creates healthier children, if it creates a more loving and sounder bond between child and its family, then it should be available as an alternative for any families who want it. But birth has not only reached the absurdity of having to be relearned, it has also reached the absurdity of becoming a criminal offense if we are to go ahead with our ideals and do things the way we desire. And so, because of the system, midwifery as practiced in this book is against the law. It has become political . . . we become criminals. (np)

The Santa Cruz Birth Center was created, in part, because in 1971 no physician in Santa Cruz County would give prenatal care to women who planned to birth at home. The seven initial members opened the center in a private house and had as birth tools "about seven empty charts to fill in, a blood pressure cuff, a stethoscope, a scale, a stack of books, photographs, a movie which we had made of a birth, and a whole lot of energy" (Lang np). A year later the group produced the *Birth Book*, secured the assistance of physician Bob Spitzer, and held a community seminar on birth.

Birth stories, narratives of the experiences, feelings, and outcomes of individual births, became an important source of information to the center and to the emerging publications generated by the movement. Although the group read medical texts, they also learned from their individual experiences with birth—and these experiences became evidence for their authoritative knowledge about birth. These stories incorporated techniques for handling difficult deliveries, reflections on emotional as well as sexual and physiological sensations involved in birth, decisions about when and how to connect with the medical community, and confirmations of women's empowerment during birth. As expressed in the *Birth Book*, birth stories were:

> Good easy labor stories and long difficult labor stories. Everyone tells their own reality. There is no censorship. Fears are openly discussed and the

childbearing couple get closer to their fears and to whether or not they have any grounds for excess concern. When a mother is not adequately prepared or in poor general health, we urge them to consider hospital deliveries. It bears out with some experience that those labors and deliveries usually end up in a hospital anyway. (Lang np)

Center members believed that the sensations of labor and birth were akin to sexual climax, that so-called civilized women had lost touch with their instincts and intuitions, and that medical intervention deprived the mother of her ability to bond immediately with her infant and the infant to "imprint" on the mother. Lang shared her own birth story as evidence of how strongly a new mother who had not been drugged during labor would bond with her new child:

> Experience. Me. Stanford Hospital, 1968. At the birth of my baby I was fully conscious. I remember a head rotating to my right leg and I saw a face in which I could recognize at least two generations of my past. A cry, forever imprinted in my mind, as clearly this minute as then. Heavy impressions . . . My perineum was stitched up and I was wheeled to maternity, my baby was sent to the nursery, my mate was sent home . . . Each time the babies were brought to their mother they would bring the babies first to the mothers who were at the far end of the maternity ward. I was in the room closest to the nursery, and so I received my baby last. . . . Later when the nursing shift changed I heard the nursery door open and a crying baby being brought out to the mother. My uterus clamped down as it had when I heard my newborn's first cry. My breasts tingled and there was a definite gush of blood from my uterus which came from the contraction caused by the sound of the crying baby. . . . My body had known this child to be mine. My self was reacting strongly. (Lang np)

The records kept at the Birth Center would supplement these birth stories to study "the relationship between birth and neurosis" (Lang np).

Midwives, "more sensitive to the woman's emotional and physical state," were essential members of the Santa Cruz Birth Center (Lang np). Herbs, such as comfrey for healing cells and shepard's purse for blood clotting, took the place of drugs. Touch determined the mother's contractions and the fetus's position. Instructions in the *Birth Book* were phrased for the general reader, with analogies from everyday life:

> When you first arrive at a labor, carefully feel the mother's abdomen and notice the hardness of the uterus during contractions. There are different kinds of contractions. Mild ones, which feel just a little bit hard; moderate ones, which feel like a cantelope [sic] that could be indented at the peak of contractions; and strong ones which are woody hard and cannot be indented. (Lang np)

Although breech delivery was not recommended for home birth, perineal massage took the place of episiotomies. Perineal tears of one-fourth to one-half-inch long were not stitched. The reader of the *Birth Book* was taught resuscitation methods and some diagnosis:

> For day three to six or seven days, there may be jaundice or a yellow coloration noticed in the baby's skin. This is a normal physiological jaundice and need not be a cause for worry. However, if the yellow coloration appears before three days or appears within the first 24 hours, this is a sign of disease and the baby should be taken to a doctor. (Lang np)

Between May 1971 and October 1972, the center gave prenatal and postnatal education for 106 women who planned home births. Out of these 106, 17 needed stitching, 2 experienced postpartum hemorrhage, 1 delivered a stillborn baby, and 2 infants needed resuscitation (Frankenberg). Finally, the center stressed that home birth was always the parents' decision.

The Farm

The Farm, started in May 1971 in Summertown, Tennessee, also responded to a community need and shared information through birth stories. Stephen and Ina May Gaskin left California where Stephen taught Zen and mysticism at San Francisco State College, and began a seven-month journey to Summertown with a caravan of roughly three hundred companions. The Farm, which still flourishes today, began as a true 1970s collective, in which the community produced its own resources, including the midwives to attend births within the group and eventually within the nearby Amish settlements. On the way from California to Tennessee, caravan members gave birth to eleven babies. Although Ina May and her collective sisters felt they had no choice but to learn how to catch babies, this decision also was confirmed by the group's philosophy of birth: "We wanted our men to be with us during the whole process of childbirth, an option that was not available in American hospitals at the time, we didn't want to be anesthetized against our will, and we didn't want to be separated from our babies after their births. We were looking for a better way" (Gaskin, *Spiritual Midwifery* 17).

Along the way, Ina May learned from a Rhode Island obstetrician and when arriving in Summertown gained the backup and support of John Williams, a general practitioner within a fifteen-minute drive from the Farm. She read Ralph Benson's *Handbook of Obstetrics and Gynecology* and Helen Varney's *Nurse Midwifery* but also modified what these medical texts had to offer based on what she learned from cultures such as the Mayan midwives in the highlands of Guatemala (Mitford 204–205).

The first two-hundred pages of Gaskin's *Spiritual Midwifery* are devoted to birth stories. Some stories, such as Mary Louise's and Pamela's, tell how the caravan and farm members came to midwifery:

> I was glad when Ina May asked me if I'd help with birthings. It was something I really wanted to do. I got to be with a lot of ladies during their labor. Later, I got to help to take care of the babies when they were born. I learned from each birth and each midwife. I hadn't really thought of be-

coming a midwife myself, but now I can't think of anything I'd rather do. There's a feeling of being One with the mother and the baby and everyone ever born that comes on strong at each birth.   (*Spiritual Midwifery* 70)

Other stories, such as Ina May's own, combine an expression of personal feelings with information on birth techniques and difficulties. Based on these birth stories, on the farm's relationship with Dr. Williams, and on self-education through reading, Ina May and the farm midwives became particularly adept at version—manually turning babies lying sideways or feet first in the womb by external touching and pushing or reaching into the vaginal aperture and helping the baby down (Mitford 204).[14] Ina May's version techniques are still taught to midwives today and have become an essential part of the midwives' authoritative knowledge about birth.

While Raven Lang and the Santa Cruz Birth Center's philosophy stressed anti-establishment activism and the imprinting experiences of birth, Gaskin's spiritual midwife combined Zen philosophy with modern medicine:

Pregnant and birthing mothers are elemental forces, in the same sense as gravity, thunderstorms, earthquakes, and hurricanes are elemental forces . . . In order to understand the laws of their energy flow, you have to love and respect them for their magnificence at the same time that you study them with the accuracy of a true scientist . . . To one who understands the true body of *shakti,* or the female principle, it is obvious that she is very well-designed by God to be self-regulating. We are the perfect flower of eons of experiment—every single person alive has a perfectly unbroken line of ancestors who were able to have babies naturally, back for several millions of years . . . The spiritual midwife, therefore, is never without the real tools of her trade: she uses the millennia-old, God-given insights and intuition as her tools—in addition to, but often in place of, the hospital's technology, drugs, and equipment.   (*Spiritual Midwifery* 276–277)

Finally, as with the Santa Cruz Birth Center, birth at the Farm proved to be quite safe. In a study of 1,707 births at the Farm as compared to the same number of physician-attended hospital births, in a 1992 issue of the *American Journal of Public Health*, Mark Durand concluded: "In this study, lay midwife-attended home births appear to have been accomplished with safety comparable to that of conventional births. Furthermore, the proportion of deliveries in which operative assistance was required was much smaller in the farm group . . . (451). Durand also speculated that interventions "may increase the risk of various adverse outcomes in low-risk women" and that the hospital setting might create an atmosphere that "undermines self-confidence and encourages passivity on the part of the laboring woman, diminishing her ability to deliver spontaneously" (452).

Legal Troubles of California Midwives

Given these positive statistics, and the emotional well-being of mothers served by the Farm and the Santa Cruz Birth Center, one might have predicted that the political and legal climate would have become more welcoming for direct-entry midwives and their home birth clients in the 1970s and 1980s. Instead, however, midwives were actively prosecuted in states such as California—arrested for practicing medicine or nursing without a license and even charged with murder.

The first arrests in California involved three midwives from the Santa Cruz Birth Center. Charged with practicing medicine without a license, the midwives were at first encouraged when the California Court of Appeals ruled that pregnancy and childbirth were not "diseases but rather normal, physiological functions of women" (*Bowland et al. v. Municipal Court*). According to section 2141 of the Business and Professional code, medicine was defined as treating or diagnosing "the sick or afflicted . . . for any ailment, blemish, deformity, disease, disfigurement, disorder, injury or other mental or physician condition." The Appeals Court ruled that the lower court should either amend the complaint or dismiss the case. However, the attorney general requested that the California Supreme Court rehear the case, and, although this specific case was eventually dropped, a precedent was set for further prosecution of direct-entry midwives. The court concluded that normal childbirth, while not a sickness or affliction, was a "physical condition" and that unlicensed persons, including midwives, could not treat physical conditions (*Bowland et al. v. Municipal Court*). Moreover, normal childbirth could not require the use of any instruments; artificial, forcible, or mechanical means; the performance of version or manual turning of the baby; or the administration of any drugs. The California midwives had not only treated their clients for the physical condition of pregnancy, but they also had represented themselves as being able to handle conditions not related to normal childbirth.

The court also dealt with what it termed the "best interests of society" and cited *Roe v. Wade*, among others, as precedents. Although a woman's right to privacy included the freedom to choose whomever she wished to assist in her delivery, the court ruled that "for the same reasons for which the Legislature may prohibit the abortion of unborn children who have reached the point of viability, it may require that those who assist in childbirth have valid licenses."[15] The state had the right to require that abortions be performed by physicians and therefore had the right to regulate who could minister to pregnant women.

In light of this legal precedent, supporters of midwifery and Governor Jerry Brown's consumer advocacy campaign, which recommended a reassessment of the monopoly held by the medical profession, argued for a Midwifery Practice Act. Beginning in June 1977, three versions of the Act were introduced by Assemblyman Gary Hart. The bill was drafted by the Department of Consumer Affairs, which argued that some counties lacked adequate obstetrical care, that midwives could provide cheaper care, and that some four hundred "black market" midwives were already practicing illegally and should be regulated to safeguard the public. The California Medical Association opposed the first version of the bill on the grounds that "less competent supervision" of birth would endanger mothers and infants. Also, the California Nursing Association opposed a revised version, which proposed that both nurse-midwives and direct-entry midwives be treated similarly as "certified midwives." This move would place nurse-midwives under the supervision of medical licensing boards rather than the Board of Registered Nursing and would rank nurses on a par with direct-entry midwives. At this time the California Association of Midwives was founded, but early on, members couldn't reach a consensus on whether licensing would raise their professional status and expand their practice or place them too soundly under medical supervision (DeVries 73–74).

A second version of the bill, introduced in April 1980, addressed only direct-entry midwives and limited their practice to normal childbirth under the supervision of a physician. Both the California Nursing Association and the California Association of Midwives supported this version, believing that it would end harassment of midwives. But once again the California Medical Association and the California chapter of the American College of Obstetricians and Gynecologists (CACOG) opposed the bill. In public testimony, Thomas O'Sullivan represented the CACOG in confirming that "it takes a lot of expertise to know which of these babies are going to be hazard" and only a doctor can do that. Senator Barry Keene asked the physician: "The bottom line is, you've got to be a doctor." O'Sullivan: "Unfortunately, yes" (quoted in DeVries 76–77). The bill was defeated in the Senate Business and Professions Committee. A third version of the bill also failed to reach the Senate floor. Again, physicians argued that midwives were "untrained practitioners" and distinguishing between normal and abnormal, low-risk and high-risk births was a challenge best met by a physician. Raymond DeVries, who provides the most thorough analysis of this legal effort, concludes that the failure of the Midwifery Practice Act "is indicative of the political and cultural power of medicine. Their political organization and the general cultural faith in their practice provides medical professionals with a power that marginal medical groups find difficult to overcome" (80).

Although California has had more legal actions against direct-entry midwives than any other state (Korte), a review of just one more prosecution of a midwife in the 1970s raises the issue of informed consent and provides another definition of the good midwife. On November 30, 1979, midwife Rosalie Tarpening was arrested for practicing medicine without a license and for murder of the stillborn infant Gabriel Villa, a child of two illegal immigrants from Mexico. This legal action was initiated by the physicians who treated Gabriel after he had been transported to Madera Community Hospital, where he was declared dead after he could not be resuscitated. Unlicensed midwives have found themselves particularly vulnerable to legal action stemming from a newborn's transport to a hospital after a difficult birth, if physicians feel a case is handled poorly at home (DeVries 120). The coroner ruled that Gabriel had died "as the result of negligence on the part of the person who delivered it." Testimony of Edith Potter, a renowned infant pathologist, proved that Gabriel had been born alive and had died as a result of "overly aggressive attempts at resuscitation at the hospital" (quoted in DeVries 121, 128). Therefore, the murder charge against Tarpening was dropped, but she was found guilty of practicing medicine without a license, sentenced to two years' probation, and had her physical therapy license suspended for six months.

In the debate over Tarpening's case, the California Association of Midwives attempted to place the choice of where and with whom to birth into the hands of parents and raised the issue of informed consent, an action that would somewhat protect the direct-entry midwife:

We believe that parents should have the right to informed choices of alternative birth settings and care. Present data and studies indicate that planned home birth is a safe and responsible alternative. We believe that state interference in the parents' choice of birth is a violation of our human and constitutional rights. We believe that this type of harassment of parents and birth attendants is indicative of medical and governmental restrictions on freedom of choice in health care and the freedom of communities to develop appropriate systems of health care for themselves. . . .

(quoted in DeVries 125–126)

A parent who was well-informed about the risks and benefits of home birth and her own physical condition had the right to choose to birth at home. The midwife might screen that parent to see if her own protocols would allow her to help the parent, but the ultimate choice and risk were those of the parents.

Moreover, in discussing the Tarpening case, the founder and director of Informed Homebirth, Rahima Baldwin, reclaimed the right of midwives themselves to define their practice and resisted the medical community's desire to define the good midwife:

What does it mean to be a "good midwife"? Good by whose standards? Since we don't have electronic fetal heart monitors, we can never be "good" by certain (obstetrician's) standards. It is our judging one another that perpetuates our being and feeling judged, results in malpractice suits, and keeps our health care system functioning the way it is today. Can we not recognize that it is adherence to the viewpoint of a good or bad practitioner and a good or bad birth that had led to compulsory hospitalization and domination by the medical profession? (Baldwin 3)

The debate over direct-entry midwifery in the 1990s, as will be seen in the Minnesota hearings, involves many of the issues raised in California in the 1970s and includes a struggle to define the good midwife.

The women's health, natural birth, and home birth movements responded to what seemed to some women an oppressive, overmedicalized society. Women claimed that birth should be within their control and that they should decide under what conditions and in what settings to give birth. The Santa Cruz Birth Center and the Farm were responses to these claims. Women who birthed without drugs and in homelike, supportive settings were more likely to bond with their infants immediately and easily and had more spiritual births, according to these communities of women, midwives, and their clients and supporters. The midwives who attended women at the Farm and through affiliation with the Santa Cruz Birth Center relied on the natural process of birth, on herbal remedies, and on touch—the midwives' hands instead of the physician's instruments. These midwives found cooperative physicians who were willing to back them up and share knowledge. However, despite a parent's right to decide to birth at home, the legal climate for the California midwives, in particular, remained oppressive during the 1970s and 1980s. Only a physician's knowledge counted when it came to distinguishing between abnormal and normal birth, high and low risk.

For the California legislature and for the California Medical Association, midwifery knowledge about birth was not legitimized until the 1990s. Although the Tarpening case raised the issue of informed consent and the question of who had the authority to define the good midwife, it also set the precedent for active prosecution of unlicensed direct-entry midwives. At present, California direct-entry midwives are governed by a new law under which they are licensed and regulated by the Board of Medical Practice. By 1998, over eighty of them had licenses and could get insurance reimbursement, order lab tests, do well-woman care, accompany women to the hospital, and even work in hospitals. The California direct-entry midwives must accept physician supervision, but as yet the board has not defined exactly what that supervision entails.

Voices and Issues from the History of Midwifery

This chapter recalls four periods in the history of midwifery in which public debate raised issues similar to those that reemerged in the 1990s. To understand the nature of the debates at the end of the twentieth century, while preserving the historical integrity of these four periods, it is necessary to understand the context in which certain warrants and rhetorical strategies were initially used.

Jane Sharp, Elizabeth Cellier, and Elizabeth Nihell were all aware of women's subordinate place in society and the somewhat tenuous claim that women had on birth. Sharp wanted to ensure safe birth by providing midwives with anatomical knowledge, but she also stressed the power of the midwives' touch and herbs and the mother's own instincts. Cellier tried to provide a way for her midwives to maintain self-determination as well as professional status, again arguing that well-trained midwives would decrease mother and infant mortality. Nihell pointed out the dangers of birth instruments in the hands of male practitioners who lacked the midwife's touch. She recognized the physician's skill and practice, but claimed a distinct and exclusive jurisdiction for her female midwives.

The invention of birth instruments such as the forceps increased the practice of the male practitioner, who could now claim to deliver, under adverse conditions, a living child from a living mother. Female midwives were more and more confined to attending normal births, narrowly defined to exclude malpresentations, multiple births, and other conditions previously within their purview. By the end of the nineteenth century, the argument for and against these instruments took place within the pages of *JAMA*. Mothers and female attendants were thought incapable of deciding on birth strategies and settings, and, although some physicians still defined birth as a natural process, that definition included fewer and fewer births.

The movement to gain state recognition for British midwives ended when the midwives accepted a distinct kind of subordination. Unlike other regulated practices, their personal conduct was scrutinized carefully, they were directly supervised by another profession, and their misconduct was cause for harsh punishment.

Moreover, all midwives had to follow the same protocols, regardless of their skill and experience. Meanwhile, in the United States, those who wished to eliminate the midwife argued (1) that she provided a double standard of care, (2) that she competed unnecessarily with physicians who, as novices, needed patients to become fully trained and who, as seasoned professionals, needed to finance their practices, and (3) that she was responsible for high infant and mother mortality rates. Those who defended her called on her long history as a caregiver and distinguished her method of practice from that of the physician. Many physicians defined birth as a pathological condition, claiming exclusive ownership of birth knowledge. In eventually overturning the Sheppard-Towner Act, physicians laid claim to preventive care, which included prenatal care of all mothers.

Finally, midwives trained at the Farm or the Santa Cruz Birth Center promoted the philosophies of the natural birth movement of the 1970s. To empower women through birth, midwives wished to turn the responsibility of birth back to the mother and her support systems. She could decide on the degree of intervention, the setting, and the attendants at her birth. Birth stories became a new genre—a narrative form that both informed women about birth and persuaded them that the experience was empowering. Birth stories shared techniques for handling difficult births as well as emotional and physiological sensations. Through birth stories, midwives and parents created a competing knowledge system about birth. However, officials in the legal and governmental structure argued that they had the right to define the good midwife and the nature of birth.

Recalling these voices and issues from the history of midwifery is essential to understanding the debates over midwifery that took place from 1991 to 1995 in the state of Minnesota and still are argued today. Often, the Minnesota midwives and their clients, supporters, and opponents were subject to similar pressures and made claims similar to those that were articulated throughout the history of midwifery. In the next chapters, a rhetorical analysis of their discursive strategies today will contribute to our understanding of the relationship among the gender of the rhetors, the status of their knowledge base, and the rhetorical and professional power they hold.

CHAPTER 4

The Minnesota Midwifery Study Advisory Group:

PROFESSIONAL JURISDICTIONS AND BOUNDARY SPANNING

In order to battle the medical establishment you have to battle in some terms that are mutually acceptable . . . because you have to acknowledge where the power is.
—*(Rita Ortiz)*[1]

So I see it happening on an individual level where people are personally out to take out their misogyny on midwives and women or whatever, but then there's this larger social system that is set up that even if people wanted to have a space for us they're not there yet. . . . And society isn't there yet . . . So midwifery is kind of always pushing the boundaries.
—*(Elizabeth Smith)*[2]

*T*his chapter traces how one faction of the Minnesota direct-entry midwives effectively raised their rhetorical status and thus influenced the recommendations produced in the first stage of Minnesota public hearings on midwifery. The chapter specifically identifies the rhetorical strategies used by these direct-entry midwives to span the boundaries of medical knowledge systems about birth, to ensure that the debate over Minnesota midwifery remained in the public sphere of discourse, and to bring midwifery knowledge about birth into the hearings. In tracing this stage of the hearings and in identifying these strategies, this chapter and the ones that follow add to our knowledge of how professional jurisdictions and authoritative knowledge systems are maintained and challenged through discourse. In particular, key rhetors such as Rita Ortiz described their midwifery practices using the vocabulary and referring to the protocols of the medical community. This strategy has been common among direct-entry midwives across the country. As Davis-Floyd and Davis say, "The fact that the legal system so completely supports the praxis of technobirth has forced those midwifery practitioners who take the risk of opposing it to become almost hypereducated in the science of obstetrics so that they can both defend themselves against legal persecution by the medical establishment and work to change the laws that keep them legally marginal" (319). Such hypereducation supports the direct-entry midwives' attempts to boundary span—a rhetorical strategy used to challenge existing professional jurisdictions.

Communication scholar Thomas Gieryn defines professional boundary work as the rhetorical strategies used by experts such as scientists to construct "a social boundary that distinguishes some intellectual activities as 'non-science'" and that excludes rivals from within "by defining them as outsiders with labels such as 'pseudo,' 'deviant,' or 'amateur,'" in order to "enlarge the material and symbolic resources of scientists or to defend professional autonomy" (782, 791–792). In turn, boundary spanning involves rhetors' attempts to establish authority within their own or another's community and often to challenge dominant jurisdictional borders. Resisting the labels of deviant or amateur, boundary spanners often attempt to prove their authority by demonstrating their ability to use the techniques and vocabulary of the dominant profession or community. If their attempt to establish such ethos is successful, they often are able to bring into that dominant community their own authoritative knowledge about a subject. However, as seen in the Minnesota hearings, boundary spanning also further encourages acknowledgment of an "other": To the dominant discourse community, the interloper might say, "It is not I, but those others who are deviant, ill-informed, amateur, or suspect." Boundary spanners may, in essence, then, do boundary work. In the case of the Minnesota hearings, that other already existed and even self-identified as independent from the Minnesota Midwives' Guild and reluctant to invite state surveillance and sanction of their practices. Key rhetors in the hearings went on to define what qualities made that other suspect in the view of the majority of hearing participants. Therefore, in spanning these jurisdictional boundaries, the Minnesota direct-entry midwives made clear that the midwifery community was divided and to some extent took advantage of that division. As those involved in the hearings struggled to define the "good" midwife, they did so by acknowledging an "other" midwife who seemed not to rely on medical knowledge to screen her home birth clients and who was, in essence, silenced in the hearings.

The identification or recognition of the other seems to be a cultural tendency, particularly during conflict. Albert Memmi characterizes the other as a "Not," a person without the qualities valued in a particular society (83). Rather than being seen as individuals, others bear "the mark of the plural" or all seem to look alike (Memmi 85; see also Hartsock 161). These others are therefore grouped according to certain self-identified or culturally identified features, regardless of differences within the group. Again, the construction of the other is part of the construction of the norm, or, as Lois McNay states, the construction of the other is central "to the maintenance of any hegemonic system of norms" (*Critical* 6). In order to assert the features that a dominant group wants to claim as normal or natural—features that give the group authority—so-called undesirable traits are assigned to the other, the deviant. However, within this identification or creation of the other, we see sites of resistance: "In this sense, it is not so much how I see myself as how I see the Other—my appropriation of an alter-ideology for the Other defines the locus of our struggle" (McKerrow, "Theory and Praxis" 95). Key rhetors' efforts before the Midwifery Study Advisory Group (MSAG) to cast the other's ideologies and practices into a certain light allow them to more effectively span the boundaries of medical authoritative knowledge about birth and suggest new jurisdictional boundaries.

In the fall of 1991, the Minnesota State Board of Medical Practice, acting with the State Department of Health, directed the newly created Midwifery Study Advisory Group to explore state regulation of direct-entry midwives in Minnesota. As a result of MSAG recommendations, the board would decide whether direct-entry midwives in Minnesota should be licensed (according to present law), registered or certified (which would require a change in the statute), or left within the present "gray" area—practicing without a license but not penalized because the board had developed no procedure for licensing. The Minnesota Midwives' Guild and its spokespersons greatly influenced the recommendations set forth in the final MSAG report, recommendations that reconciled conflicting definitions of normal and abnormal birth and that acknowledged the midwives' knowledge systems. The final recommendations in the MSAG report shifted the emphasis from state surveillance of individual practitioners to midwifery practice in general, and suggested lines of cooperation and communication between midwives and physicians and between midwives and the state. Midwives would be allowed to sign birth certificates; a midwifery advisory council would present midwifery as a viable birth choice to the public; and physicians who provided backup for midwives' patients would have limited liability as a result. These recommendations seemed to pave the way for direct-entry midwives eventually to have legal sanction to use medical procedures and tools, such as drugs, to control postpartum hemorrhage and to have permission to perform episiotomies and to suture. Yet, when the recommendations of the MSAG report were later proposed to the state legislature, they were considered too controversial even for discussion. Although at the end of the MSAG hearings, the guild direct-entry midwives did not change their social or legal status outside the local center of the MSAG community, they gained the rhetorical status within the hearings to contribute to authoritative knowledge about birth.[3]

Therefore, this chapter concentrates on specific rhetorical strategies of two key rhetors from the midwifery community, Mary Emerson and Rita Ortiz, and one rhetor from the medical community, Rachel Waters. These midwife rhetors, to use Raymie McKerrow's terms, entered "into a scene while being a part of that scene" and changed "the social practices within that context"; in the process, they overcame the assumptions about midwifery and birth that were posed by the medical specialist ("Possibility" 61). As expressed in the opening quotations to this chapter, the direct-entry midwives chose their rhetorical strategies with much consideration of their social and professional status. Finally, this chapter not only introduces the reader to the Minnesota public hearings but also establishes the framework for chapters that follow—chapters that trace how the status the direct-entry midwives gained in the first set of hearings was lost in the second, how the rhetorical strategies that worked in one context failed in another. Again, tracing these initial rhetorical strategies and their effects suggests that when rhetors span boundaries to gain credibility in a communication situation, and when they demonstrate shared values, knowledge, and ideologies in order to do so, they may create or acknowledge factions within their own communities. These factions might arise because community members simply disagree with the strategies and goals of boundary spanning or because rhetors deliberately divide the community in order to move certain members into a more powerful position and leave others behind. One important feature of that power position is a legally sanctioned and socially accepted claim to scientific knowledge and procedures. Initially, all midwives were cast in the role of "other" by the more socially and professionally privileged medical community, but during the first stage of the Minnesota hearings, key rhetors for the direct-entry midwifery community convinced hearing participants that only one faction of midwives deserved this characterization.

The MSAG Conversations: Rhetorical Strategies

Participants in the MSAG conversations included a representative from the Minnesota Department of Health, Tom Hiendlmayr, who would write the final report on behalf of MSAG and submit it to Leonard Boche, executive director of the Board of Medical Practice; Joan Montgomery, a former citizen member of the board and chair of the MSAG discussions; two senior members of the Minnesota Midwives' Guild; the chair of the Parents' Coalition for Homebirth; an associate professor of sociology; four certified nurse-midwives; the president of the International Cesarean Awareness Network/Cesarean Prevention Movement of Southwest Minnesota, who was also a home birth parent and lobbyist for the guild; a certified child-birth educator; two family physicians; a perinatologist practicing in a major hospital; a member of the Minnesota Board of Nursing; a member of Blue Cross/Blue Shield/Blue Plus of Minnesota; an attorney practicing in medical malpractice; and a home birth parent who was executive director of the B'nai B'rith Hillel Foundation at the University of Minnesota. This group was chosen by Leonard Boche and Joan Montgomery to represent the diverse voices in the medical and home birth communities, and the majority of these members went on to constitute the licensing rule writing group that conducted the second set of public hearings. Finally, because the hearings were open, an audience was usually present but consisted, for the most part, of other members of the medical or home birth communities.

As the Midwifery Study Advisory Group hearings got under way, the chair, Joan Montgomery, articulated an essential part of the charge given to MSAG by the Department of Health and the Board of Medical Practice—protection of mothers and infants: "We need to assess what is the potential harm to the public by not regulating [the direct-entry midwives]" (October 23, 1991, MSAG hearing).[4] In affirming the state's right to protect its citizens and in acknowledging that the public, because of its limited knowledge, needs protection in making decisions about how to birth its children, Montgomery also affirmed that the subject of birth was an appropriate topic for public debate. The debates within MSAG were to focus on that common good, and those rhetors who were able to identify with that common good within their arguments were more likely to be persuasive.

Raising Rhetorical Status through Boundary Spanning: The Testimony of Mary Emerson

The first speaker before the Midwifery Study Advisory Group, Mary Emerson, the representative from the Parents' Coalition for Homebirth and a lobbyist for the Minnesota Midwives' Guild, was well aware of the social status of direct-entry midwives at the beginning of the MSAG hearings. Again, social status depends on typing and ranking; we esteem and believe others and predict their behaviors according to how we type and rank them by their gender, age, occupation, and such. In communication interaction, such as the MSAG hearings, rhetorical status can initially be based on social status. Emerson began by questioning the low social status of the direct-entry midwives. She said that the first thing she thought to do in preparing her talk was to "button-hole" some legislators to "find out what their biases were and meet them head on"; in so doing, she found that there was "always a personal issue [or prejudicial assumption] that needed to be uncovered before you could find out what their attitudes toward home birth and midwifery were." "People may imagine herbs and candles . . . that's not so," said Emerson. Although Emerson was aware of the direct-entry midwives' lower social status in contrast to those who would not appreciate the midwives' knowledge system, she could not immediately level that field. Instead, she wanted the MSAG participants to acknowledge publicly their suspicion of direct-entry midwifery and, in so doing, make this suspicion a matter for discussion. As Emerson admitted outside the hearings: "I have known since 1988, it's a guerrilla war and just surviving is a subversive activity and a wonderful thing . . . becoming a little more open and out there—so the opposition has someone to talk to and you become not a 'them.' "[5] Thus, as their first spokesperson, Emerson began the careful task of raising the rhetorical status of the direct-entry midwives within an initially suspicious environment and giving a positive and personal face to direct-entry midwifery.

Lobbyist Mary Emerson believed that she could turn the hearings into a forum to create awareness and understanding of the home birth community and midwifery in general. In her view, the direct-entry midwives were not necessarily disadvantaged by the biases that MSAG members might bring to the hearings, because these very biases—which she planned to debunk in the hearings—presented an opportunity within the MSAG community for the midwives and those suspicious of midwifery to enter into a conversation or even a relationship. Through this relationship and the discourse within the hearings, then, jurisdictional boundaries could be altered and the midwives' knowledge could come to be valued.[6] If the direct-entry midwives could overcome the biases brought to the hearings and raise their rhetorical status to enhance open discourse about birth, then their knowledge about birth could contribute to MSAG's final recommendations to the Department of Health and Board of Medical Practice. Moreover, the midwives needed to be aware of their present relationship with the dominant medical community.

Therefore, to span the boundaries of the medical community, Emerson had to convince the MSAG participants that midwifery knowledge contributed to any discussion about birth and should not be cast into the role of deviant or other.

Emerson was well aware that this impulse to define the normal in relation to the abnormal or other was also seen in other states' efforts to define and regulate midwifery. She and Ortiz had conducted a survey of state regulations for the Minnesota Midwives' Guild. For example, the definitions of direct-entry midwifery, represented by the Florida, Arkansas, and Alaska statutes discussed in the first chapter of this book, were established in relationship to what the state considered "normal" medical care of pregnancy and birth. Midwifery in these states was defined as other than nursing or medicine. If the normal is established in relation to the abnormal, then for direct-entry midwifery to be considered normal, Emerson and other spokespersons for the midwives would have to lead the hearing participants in acknowledging a different so-called abnormal practitioner (Foucault, *Sexuality* 94). Therefore, part of Mary Emerson's strategy was to make the direct-entry midwife—the member of the Minnesota Midwives' Guild—appear to be normal in relation to safe birth practice and to invite MSAG to engage in discourse that would create knowledge about birth that included both medical and midwifery experiences and values.

Thus, Emerson, as the first person to testify on behalf of direct-entry midwifery before MSAG, celebrated the midwives' knowledge about birth and called on MSAG members to question their own suspicions about home birth. She focused on the emerging character of the home birth community after 1973, when the last licensed direct-entry midwife, Ebba Kirschbaum, retired and left the state. Emerson explained that the home birth community developed its knowledge through an oral tradition that became a form of peer review. In the absence of Kirschbaum's leadership, women began sitting together to learn from the home birth stories of others. Emerson testified, "To consult with someone who was practicing in a hospital would not have been very relevant." Rather, women interested in home birth needed to learn from people practicing in the "same way." Direct-entry midwives shared birth stories to educate each other—"This is what happened . . . this is what I saw. This is what's going on with this woman . . . what do you expect?" Emerson attempted to legitimize birth stories and their contribution to midwifery knowledge by comparing them to medical education: "I have been privileged to sit in on some of these [peer review sessions or the telling of birth stories] . . . and I have learned a great deal. It's a very useful way of teaching. It's very similar to the way the doctors used to teach in many ways, an anecdotal, case by case tradition." Emerson drew a telling analogy: Physicians' authoritative knowledge about birth derived from medical case histories, just as midwives' authoritative knowledge derived from midwifery birth stories and peer review. Therefore, the midwives' knowledge had comparable legitimacy.

The peer reviews to which Emerson alluded were, at the time of the hearings, conducted yearly by the Minnesota Midwives' Guild and when needed to discuss special circumstances. For example, at the January 18, 1997, peer review session, one guild midwife discussed the forty births she had attended that year. She shared with her midwife sisters not only how she handled such difficult cases as shoulder dystocia and postpartum hemorrhage but also how she managed emotional demands, such as the mother who called her three times a day for support and the mother with a history of premature babies who wanted a home birth for her eighth pregnancy (see appendix B for definitions of birth terms). The midwife also explained how she used external bi-manual compression and pitocin for one postpartum hemorrhage. After hearing the case review, the guild members questioned her handling of a few difficult cases. When one mother's membranes ruptured but her labor did not start for five days, the midwife advised the couple to go into the hospital. But they assumed the responsibility to stay home, signed a second informed consent form, and argued that they had a "spiritual belief in what they were doing." They had a "lovely birth," "such a gift." Peer review sessions challenge each midwife to describe her cases, defend her decisions, and educate her sister midwives but also give her an opportunity to share emotionally difficult decisions and to receive feedback and support.

By comparing birth stories and guild peer review to medical case study, Emerson was engaging in boundary spanning. Emerson questioned or spanned the boundaries between medical and midwifery knowledge about birth, between formal medical education and birth stories told during peer review. She challenged the boundary work done by medical practitioners to exclude those without formal training and education. In doing so, she also gave voice to the direct-entry midwives' knowledge systems. Such discussions about women's ways of knowing have generally been raised because, as Sandra Harding says, women have "not been given voice of authority in stating their condition or anyone else's or in asserting how such conditions should be changed. Never was what counts as general social knowledge generated by asking questions from the perspective of women's lives" (*Whose Science?* 106). The birth stories told at the Farm and the Santa Cruz Birth Center in the 1970s, and offered in the 1990s by rhetors such as Rita Ortiz and Mary Emerson, reflect a claim to knowledge based on women's perspectives and experiences. Again, even though Emerson claimed that birth stories demonstrate common ground between the home birth and medical communities, these birth stories also question dominant knowledge claims or those pictures of "nature and social life provided by the natural and social sciences" and created in particular cultures such as the medical community (Harding, *Whose Science?* 121).

Through her description of birth stories and peer review, Mary Emerson not only spanned boundaries but also reconstructed the image of midwifery within MSAG by arguing that direct-entry midwifery, rather than relying on candles and herbs, offered a high degree of personal trust, intimate knowledge, and intuition, which, in turn, created a safe birth environment:

> The relationship with the midwife is very intimate and very personal. The birth takes place in the context of the woman's whole life. Part of that is a degree of trust that is incredible. The midwife has access to information that the medical caregiver does not have. For instance, you can do a dozen of your nutritional diaries, and you don't have the same information you have by opening the woman's refrigerator.

Significantly, Emerson did not seek to address all of direct-entry midwifery but focused instead on an image of the midwife as a member of the Minnesota Midwives' Guild. Because guild midwives spend about one hundred hours per birth with a pregnant woman and her family, Emerson noted, they can learn about those aspects of the woman's personal life that might affect her health. Their practices are different—not inferior—to that of the physician; their authoritative knowledge about birth, gained through these experiences and reflected in their standards and protocols, is fully legitimate.

However, as she was spanning these jurisdictional boundaries, Emerson did not attempt to move guild midwifery too far into the medical realm. She asserted that the direct-entry midwife needed medical knowledge not to treat but to discern medical conditions that rule out a safe home birth. Emerson created a taxonomy, distinguishing between what is medical and what is nonmedical and therefore can be practiced safely by midwives. Emerson wanted direct-entry midwives to be able to carry antihemorrhagic drugs, to suture, and to use a local anesthetic and simple suction devices at home. On the other hand, she defined drugs to induce labor, forceps, vacuum extractors, and non-emergency episiotomies as medical and invasive. Because the direct-entry midwife faced a special challenge in practicing nonmedical, non-invasive care, she must be extra attentive, according to Emerson: "Since she cannot rely on a fetal monitor, she must be highly trained in how to listen to and interpret fetal heart tones. Because she does not have at her disposal the use of antibiotics, should uterine infections ensue, she cannot perform invasive procedures which place the mother at risk of infection." Emerson combated cultural constructions of the direct-entry midwife that placed her outside the norm and therefore disqualified her knowledge. To combat this pejorative judgment of the direct-entry midwife as practicing outside the norm, Emerson differentiated between the degree and kind of care a direct-entry midwife and medical caregiver offered by stressing the quality of care the midwife could provide in a low-risk birth. Thus, she began to sketch for MSAG participants a picture of low-risk birth as the norm and home birth as appropriate for that norm. Again, she spanned the boundaries between the medical and home birth communities by noting their common concern with safety. In essence, she argued to expand the boundaries of normal birth, boundaries that were narrowed beginning with the invention of the forceps by the Chamberlen family in sixteenth-century England and continuing throughout the twentieth century in the United States.

Moreover, Emerson continued to question the strict jurisdictional boundaries between the medical and home birth communities by stressing their relationship, one that must be maintained for the midwife who might have to transport a distressed mother in labor: "There is a lot of harm that can be done in a transfer of care that's not diplomatically done and frightens the [hospital] staff—they expect the worse and they would treat for the worse." Emerson's testimony was designed to counter conventional notions of direct-entry midwives as emotional amateurs by describing instead the potential for medical caregivers to overreact to a home-birth transport unless the physician and midwife are in touch with each other.

Additionally, Emerson argued that, if both medical and midwifery knowledge were indeed legitimate, the relationship between the medical caregiver and the direct-entry midwifery must be nonhierarchical: "I would assert that for home birth to be safe, it must be nonmedical, and I feel very strongly that the traditional midwife is the one to provide nonmedical birth services at home. . . . No other profession is sufficiently independent." Any disciplinary power granted to the medical community would not only normalize medical knowledge about birth but also create a hierarchy or a supervisory relationship between medical and midwifery practitioners (see, for example, Foucault, *Discipline* 170). Nurse-midwives, Emerson pointed out, were under the supervision of doctors, and doctors were subject to peer pressure and review as well as malpractice insurance restrictions. If direct-entry midwives were to become medical, which Emerson equated with the use of invasive procedures, then they would give up their independence and would introduce, rather than screen out, risk. Emerson also undermined any cultural convention that equated birth technology with safety by reminding the MSAG members that the midwife "has no forceps, so there are no cervical or vaginal wall lacerations, no bruising or lacerations to the baby's head."

Emerson concluded her presentation by arguing that home birth and safety were linked, not mutually exclusive: "Safety is the top priority; home birth is the second priority. As a childbirth activist, I want traditional midwives to be available in this state. And the midwives in this state are concerned with the integrity of their profession . . . Even at its worst, traditional midwifery and home birth are very, very good." By making this link, Emerson aligned direct-entry midwives with MSAG's public goal—the protection of those who choose home birth—and established midwives as sharing with the state its concern for the well-being of its citizens. Thus, Emerson raised the rhetorical status of the guild direct-entry midwives as a group, extended the possible boundaries of their expertise, and reminded MSAG of the midwives' experiential knowledge of birth gained in the private sphere. But she also acknowledged that the issue of birth would be debated in the public, not the private, sphere.

To appreciate the rhetorical strategies that Mary Emerson used to span boundaries and yet maintain a distinction between midwifery and medical care, it is useful to recognize the effects of what feminist scholars call a "bifurcated consciousness" of women's understanding of their own experiences and knowledge and to acknowledge that knowledge systems are complex and changing. A bifurcated consciousness potentially affects a woman's ability to appreciate her own experiences and to interpret their meaning outside the gender role assigned to her. For example, Sandra Harding defines bifurcated consciousness as follows:

> It is a struggle to articulate the forbidden, "incoherent" experience that makes possible new politics and subsequent analyses. On the other hand, this theory holds that our actual *experiences* often lead to distorted perspectives and understandings because a male supremacist social order arranges our lives in ways that hide their real nature and causes.
>
> (*Whose Science?* 282)[7]

Emerson herself acknowledged the deliberate rhetorical positioning she established through her testimony, given the broader cultural assumptions about midwifery and women's experiential knowledge. Although the direct-entry midwife might claim that her experience with birth grants her special knowledge, her own view of these experiences is formed and potentially distorted by her experiences in a system that undervalues her knowledge. For example, Gloria offered the following story to the Midwifery computer listserv in a discussion thread about tying or cutting umbilical cords:

> When I was apprenticing many years ago I was in the room a few hours after the birth of the baby; the cord had been tied with tape. Everyone was resting and I was the watcher . . . The baby wimpered and I went to check on him; I noticed blood on his blankets and when I unwrapped him I found his cord-tie had slipped and the cord was SPURTING blood with a great deal of pressure! I grasped it between my fingers (very slippery and hard to hold) and hollered for help! We got his cord retied. I'll bet he lost 1/4 cup or more, but he handled it well, though. I don't like to think what might have happened if someone hadn't investigated the little noises he was making!   (listserv communication, July 16, 1996)

We might speculate that Gloria was the watcher because she was the apprentice among more experienced care providers. She saved the baby's life because she was attuned to his cues, but still called these cues "little noises" and defines herself as a "someone." She expressed her fear about "what might have happened" had she not noticed, but she didn't claim the credit for her act or celebrate her ability to pay careful attention to such cues. Her birth story offered her readers advice and knowledge about how to secure the umbilical cord, but she undervalued her own role. Emerson's challenge, then, before MSAG was to legitimize midwives' knowledge, to establish the midwives as knowers despite cultural assumptions and individual perceptions that might discredit their knowledge based on experience.

Moreover, Emerson celebrated direct-entry midwives' experiences within a knowledge system that is complex, changing, and multiple. The midwives' experiences and their protocols are not uniform and to present them as such might invite dispute within the midwifery community. For example, knowledge over what might seem basic—such as securing the umbilical cord to prevent the baby from bleeding to death—appears as something complex and changing in the midwives' birth stories. Peg confirmed to the listserv that, regardless of what current theory recommends about securing that cord, particular experiences demand refinement and rethinking:

> I had a cord just break for no reason on me one time. It had been a shoulder dystocia for an 11 pound baby and as I was finally handing the baby to the mom after working on him a little while, it just snapped. Blood does shoot everywhere. Twice now I have also cut a cord with only clamping one side of it hoping that it was clamped on the baby's side. Both times it was. I had a cord so tight I could not get two hemostats in there so I clamped with one and cut. I hate cleaning up bloody messes.
>   (listserv communication, July 17, 1996)

If Emerson was to be successful in raising the rhetorical status of direct-entry midwifery by boundary spanning, she had to find a commonality between changing knowledge systems while avoiding too much detail about specific practices that may vary among midwives. Therefore, she portrayed direct-entry midwives as having definite and universal characteristics: intuition balanced by experience, trust supported by intimate knowledge of their clients. In her telling, they shared with physicians concern for safety but had distinct skills that offered an alternative approach to birth. There may be a deviant birth practitioner who deserves the skepticism of the medical community, but it is not the direct-entry midwife, who creates and shares knowledge about birth through peer review and birth stories, who practices according to the traditions and standards of the Minnesota Midwives' Guild, and who possesses the ability to use medical technologies but only those appropriate for assessing the safety of each home birth.

Asserting Medical Authority: The Testimony of Rachel Waters

The next spokesperson for direct-entry midwifery continued Emerson's portrayal of the direct-entry midwife but had to follow a rhetor whose testimony carried much authority in the Midwifery Study Advisory Group. That authoritative rhetor was Rachel Waters, a pathologist in the Department of Laboratory Medicine, Pathology, and Ob/Gyn at the University of Minnesota, who challenged the image of the direct-entry midwife as constructed by Emerson by reasserting before MSAG that the majority of births were risky and therefore best managed in the hospital by medical caregivers. In her testimony, Waters asserted that birth was a proper subject for debate in the public sphere as long as authoritative knowledge about birth was created by the medical community in the technical sphere. Waters, a member and eventually vice president of the Board of Medical Practice, also spoke before MSAG as a medical authority for the state.

Again, direct-entry midwifery at the time of the Minnesota hearings (1991–1995) was legally defined by exclusion or exception in most states—midwives could assist or attend births *only* if they did not engage in certain medical procedures. When the MSAG hearings began, the state of Minnesota defined direct-entry midwifery as "the furthering or undertaking by any person to assist or attend a woman in normal pregnancy and childbirth," but it excluded certain practices:

> [Midwifery] shall not include the use of any instrument at a childbirth, except such instrument as is necessary in severing the umbilical cord, nor does it include the assisting of childbirth by an artificial, forcible, or mechanical means, nor the removal of adherent placenta, nor the administering, prescribing, advising, or employing, either before or after any childbirth, of any drug, other than a disinfectant or cathartic.
>
> (Minnesota State Legislature)

Minnesota direct-entry midwives (should licensing become available through this statute) were to be examined on a number of aspects of pregnancy, labor, and delivery, including "abnormal conditions requiring attendance of a physician" and could lose their licenses for "unprofessional or dishonorable conduct," including performing abortions or failing to "secure the attendance of a duly licensed physician" when needed. The law dictated that direct-entry midwives were to prove their knowledge of such techniques as "management of the puerperium" and "cause and effects of ophthalmia neonatorum" through examination, but midwives were not asked to demonstrate their knowledge of how to ease a mother's pain and fears or integrate the birth experience into the family environment. Up to the point of the MSAG hearings, those rhetors who were "given legitimacy and status to engage in discourse" on the legal status of midwifery, to use Carole Blair and Martha Cooper's terms, were primarily officials in state legislatures and agencies (165).

Therefore, to understand the complex legal status of direct-entry midwives at the time of the Minnesota hearings, one has to understand how their status was interpreted in other states. In some states, the direct-entry midwives seemed to provide an acceptable alternative to hospital birth. For example, New Mexico's statutes referred readers to the *New Mexico Midwives' Association's Policies and Procedures* manual, a formal recognition of that state's direct-entry midwives' guild. In Florida's accepting climate, by the summer of 1995, thirty-three direct-entry midwives had been licensed and the state had established or recognized three midwifery schools. Although South Carolina and Louisiana provided a route to licensure, the required physician backup and supervision prevented the direct-entry midwives from being independent. In Wyoming, licensed direct-entry midwives were prohibited from offering prenatal and postnatal care, an indirect means of requiring physician supervision. And in Colorado, direct-entry midwives had to graduate from an accredited school to be registered; the certification program of the Colorado Midwives' Association (a group comparable to the Minnesota Midwives' Guild) had not been approved because the program was not a "school" as defined by the private schools act (Colorado; Carrie Abbott).[8] Thus, even in states that sanctioned direct-entry midwives, the limits on their activities were not immediately obvious by their legal status.

In addition, MSAG and subsequent public hearings in Minnesota were created because legal agencies such as the Minnesota Board of Medical Practice and the Minnesota Department of Health were authorized by state legislatures to investigate and possibly regulate direct-entry midwifery. Therefore, to a great extent, when Rachel Waters began her testimony, she spoke not only with the voice of medical authority but also with legal authority granted by state agencies. Studies such as Vicki Bell's of incest and Carol Smart's of rape, pornography, and child abuse are useful in understanding the social, professional, and rhetorical status of medical spokespersons such as Rachel Waters. As Bell states, "How law comes to be regarded as having access to the Truth, the processes by which law allows or disallows interpretations of events, and how law extends its terrain into traditionally non-legal discourses—these are the questions which need to occupy feminist perspectives on the law" (11). As Bell and Smart explain, the law often exercises power—often through those whom it recognizes as having expertise—to disqualify other knowledge systems. For example, Smart argues that alliances between law and medicine have extended "the potential for the legal regulation of women's bodies" (3). Thus, rhetors whose discourse appears to have legal sanction may claim to know the truth about a subject, such as the risks encountered in birth.

The law imposes definitions and interpretations on everyday life and asks experts such as medical professionals to help it decide how to judge issues such as safety, prevention, and risk. As Smart says:

> If we accept that law, like science, makes a claim to truth and that this is indivisible from the exercise of power, we can see that law exercises power not simply in its material effects (judgments) but also in its ability to disqualify other knowledges and experiences. Non-legal knowledge is therefore suspect and/or secondary. . . . So the legal process translates everyday experience into legal relevances, it excludes a great deal that might be relevant to the parties, and it makes its judgment on the scripted or tailored account. (11)

It was that power to translate, to exclude, and to judge that Rachel Waters brought to her MSAG testimony. And the legal authority of the public hearings on midwifery had the potential to exclude the knowledge systems of the home birth community.

Rachel Waters reported to MSAG on the Minnesota Obstetrics Management Initiative or MOMI project study with both legal and medical authority. To a great extent, the MOMI project excluded the knowledge of the direct-entry midwives and the home birth community. The project's objectives, as Waters explained them, were to

> look at the aspects of risk in pregnancy and obviously to separate out the aspects of high and low risk by risk scoring. We knew that outcome analyses are extremely important, and we capsuled that in relationship to risk. We knew from the claims, the closed claims, in malpractice . . . the use of risk scoring formats or some assessment . . . determined the risk factors that could be managed to minimize the bad outcomes that we'd seen in over half of the malpractice claims.   (November 7, 1991 MSAG hearing)[9]

Waters redefined the majority of births as high risk and described how the hospital setting recognized risk and controlled birth. Birth was not a private but a medical event, one informed by the scientific knowledge and controlled by the technology claimed by the medical discourse community.

Waters's knowledge about birth stemmed from data gathered from large numbers of participants, analyzed mathematically in the technical sphere, and intended for publication in the *Journal of the American Medical Association*. Waters's statistics were gathered from hospital births only. In describing the MOMI project, she linked risk scoring with outcome in pregnancy; the more risks in a mother's health profile, the more likely a "compromised outcome" for mother and baby. MOMI was "essentially a systems analysis," according to Waters, but she became enthusiastic about its possibilities: "[T]his study is really unique in the nation in that it starts out in the prenatal period, goes through labor and delivery, goes up through the postpartum period and six months of the infant's life. It's a research tool; it's not a quality assurance tool yet at least, and it's very detailed." By mentioning "quality assurance" and risk assessment and management, Waters suggested that although no one can prevent all bad outcomes, medical experts could define, detect, measure, and manage risk to ensure quality care.

Using MOMI project data, Waters argued that normal or safe pregnancy was limited to a small number of births. Again, out of a random sampling of five thousand hospital births from May 1988 to May 1989 in Minnesota, the MOMI project identified and ranked twenty-five thousand risk factors. The median number of risk factors per birth was four and included characteristics ranging from the age and income of the mother to the presence of diabetes or anemia. Although Waters admitted that the standards of care used to assess risk were high, the preliminary conclusions of the MOMI project indicated that identification and management of risk factors—surveillance best done by medical personnel—would help prevent bad outcomes.

Waters described how the medical community could assist the state in protecting children from parents who exhibit "real irresponsibility" during pregnancy and delivery by choosing home birth without taking into consideration the degree of risk involved. The knowledge about birth created in the technical sphere must inform the public:

> It is important that the public, that the mom and dad, it's just all so terribly important, that we be honest and truly inform people about the aspects of risk in pregnancy and that the outcome can be poor, that outcome can be affected by non-preventable aspects, and tell them about them. So in terms of our own sense we are now at a point where we can measure with the data the quality of care and risk-management with quality assurance.

Therefore, Waters aligned the MOMI project with the goals of MSAG—the protection of public citizens as they made decisions about where and with whom to birth their children.

At the end of her presentation, Waters alluded to her own image of the direct-entry midwife. She assumed that direct-entry midwives handled high-risk mothers and that the resulting births were more likely to be compromised:

> The poor in Minneapolis/St. Paul are those who have risk and have possibilities in terms of compromised outcomes. And I just wanted to share that great concern. . . . It is so very clear from this high-risk group that again what I am saying I guess is that these women have risk in beginning . . . the anemia, poor nutrition, great number of infections, the whole environment . . . they certainly have the outcomes that are much more significantly compromised.

In this last statement, Waters asserted another damaging "truth" about the risks of home birth and countered Emerson's careful portrayal of the intuitive and conscientious midwife who screened out high-risk clients.

Thus, with Waters's testimony, direct-entry midwives were reminded of how medical authoritative knowledge about birth informed their legal status. Throughout the country in the mid-1990s, other direct-entry midwives also struggled with the relationships between medical practice and the law. For example, when the participants of the Midwifery listserv discussed the issue of carrying outdated drugs, they identified the differences between their legal status and their everyday practices. For example, Sara, a licensed direct-entry midwife in Washington, proposed that outdated pitocin is probably still effective in controlling postpartum hemorrhage but not in creating positive impressions of direct-entry midwifery:

> As a group we feel misunderstood by the medical profession, ignored by payors (ins & managed care organizations), and unknown to or unappreciated by the majority of pregnant women. Some things we can do little about but there is one thing we do have control over and that's practicing safe, quality midwifery care. Along with the actual practice of good care is the perception of quality care that our "public" has. We also can effect this by our attitudes and actions. This is where carrying outdated meds falls in. Yes, PERHAPS the US outdates too soon, and MAYBE we can still use the meds and control for lowered doseage [sic], but, for the cost of a little more time and money obtaining current meds we can enhance not detract from our image. To put it bluntly, I would not want to be transferring a mother for PPH [postpartum hemorrhage] and wondering if my outdated Pit contributed to the transfer . . . We could approach this conversation like . . . how can we alter the prevailing attitude about midwives and out of hospital births?? (listserv communication, July 17, 1996)

Joan then reminded Sara how the law in many states either restricts all direct-entry midwives from carrying drugs or restricts those who are not supervised by a physician:

> Sara, I totally agree with you, as I too am very passionate about both the giving of safe care and the perception that we give safe care. I have spent many years promoting safe midwifery. I do feel though, the need to address the issue of carrying outdated medications. Doctors and pharmacists I have discussed the issue of outdated medications with have all agreed that meds such as pitocin are good for at least one year after the expiration date stamped on the ampule. I personally have never seen a lack of effectiveness in their use. You are practicing in an area where certain medication are available for the asking. Many midwives in this country do not have that privilege. They do the best they can with what they have available. I would much rather see a midwife attend a birth with six month outdated pitocin than with none at all. Hopefully one day all midwives across the country will have the luxury of calling their medical supply and ordering what they need. In the interim they must do the best with what they have available without being criticized. (listserv communication, July 17, 1996)

Medical authority claims jurisdiction over drugs, the law determines whether a direct-entry midwife can carry and administer drugs, but the midwives quite often feel that they must carry drugs such as pitocin to ensure safe home births. Rachel Waters's testimony reminded MSAG and the direct-entry midwives that authoritative knowledge about birth dictates that only medical professionals have the established diagnostic procedures necessary to predict and control risk in birth. Such an exclusive claim to scientific knowledge confirms a profession's jurisdictional boundaries. Placing the direct-entry midwives in a kind of double bind, medical professionals such as Rachel Waters suggest that birth practitioners offer safe care only if they have scientific knowledge but then deny that those practitioners outside the medical profession might have the ability to diagnose, treat, and screen their clients.

Identifying the Other: The Testimony of Rita Ortiz

Minnesota Midwifery Guild member Rita Ortiz, who followed Rachel Waters in testifying before the Midwifery Study Advisory Group, had to regain the rhetorical status that Mary Emerson had established for the direct-entry midwives by bringing the debate back into the public sphere and reidentifying a place for midwifery among birth practitioners. Rather than accepting the knowledge from the technical sphere generated by the MOMI project, Ortiz had to reestablish MSAG as a forum in which to create knowledge about birth so the direct-entry midwives could resist narrow definitions of normal birth and the characterization of most births as risky. This challenge for Ortiz was great, in light of Waters's testimony and her medical and legal authority.

Ortiz followed the lead of Mary Emerson by using a rhetorical strategy that allowed her to retain a credible voice without sacrificing her belief in midwifery practice as a viable alternative to medical care in certain cases. Ortiz continued to identify the distinctions among direct-entry midwives, casting some in a less favorable light than others and creating a hierarchically subordinate group. In essence, much as Emerson did, Ortiz defined the guild midwife as the normal and competent home birth care provider and the non-guild midwife as abnormal or deviant. To do so, she built on the boundary spanning work done by Emerson and demonstrated how midwifery systems of knowledge included knowledge of medical techniques to screen for risk.

Ortiz began by creating a very concrete and very private picture of her own birth and that of her children, the beginning of her own embodied knowledge, in the testimony discussed in chapter 1. Although Ortiz was also a registered nurse, and several MSAG participants knew that shortly she would begin nurse-midwifery study, she did not claim that professional status to gain rhetorical status. Instead, she created a concrete image of a certain direct-entry midwife, one who was self-educated but still competent to screen out high-risk and attend low-risk or normal birth. That image was exemplified by the Minnesota Midwives' Guild midwife.

Picking up on Emerson's refutation of the myths about midwifery, Ortiz laid out for MSAG her own education as a direct-entry midwife so as to defuse the notion that Minnesota Midwives' Guild midwives were in some way fanatical. Ortiz stressed her reluctance and sense of inadequacy in coming to midwifery, sketching for MSAG an image of the direct-entry midwife as filling a necessary gap, but avoiding hubris. Because the few birth books available to her in the 1970s were written in "medicalese," she had to study to understand them. Even during this self-education, Ortiz waited for a "qualified practitioner who would come on the scene and start attending to the needs of home birth women . . . whether that was to be a friendly physician or a nurse-midwife who was going to budge from the system . . . I waited for the person to come and rescue me from myself. . . . It took a number of years before I realized that . . . I had become the person I was waiting for" (November 7, 1991, MSAG hearing)[10]

Ortiz then described how safety in birth was less a matter of private decision by parents and more a result of midwifery knowledge. Although the births she attended early on were simple and many of them took place in Mexico, where the culture prepared women for self-sufficiency during home birth, she soon realized that "certain things," ranging from "attitudes toward health and medical history" could affect a woman's "ability to give birth at home." She reaffirmed that guild midwives used their knowledge of these "certain things" to screen out high-risk mothers. Ortiz stated that she accepted only 10 percent of the calls she received and eventually attended the births of only 75 percent of those she interviewed. Her practiced assessment of the mother's physiological and psychological state guided her choice of which women she could safely assist.

Quoting often from the guild's *Standards of Care*, Ortiz asserted that the guild midwife was responsible for limiting the number of births she took on and assessing her own level of stress. Ortiz used her knowledge not only to monitor the safety of others but also to help her conserve her own energy: "Every woman who wants to have a home birth does deserve to have a home birth, but she doesn't necessarily deserve to have me. I have learned that in order to take care of other people, I also have to take care of myself." Ortiz took pains to correct Waters's impression that direct-entry midwives in Minnesota treated the economically deprived; in fact, the mother who has no money comes to the midwife, Ortiz said, "in the position of victim and powerlessness. For a woman to have a home birth, she has to be in a place of power. . . . A woman who feels powerless is setting herself up for complications." For more than an hour, Ortiz read from the long list of the contraindications for home birth in the guild's *Standards of Care*, the conditions requiring medical consultation, the conditions requiring consultation with other direct-entry midwives, and the conditions established by the guild that required immediate hospital transport. As Ortiz said, "Unlike most other caregivers, we try to send people away as opposed to get them to come to us." Thus, Ortiz evoked the image of the Minnesota Midwives' Guild midwife as reluctant but necessary, informed but humble, selective and careful. She demonstrated that the special place of guild midwives in birth came both from their knowledge about birth, created in the private sphere—within their peer review sessions, birth stories, apprenticeship experiences, and self-education—and from a concern for safety that they shared with medical caregivers.

The Minnesota Midwives' Guild had decided that Emerson and Ortiz "were to present a united front and control the flow of information" within the MSAG hearings.[11] Ortiz believed that this dividing strategy was rhetorically sound: "I come from generations of very political people. I knew politics as a little kid. I understand the difference between what you believe and what you can say and whom you can say it to. There is a difference between the *us* crowd and the *them* crowd and how 'us' presents ourselves to 'them.' And somehow this us crowd thinks that everyone can be part of us—no!" If the guild midwives could distinguish themselves uniformly from the direct-entry midwives about whom the medical community and the Board of Medical Practice had heard stories of poor outcomes and disastrous transports, then Ortiz could convince MSAG that some home births were safe, despite Waters's testimony.

This analysis of Rita Ortiz's and other rhetors' testimonies in the Minnesota hearings raises the question of whether rhetors are free to choose their own rhetorical strategies and to change the way that self might be socially defined, controlled, encouraged, or silenced. Theorists have questioned this rhetorical freedom and choice. Much as feminist theorists have recognized the bifurcated consciousness that might affect women's ability to interpret their own experiences, rhetorical theorists have wondered if, given the social construction of the self, rhetors can so carefully plan their persuasive strategies as Ortiz and Emerson claim they have. Foucault seems to turn away from the "choice and decision of an individual subject" to discourse "in which the speaking subject is also the subject of the statement." When the rhetor is the subject of the statement, the rhetor's sense of self is constructed by the discourse itself and not by the rhetor's conscious choices (*Sexuality* 61, 95). However, in considering resistance, Foucault and other theorists provide us with a means of identifying, first, the persuasive strategies designed and selected by the individual and, second, limiting and silencing definitions socially imposed on the individual. In particular, Foucault recommends "taking the forms of resistance against different forms of power as a starting point," to bring to light power relationships, their locations, their "point[s] of application," and their methods. He mentions sites of resistance where individuals or groups are disempowered, such as when men dominate women or medicine influences the general population ("Subject and Power" 211). When rhetors resist, they both assert their right as individuals to be different and attack "everything which separates the individual, breaks his links with others, splits up community life, forces the individual back on himself and ties him to his own identity in a constraining way" ("Subject and Power" 211–212). The power relations that the rhetor resists might categorize the individual by imposing "a law of truth on him which he must recognize and which others have to recognize in him"; they are forms of power that make "individuals subjects" (212).[12] The Minnesota direct-entry midwives had been made into subjects by cultural norms that considered birth risky, the physician in the hospital as the appropriate caregiver, and the midwife as irresponsible, suspect, or invisible. However, rhetors such as Mary Emerson and Rita Ortiz seemed to exercise rhetorical choice as they resisted the efforts of MSAG rhetors such as Rachel Waters to cast them into this derogatory role or image. They planned their strategy carefully, and it began to be successful.[13]

Following Ortiz's presentation, several MSAG members confessed that they were "getting warm" toward home birth, letting go of those "personal issues" that Emerson had brought to the fore. One such member was a medical malpractice attorney, who confessed, "I would be pleased as punch to be involved in a home birth with *some* lay midwives now, and I didn't feel that when I started this process." He then offered a definition of "good" midwives, one that he created after Ortiz's testimony:

Good lay midwives offer time and thoroughness in developing rapport with patients [Emerson reminds him at this point that women are "mothers giving birth," not "patients"], a probable enhanced psycho-social evaluation and support, more than some traditional medical providers. . . . Women desire, need, or benefit from this component of care and perhaps cannot avail themselves of it as well in traditional [medical] systems. Some women are going to deliver at home irrespective of the decisions of this group. . . . Medical knowledge is desirable in the care given at home. . . . There may be some lay midwives in certain communities who do not agree with this.

(November 22, 1991, MSAG hearing)

This definition depicts the good midwife as knowing when to call in the physician, how to screen out high-risk mothers, and how to distinguish her practice from other practitioners with a more medical bent. Despite Rachel Waters's legal and medical authority, Ortiz appeared to have refuted a great part of Waters's "truth" about birth and to have contributed to a new definition of the good midwife that would honor the practices of the Minnesota Midwives' Guild. Emerson and Ortiz accepted this definition of the good midwife because it confirmed a place for home birth in Minnesota.

Confirming the Other: The Testimony of Kris House and Karen Mist

The effectiveness of Ortiz's rhetorical strategies was also confirmed when two non-guild midwives, Kris House and Karen Mist, testified before MSAG. Although House and Mist presented themselves as individuals, they were already cast as different from the guild midwives and therefore suspect in the final MSAG report. To the majority of MSAG participants, House and Mist seemed not to follow the screening process that Rita Ortiz described or that was encompassed in the definition of the good midwife. Emerson and Ortiz had focused on this division to persuade MSAG members that, by identifying "unsafe" midwives, MSAG could recommend the practices of "safe" midwives. However, regardless of the nature of the Minnesota hearings, House and Mist had long identified themselves as resisting the guidelines of the guild; instead, they gave priority to the religious beliefs of their home birth clients. An important part of their identity as midwives was tied to supporting the faith of their clients to birth safely at home; therefore, this division within the Minnesota direct-entry midwifery community existed before MSAG. Mist and House believed that their practices were indeed safe, but that their clients— not they themselves—were responsible for weighing advice about risk against their faith to home birth. However, because of the focus that Emerson and Ortiz cast on the other midwife in contrast to the good midwife, Mist and House failed to gain rhetorical status before MSAG.

Karen Mist began her testimony by saying she had a "real deep feeling inside" that she was meant "to participate in birth" (December 3, 1991, MSAG hearing).[14] And Kris House got a call from an old friend who said that "she had been praying and the Holy Spirit put it on her heart to call me and tell me that there was a midwife meeting in a Quaker meeting house" and that Kris should attend. For

Mist and House, birth was always a private matter, not a subject for public debate before MSAG, a stance that affirmed the distinction between the guild and non-guild midwives.

Similar to Ortiz, Kris House began her testimony with a description of her own hospital births:

> My first baby was born prematurely. I was in the hospital twenty minutes, and in that time, they had time to prep me, which back then meant complete shaving and enema . . . major episiotomy to get a five-pound, four-ounce baby out. . . . All I needed really was someone to say, "You're OK, and your baby is OK." But their response was what was then high-tech stuff. . . . With my eighth baby, she had a severe problem with jaundice. . . . After reading some articles in the newspaper, I began to realize that it was medically induced.

Kris House noted that this experience caused her to reject the knowledge about birth claimed by the medical community and to find authority within herself: "They told me what to do and I listened to them. And I began to realize through the years that they didn't always have the right answers for me. I began to realize who I was." Her twelfth pregnancy was high risk, and she praised her own midwife for supporting her decision to stay home: It was an "honor to have someone else let me be who I was, to have someone else encourage me, to let me know that I could make choices, that I knew my body better than someone else did. . . . If the same circumstances were to happen today, I would not find anyone to help me. . . . It was a twelfth baby, I was RH negative, I was close to forty years old." Although House's birth story was indeed similar to Ortiz's, rather than using the story to span boundaries, House affirmed her own personal authority to make choices about birth.

House's journey to midwifery was as personal as Ortiz's, somewhat accidental and designed to fulfill a community need:

> In 1983 I got a call from a couple who wanted to birth at home and one of the midwives had given my name, and I just said WOW. I haven't caught any babies; I have just observed. I made it really clear how many I had seen and what my participation was, and they said, Kris, we have prayed about this, and we really are going to stay home, and we want someone to stay home with us. Would you do that? I was able to find another midwife who felt responsible that my name had been given out, and she felt like she would be a backup. She hadn't yet met the couple when they went into labor, but she was available by phone throughout the day. She was ready to come over any time—I had a friend with me from my [Christian] fellowship who was around for support. But the most important thing was that this couple had made this determination—and that will be 11 years in March. I helped them with five babies. And that's how it started happening. . . . I help a lot of families who are in Christian community groups, whether it's a formal church or organized church or whatever. They have their own communities—they had their women who will come and be there.

And that's all they want at the birth. Probably comparable to [the] Amish situation, just not recognized in the same way . . . The couples we [Kris and Karen] are helping now primarily feel like spiritually they have come to a place where they want to take responsibility for themselves. They don't want the state to do it for them—yet they are open to the medical community in emergency situations.[15]

However, again, House did not use her story to establish common ground with Ortiz and Emerson, and MSAG members did not seem to appreciate any similarities. Although Emerson and Ortiz both cited values, such as safety, that the midwifery and medical communities share, they distinguished between what midwifery and medical practice can bring to the birth experience. By contrast, House focused almost exclusively on the spiritual nature of birth, perhaps reminiscent of the image of herbs and candles that Emerson worked to overcome in describing direct-entry midwifery. House and Mist granted the parents whom they attended almost absolute authority to make decisions about the safety and risk involved in their pregnancies and births, while, again, guild midwife Ortiz described in detail how she screened out a high proportion of her potential clients.

Therefore, MSAG participants questioned Karen Mist and Kris House almost exclusively about their screening practices, their knowledge about contraindications for home birth, and how they fit into the definition of the emerging MSAG definition of the good midwife. Karen Mist was asked what her role was in informing home birth parents of their risks, what she did if she felt the parents did not make good choices, what things she might ask of parents, what physical signs she looked for to determine risk, and what training she had. Her answers confirmed that she and the parents decided how to handle risk together but that she relied on the good judgment of the parents:

We talk about complications that can come up. . . . I ask them to tour some hospitals. I also share with them some stories. I'll give them names of some women they can talk to who have maybe experienced that. . . . So they can get a good range of how they feel about that, that they are basically taking that responsibility at home. And ultimately it's their decision what they choose to do about that.

Kris House became somewhat impatient with the questions that asked her to defend her ability to handle risk. Ultimately, House's belief in women's rights, her own personal calling, and the specificity of her cases caused her to resist MSAG's growing regard for the active screening done by guild midwives. House stated that regulation "scared" her, as "every woman should have the choice to stay home or not. . . . We talk about protecting the public but to tell a woman she cannot stay home, I do not know how that is protecting her [women will stay home anyway] . . . Home birth needs to stay an option for women. It's a beautiful way to birth your baby." House defined screening quite differently from Ortiz:

Screening? Screening to me, and it goes back to my whole philosophy, and I am not the one dictating to this couple about where they are going to birth,

who they are going to have at their birth, how they are going to maintain
themselves nutritionally, and whether they are healthy or not. In other words,
when they come to me, I am not the one saying this is what you have to do,
you have to take my pre-natal classes, have a back-up doctor . . . And they
will say "well, we really feel like this baby is OK," I am not going to *not*
help them.[16]

Thus, although she might give advice regarding medical conditions, House allowed
the home birth parents to make the final decision to birth at home if their personal
faith determined that their baby would be safe there.

When one MSAG member asked them how the state could protect the public from someone who just "wakes up one morning" and decides to become a midwife, Mist countered with this statement: "I really think that women themselves
when they sit down to talk to someone about staying home for birth they are being
real careful, they are asking questions they feel are important, and they want to
know who you are. I do not see [what you're saying] as happening." She resisted
MSAG's notion, as did House, that home birth parents need protection from their
own irresponsible decisions and unsafe practitioners, and, in so doing, she distanced
herself from MSAG's charge and excluded herself from the emerging MSAG definition of the good midwife—the direct-entry midwife who acknowledged that high-
risk home births must always be screened out and respected medical jurisdiction
over high-risk birth.

The MSAG Recommendations: The Rhetorical
Effectiveness of the Guild Midwives

In the final MSAG report, the non-guild midwives were singled out for
scrutiny: "Not all homebirth attendants meet MMG [Minnesota Midwives' Guild]
standards, and members of the Midwifery Study Advisory Group expressed serious
concerns about the practices of these other 'midwives' " (Minnesota Department
of Health, *Regulation* ix). Moreover, MSAG recognized the standards of guild practice: "The unsafe practices occurring within the [home birth] community are not
always performed by traditional midwives, but may be performed by other individuals attending homebirths" (Minnesota Department of Health, *Regulation* 54).
The list of prohibited practices MSAG produced matched those prohibited within
the Minnesota Midwives' Guild's *Standards of Care*. MSAG recommended that an
advisory council oversee complaints about home birth practices, that direct-entry
midwives serve with medical caregivers on that council, and that the midwives sign
birth certificates, thus not only acknowledging their care but also allowing them to
contribute to statistics about birth. Finally, the MSAG report recommended limited
liability for health care providers accepting transports from direct-entry midwives,
a recommendation which, although unacceptable once the MSAG recommendations were written into proposed legislation, also reflected the rhetorical status
gained by the Minnesota Midwives' Guild.

Ortiz and Emerson accepted, for the guild midwives, that birth was a subject for discussion in the public sphere and used this discussion to counter images of deviance and carelessness imposed on direct-entry midwives. Even though the guild midwives' knowledge about birth came from very private birth experiences, peer review and birth stories shared in guild meetings, apprenticeship training, and self-education, through their key spokespeople—Ortiz and Emerson—guild midwives stressed the concern they shared with the state for the safety of its citizens and with the medical community for ensuring that safety by screening out high-risk mothers. The common good was the accepted goal of the guild midwives as well as of the MSAG discourse community. Participating in the public debate enabled the guild midwives to contribute to MSAG's eventual acceptance that, with proper screening by a careful and scrupulous direct-entry midwife, home birth could be a safe choice for many mothers. Thus, the guild midwives questioned certain medical attitudes toward birth as a high-risk condition best handled in the hospital but agreed that those midwives who could not or did not identify risk according to guild standards were deviant, to be subjected to future scrutiny and observation. Knowledge not only about birth, safety, risk, and normalcy, but also about direct-entry midwifery, was produced in the MSAG conversations and reflected in the MSAG recommendations. However, this knowledge about birth established within MSAG focused negative attention on non-guild midwives, such as House and Mist, who would have preferred to function outside state sanction and surveillance.

Therefore, using discourse to span the boundaries of the dominant medical community, Ortiz and Emerson recast the image of the "other." Not all direct-entry midwives, but some other direct-entry midwives, were deviant and abnormal; midwifery knowledge systems, as represented by Ortiz and Emerson, gained legitimacy through this distinction. Through discourse within MSAG, Ortiz and Emerson not only performed boundary spanning but did boundary work to create an image of direct-entry midwifery that empowered the Minnesota Midwives' Guild, to challenge the existing jurisdictions of the medical community represented in Rachel Waters's testimony, and to further an understanding of midwifery knowledge that garnered respect. The guild midwives needed that empowerment and respect to argue eventually for legal sanction to administer antihemorrhagic drugs, perform emergency episiotomies, and suture, but still remain autonomous. States that had granted those practices to direct-entry midwives usually required medical supervision going beyond the cooperation that Minnesota midwives would welcome. This rhetorical move on the part of the guild, to so pointedly separate guild midwives from their non-guild counterparts, seemed the best option considering, first, that the catalyst for forming MSAG came in part from the stories of poor home-birth outcomes that had reached the ears of the Board of Medical Practice; second, that the Board of Medical Practice had the statutory obligation to regulate direct-entry midwifery, even though they had not elected to establish the required examination; third, that the direct-entry midwives had a strong desire to practice independently with certain "medical" tools to ensure the safety and comfort of home birth; and, fourth, that the midwives had a keen awareness of the licensing practices in other states.

However, to argue effectively for the kind of midwifery care that included both autonomy and expanded practices, the direct-entry midwives needed a solid, consistent, and unified front. Outside the hearings, the midwives, both within the guild and outside it, revealed how divided they were about the rhetorical strategies used by Ortiz and Emerson. Guild member Susan Olson strongly disagreed with boundary spanning strategies that established common ground between midwifery and medicine:

> Coming from a poor, inner-city family, working class, uneducated, white trash background, my interest in midwifery has gone hand and hand with my evolving education . . . I realize that I always had a place, I haven't acquired this place because of my acquired education. And . . . I used to feel that same [way] about midwifery—that we had to keep it underground and protect it and that we were lucky that we found this dark little niche where we could do our women thing. I have evolved to the part where I think that we are entitled to our women culture, to support women in having respectful health care . . . I do feel [that] . . . if we are not acceptable as women practicing a feminine art, if we have to pretend that we are men practicing a medical art, then I don't want to do it. I am not going to do in and speak in medical terminology or speak like a privileged middle or upper class white person when I am not.[17]

Also, Greta Godwin, a direct-entry midwife who did not belong to the guild, revealed that she was quite aware and remained suspicious of these boundary-spanning strategies that standardized the relationship between the midwife and medical caregivers:

> It's important for me if I help someone who wants to have a birth outside of the medical community to not confuse them that I am part of that community because I am not. So, if a medical need comes up, CBC [complete blood count] for instance, or a question, then we will figure out whom they can go see in the medical community. Because I think that having communication is appropriate. A few women don't want anything to do with that. I don't think they should be refused—I wouldn't refuse a woman to help her only on the basis that she doesn't want any contact with the medical community. Of course, I would if she said she wouldn't go to the hospital no matter what. But say she didn't want to have lab work; you know, I might help her and I might not, depending on the whole picture, her lifestyle and past, and depending on what she was willing to do in place of that.[18]

Both Olson and Godwin became key rhetors in the next set of public hearings, and their comments foreshadow the conflicts and problems that emerged as the MSAG group was reconstituted into a collaborative writing team, charged with writing licensing rules and regulations for Minnesota direct-entry midwives.

CHAPTER 5

Licensing Rules and Regulations:

NORMALIZING THE PRACTICE OF MIDWIFERY

[Licensing will mean] just an easier way to find midwives and a lot cleaner. People will have more choices. A new group of people will want to become midwives—they'll see that as an option. I would love to have it be like the Netherlands where home birth is the norm. That's my vision. That traditional midwifery care is an option.
—*(Julia Dylan)*

A lot of people just like to practice on the fringe and maintain that fringe identity. And there is a certain amount of personal power in that. And you don't have the pressure of choosing whether you are going to help someone based on an abstract or exterior doctrine. You can make your decisions based on your heart and your intuition.
—*(Elizabeth Smith)*[1]

$\mathcal{T}$he first stage of the Minnesota hearings on direct-entry midwifery, as analyzed rhetorically in chapter 4, illustrated how, through discourse, professional boundary work might label those whose knowledge systems and practices fall outside these boundaries as deviant and amateur—as the suspect "other." To some extent, the boundary work of the dominant medical profession was exemplified by Rachel Waters's testimony before the Midwifery Study Advisory Group (MSAG). In turn, to gain legitimacy for the marginalized, experientially based knowledge systems of midwifery, the key rhetors for the Minnesota Midwives' Guild, Rita Ortiz and Mary Emerson, overcame Waters's boundary work by delineating a certain category of others. These others were those within the Minnesota midwifery community who might not follow the standards of the guild, standards that relied on medical knowledge as well as experiential knowledge and intuition, used by guild members in screening and treating home birth clients. To some extent, those others, represented by Kris House and Karen Mist, had already self-identified as having ideologies grounded in personal faith as well as experiential knowledge and intuition.

This chapter focuses on the second stage of the Minnesota hearings and illustrates how one genre or form of communication created by and for the hegemonic, technologically based knowledge systems of medicine supported existing jurisdictional boundaries of the medical profession. The conventions of the genre of licensing rules and regulations normalize competing professions and, in the case of the Minnesota direct-entry midwives, narrowed the parameters of the practice of midwifery. The conventions also dictated a hierarchical relationship with the dominant medical profession, spelled a potential loss of autonomy for the midwives, and caused further division within the direct-entry midwifery community at a time when the community needed to maintain a united front. In this chapter and the next, we explore the direct-entry midwives' accommodation or resistance to the conventions of the genre of licensing rules and regulations, and we see how this genre provides a discursive means of maintaining the medical profession's culturally accepted appropriation of scientific discourse and claims to exclusive authority over scientific knowledge.

As mentioned in chapter 2, during interprofessional competition and conflict, we often see systems of knowledge publicly articulated when professions debate what counts as evidence, identify abstract norms in standards and practice, discuss educational and examination routes to professional standing, and defend or challenge jurisdictional boundaries. As Andrew Abbott has noted, interprofessional competition is a "fundamental fact of professional life" and "control of knowledge and its applications means dominating outsiders who attack that control" (2). Specifically, during interprofessional competition, the ability of a profession to abstract its system of knowledge often helps the profession maintain its jurisdictional boundaries; for example, "It is with abstraction that American medicine claims all of deviance, the abstraction of its all-powerful disease metaphor" (Abbott 30). Another response to interprofessional competition might be an attempt by the incumbent or dominant profession to reduce the practice of a competitor into a version that resembles its own. Again, these discursive responses may take place in the broader public arena and in the legal system. Before the public, a profession can claim the right to practice as its members see fit, to exclude other practitioners, and to dominate public definitions of the tasks of the competing practices. In making these claims, the dominant profession reveals and asks for public support of the professional terminology and knowledge that define its tasks and problems and its means of undertaking and solving them. In the legal arena, the claim of jurisdiction might include not only a monopoly of certain practices but also the "formal control" of language, the language that describes tasks, that identifies the practitioners performing these tasks, and that is used to conduct the work within the profession (Abbott 62). Andrew Abbott summarizes the contribution that language makes to legally established jurisdictions as follows:

> Since all terms must be rigidly defined, reification is absolute. All members of the legal category of doctor are indeed exactly the same in legal eyes. All tasks are rigidly defined as well, with definitions normally taken from the dominant professions involved. This absolute necessity to abolish uncertainty leads to virtually arbitrary definition of the margins of professional jurisdiction. Boundary areas are firmly delineated with formal definitions that are in fact uninterpretable in actual situations. (63–64)

Because the incumbent profession's definitions of problems and tasks have already been accepted in the public arena and the legal setting, the incumbent has an advantage over the competitor who must make a case based on definitions perhaps new to the public or legal arenas. This chapter gives us an opportunity to see how that discursive power is usually exercised through licensing boards and by statutory or judicial monopoly of practices, and by legal prosecution of unauthorized practitioners.

A genre such as licensing rules and regulations contains the terminology, reflects the abstractions, defines the parameters of practice, and prescribes mechanisms for punishing unauthorized practitioners. Again, an incumbent profession might call upon these genres to limit the ability of a competing profession to absorb any portion of the incumbent's jurisdiction or even to prevent the competing profession from emerging. Because genres are dynamic, each new reading of a text, as Charles Bazerman says, "reshapes the social understanding." "The genre does not exist apart from its history, and that history continues with each new text invoking the genre" (*Shaping* 8).[2] Thus, rhetors can manipulate genres for rhetorical purposes. Genres develop as dynamic community responses to communication needs and become common rhetorical strategies, "enacted, collectively, by members of a community in order to create knowledge essential to their aims" (Graham Smart 124).[3] Thus, genres also provide the rhetor with a way to respond to conflict and to take action, as the rhetor within a dominant or incumbent profession can defend knowledge systems, call upon reified definitions and categories, and claim exclusive control of practices. The genre of licensing rules and regulations, then, can become an important rhetorical tool for incumbent professions during interprofessional competition, and an essential text for the competing practice to resist or modify in defining its own jurisdiction and gaining legal or public approval.

The second stage of the Minnesota direct-midwifery hearings provides a way to assess how, through the discursive practice of imposing the conventions of a genre upon a competing profession, jurisdictional boundaries are defended. Again, because the genre of licensing rules and regulations impacted the public and legal discussions of midwifery, the Minnesota hearings reveal the uneasy relationship between medical and midwifery systems of knowledge. That uneasy relationship becomes even more apparent because of the collaborative process hearing participants used to draft the licensing rules and regulations. The Minnesota Midwifery Study Advisory Group, as it functioned between October 1991 and May 1992, used a teamwork collaborative process; the teamwork collaborative gave one author, in this case Tom Hiendlmayr from the Department of Health, authority over all writing decisions but assumed that this author would receive input from others (Van Pelt and Gillam 173). The MSAG members reached agreement on and recommended the content of the report; in essence, MSAG served as advisors to Hiendlmayr. However, during the second set of hearings, from December 1993 to June 1995, the participants employed a shared-document collaborative process to write the licensing rules and regulations. This process assumes that the contributions of one person or discourse community are of equal value to those of any other and that the writing process will generally not reflect a hierarchy or levels of authority. The goal of this type of collaboration is intellectual negotiation (Van Pelt and Gillam 175).[4] In the second stage of the Minnesota hearings, direct-entry midwives were invited to write collaboratively with nurses, physicians, and nurse-midwives the licensing rules and regulations that would define direct-entry midwifery practice. Because each participant was granted an equal voice, the ways in which the conventions of the licensing rules and regulations enabled the incumbent medical profession to maintain jurisdictional boundaries were clearly illustrated as the midwives' suggestions of alternative language exposed the rigid definitions and categories of the genre and so escalated conflict. This conflict exposed the culturally accepted and legally sanctioned hierarchical relationship between medical and midwifery knowledge systems that Rita Ortiz and Mary Emerson had worked so hard to overcome during the MSAG hearings.[5]

This chapter first describes the legal catalyst that led to the next set of hearings on direct-entry midwifery in Minnesota and the difficulties that the midwives had in agreeing whether to seek state-sanctioned professional status in the first place and then how much they would accept the normalization and narrowing of their practices. Then the chapter analyzes how the participants' responses to the genre of licensing rules through the collaborative process illuminates interprofessional conflict and sets the framework for understanding the medical profession's claims to exclusive authority over scientific knowledge studied in the next chapter.

The Legal Catalyst for the Licensing Rule Writing Group

As mentioned in chapter 1, in the spring of 1993, Minnesota State Senators Sandra Pappas and Carol Flynn and House of Representatives member Kay Brown wrote companion bills to repeal present midwifery laws and to enact the recommendations of the Midwifery Study Advisory Group (MSAG). The bills, to be heard in the 1993 session of the Legislature, would have provided the direct-entry midwives with more professional status but would also have allowed them to maintain much of their autonomy. To add further protection for direct-entry midwifery, the bills placed much of the responsibility for weighing the risks of home birth on parents' shoulders as they consulted with their midwives.

Specifically, the Pappas-Flynn-Brown bills would have created an office of midwifery practice in the Department of Health, taking surveillance of direct-entry midwifery out of the hands of the Board of Medical Practice. Not only would the office of midwifery practice have investigated complaints and taken disciplinary action against midwives who violated conduct regulated by the new bills, the office would also have disseminated what it determined was objective information about direct-entry midwifery to the public. The bills would have established a midwife practitioner advisory council to advise the Commissioner of Health. Consisting of three direct-entry midwives, one certified nurse-midwife, one physician, and two members of the public, the council could have been dominated by members of the home birth community. Moreover, the writers of the bills assumed that professional liability insurance would be available to direct-entry midwives.

Also important in the bills was the statement that the Commissioner of Health "may not adopt rules that restrict or prohibit persons from providing midwifery services on the basis of education, training, experience, or supervision" [Minnesota Statutes, Chapter 148 (proposed), Subdivision 2]. Direct-entry midwives, such as Rita Ortiz, who had taken self-education or apprenticeship routes to midwifery, would have been free to practice.

The bills would have prohibited some conduct on the part of direct-entry midwives—including some of the specifics that became important in later hearings about midwifery. For example, Section 148.498 of the proposed bills included a list of unsafe practices, including "attending births of women who have been diagnosed with a medical condition which requires medical supervision" such as diabetes mellitus and Rh negative sensitivity and "failure to refer or to transport a client" in such situations as "uncontrolled maternal hemorrhage." The midwife also would have had to provide clients with a Bill of Rights that included a statement of her credentials and fees and the risks of home birth. The client would then have to sign an informed consent form. Midwives who failed to follow these guidelines could be fined or prohibited from practicing. But most important to the direct-entry midwives, conditions such as malpresentation, twins, and vaginal birth after cesarean section (VBAC), conditions that became the focus of controversy in later public hearings, were not on the unsafe practices list in these bills (see Appendix B for descriptions of these conditions). Also, this list seemed to assume that the direct-entry midwife had access to some means of responding to emergencies, such as pitocin for postpartum hemorrhage.

However, in the end, the Pappas-Flynn-Brown companion bills were considered "too controversial" even for discussion. The bills never reached the floor of the House or the Senate. Consequently, direct-entry midwives were left in that gray area of the law—unable to become licensed but not outlawed from practicing. Desiring not only autonomy but also backup from the medical community and access to its tools, the direct-entry midwives were left uncertain about what procedures they could perform legally.

After the proposed Pappas-Flynn-Brown bills failed and the direct-entry midwives continued to practice underground or a-legally, in the summer of 1993 the Board of Medical Practice was again challenged to meet its responsibilities to regulate direct-entry midwives and to again curtail what some legal officials considered unsafe practices. The board received a copy of a letter to the Speaker of the House from an Assistant Steele County Attorney asking that the House " 'review refusal of the Board of Medical Practice to register midwives as required by law' " (quoted in McAfee 1). Phillip McAfee, the board's policy analyst, recommended that the board proceed to set up the process to license direct-entry midwives in Minnesota as dictated by the current Minnesota statute (McAfee 4). McAfee's task was to weigh the benefits and problems with licensing the midwives, to assess the board's legal responsibility to do so as required by the current statute, and to recommend a way to license the midwives if the benefits outweighed the problems or to repeal the statute if the problems outweighed the benefits. In his report to the board, McAfee noted what he called the Department of Health's worry about "the inherent conflict of interest between physicians and midwives, in that they are competing for patients and have somewhat divergent practice styles" (4). But he felt that with licensing the board could again address the issue of regulating the midwives and continue to protect the public "in an unbiased fashion," particularly given its five public members and "gender balance" (4).

Moreover, McAfee recommended that the board consider the North American Registry of Midwives (NARM) exam an appropriate licensing exam. He predicted that, with some minor revisions, the present statutes and rules would be adequate to license direct-entry midwives. For example, he cautioned that in the present Minnesota rules the midwives were required to have a diploma *and* pass an exam, a problem in that the midwives were "not likely to be formally schooled" so the "and" would have to be changed to an "or" (2). He noted the prohibitory "language relating to instruments and drugs" in Rule 5600.2000, even though he acknowledged that "midwives use clamps and other substances to stop bleeding incident to normal childbirth" (2). McAfee's involvement in direct-entry midwifery was short-lived he attended only the first few Minnesota licensing rules and regulations hearings, and he did not foresee the controversy that would eventually engulf these issues. McAfee underestimated the birth technologies that some direct-entry midwives already used, even without legal sanction, just as he underestimated the difficulty in asking members of the medical profession to accept the knowledge systems of the direct-entry midwives.

However, McAfee's recommendations to the board did set the stage for the second set of hearings. In making his recommendation to license using the NARM exam, the McAfee report rejected the board's other two options—to turn regulation of direct-entry midwifery over to another government agency or to not regulate midwifery at all. He felt that supporting the MSAG recommendations, repealing the board's authority, and supporting another discussion of the Pappas-Flynn-Brown bills would not provide "the same level of supervision that BMP [Board of Medical Practice] could provide through its physician review. It would result in MDH [Minnesota Department of Health] increasing its licensing activities. Finally, it is unclear what kind of a reception this legislation will receive if it is heard this session" (3). Thus, besides being politically controversial, this option would decrease the surveillance activities of the board and increase those of an agency less dominated by medical authority.

The second option—repealing the Minnesota statute that determined that the board must license direct-entry midwives, and supporting legislation waiving malpractice liability for attending home births—would "shield the BMP from criticism for not licensing midwives, while at the same time encouraging physicians and nurse midwives to attend home births." But this option would be "a difficult sell," predicted McAfee, and "without the encouragement of physician or nurse midwife attendance at home births, this option may fail to protect the public and open the door for attack on the current (fragile) legal status of traditional midwives" (3). With this option, the direct-entry midwives, unlicensed and unregulated, could be prosecuted for practicing medicine or nursing without a license, as they were in states such as New York. But McAfee also assumed that without surveillance from the medical community, home births would be more dangerous for mothers and infants. Thus, inherent in his final recommendation was supervision of direct-entry midwifery by state and medical authority represented by the Board of Medical Practice.

The existence of the NARM exam, then, seemed not only to relieve the board of the burden of creating its own exam but also to provide a way of normalizing home birth and exercising disciplinary power through examination. Thus, regardless of the origins of the NARM exam, whose later forms were determined by a survey sent to more than eight hundred practicing home birth midwives, the board seemed to want the NARM exam to function much as Foucault found that such examinations function in general, as procedures that combine "hierarchical observation" and "normalizing judgement" (*Discipline* 170). In particular, Foucault noted that the examination

> is a normalizing gaze, a surveillance that makes it possible to qualify, to classify and to punish. It establishes over individuals a visibility through which one differentiates them and judges them . . . In it are combined the ceremony of power and the form of the experiment, the deployment of force and the establishment of truth . . . The superimposition of the power relations and knowledge relations assumes in the examination all its visible brilliance.   (*Discipline* 185)

Therefore, the board decided to rely on its genre of licensing rules and regulations, and on the NARM exam, to maintain its "interest in parents who choose home birth having safe births" and to fulfill its obligation to license direct-entry midwives (Minnesota Board of Medical Practice, Public Policy Committee). The board counted on the NARM exam to enable it to distinguish between safe and unsafe practices—to determine the definition of normal and abnormal births—and counted on the licensing rules and regulations to affirm the board's authority to discipline unsafe practitioners. The board's choice of the NARM exam in and of itself was not unusual; among the states that had licensed direct-entry midwives by November 1994, eight had adopted the NARM exam (Pulley, "Legislative Committee Report"). Only those midwives who demonstrated proficiency in particular protocols, including screening out home birth mothers who had certain risk factors, would be licensed by the board. Others would be prohibited from practicing. However, the board did not foresee an important complication with this recommendation. Unlike later versions, this early version of the NARM exam did not address strict screening. More important, although the NARM exam was meant to "be an objective measure of basic knowledge" of MANA's core competencies for midwifery, the exam embraced the following ideologies:

- Midwifery practices vary in style and means of training, and many routes to excellent midwifery practice are acceptable.
- Academic, or written, knowledge alone does not determine midwifery competence.
- Use of the Registry Examination in no way suggests that the physical, psychological, emotional or spiritual skills of a midwife are less important, only that these qualities are not measurable on paper. (Sullivan 1–2)

These ideologies confirmed a certain autonomy of practice and variation in education among direct-entry midwives. The NARM exam clearly celebrated the knowledge systems of direct-entry midwifery.

The board gathered together once more direct-entry midwives, nurse-midwives, nurses, physicians, and home birth parents, many of whom had participated in the Midwifery Study Advisory Group. The Licensing Rule Writing Group (LRWG), chaired again by Joan Montgomery for the majority of the hearings, was formally charged by the Board of Medical Practice to write the licensing rules and regulations for direct-entry midwifery.

Professional Standing: Advantages and Disadvantages

Although studies of professionalization have focused on interprofessional competition and have assumed the desirability and advantages of professional standing for the emerging profession, few have addressed the losses practitioners might realize when their practice is normalized—defined legally along discrete jurisdictional lines. Licensure through such an agency as the Board of Medical Practice brings to the emerging profession the advantages of state sanction but also the disadvantages of state surveillance. Elizabeth Cellier sensed this tradeoff when she proposed her independent midwifery corporation in 1687; British midwives realized this too as they debated the 1902 Midwives' Act. For Minnesota direct-entry midwives engaged in the hearings in the mid-1990s, licensure meant a potential increase in social and professional status but loss of autonomy when midwifery practices were normalized. Jurisdictional boundaries usually imply what Foucault would call normalization, which not only "imposes homogeneity" but also makes it possible to classify and rank, "to measure gaps, to determine levels, to fix specialties" (*Discipline* 184). These gaps, levels, and specialties include, according to Foucault, the "medical bipolarity of the normal and the pathological" (*Clinic* 35). Normalization through licensing would make home birth a more visible and acceptable option, as Julia Dylan noted in one of the epigraphs to this chapter, but it would also standardize direct-entry midwifery practices, as Elizabeth Smith cautioned, in her epigraph.

If the direct-entry midwives were to avoid being silenced during the interprofessional competition that might emerge during the licensing rule writing process, they had to fit into the existing system of the professions, which granted authority over scientific discourse and knowledge to the medical profession. Moreover, to be licensed by the Board of Medical Practice, their knowledge systems, practices, and ideologies had to be described in the genre that defined such diverse professions as athletic trainers and physicians' assistants. This genre usually placed these practices under the supervision of physicians. Direct-entry midwives, on the other hand, were involved in the practice of birth—already claimed professionally and culturally as within the jurisdictional boundaries of obstetricians and some family practice physicians. Finally, many of the Minnesota direct-entry midwives struggled with the knowledge that professional standing would entail a loss of potential autonomy through the normalization of their practices.

Loss of Autonomy Through Normalization

Although the Minnesota Midwives' Guild as a group decided to support licensing, individual members were wary about the eventual effect on the autonomy of their practices. For example, Julia Dylan, a guild midwife, described this prospective loss of autonomy as follows:

> [It means] losing out on certain ways of practicing. Having to practice in a real strict form. I just know that like in Arkansas—some of their parameters of keeping their license are really strict. There are just certain people who aren't going to fit those guidelines who would be ideal home birth candidates. Like being pregnant with your sixth or over or under a certain age . . . Licensing would lose out on things that are beautiful about midwifery. Now you can do things that are in that blurry gray area—licensing would make things much more black and white.[6]

One of the more experienced guild midwives, Gloria Olson, agreed: "You get more regulated and monitored, and there is a constant move to oppress you more, to shut you down, to give you the ability to do less and less."

Some Minnesota direct-entry midwives resented the very philosophy of normalization—of inclusion and exclusion, the ranking and classification, of types of midwives as well as kinds of practices that professionalization seemed to impose. According to one guild midwife, Connie Baker, who had worked in South America,

> Every little town [in Mexico and Central and South America] has lay midwives, and they are easy to find. At any house you can just ask and they will say "Oh, here and there." I have talked to a lot of women, and more often than not they are not educated women, but they are the women who for whatever reason other women have gone to and trust and get their needs met by. I just feel like with the shrinking world that it would be just terrible to define midwifery that would not be inclusive of women in the world . . . And then here in Minnesota we would have this definition that would say they're not real midwives.[7]

Two of the non-Guild midwives admitted that they might not become licensed but would work entirely underground and illegally because of the potential changes in the midwife-client relationship and the degree of government involvement. For example, Greta Godwin noted:

> But I feel that licensing will change midwifery and the relationship you have with the parent. With licensing, women are again birthing under a professional—a so-called expert. Someone stands "above them" at their births. A direct-entry midwife is chosen by the community and should sit as an equal with the laboring women. Moreover, a professional has to put their professional organization before their client.[8]

Kris House believed that professionalization would limit, not affirm or extend, basic human rights, such as the right to choose how and where to birth:

This really falls into line with what is happening politically in this coun-try—a lot of folks are questioning government involvement. And so there are a lot things, constitutionally; it [the government] is supposed to protect us, not license us to give us rights. I feel like we already have the right to birth when, where, and with whom, and why do we need anyone's per-mission to do that . . . the purpose of this [Licensing Rule Writing Group] committee was for the safety of the moms and the babies, not just licens-ing midwives.[9]

Finally, other direct-entry midwives such as Elizabeth Smith feared the financial burdens that professionalization might bring: "If you have to pay a lot of money for them to tell you that you cannot do anything, then who needs it?"[10]

The Advantages of Visibility and Clear Professional Boundaries

However, despite the problems with normalization, for many of the direct-entry midwives, the idea of state-sanctioned professionalization remained attrac-tive. Licensing would increase their confidence and reduce their fears of legal harassment; licensing could also increase the number of direct-entry midwives and home births.

Several direct-entry midwives who were apprentices during the time of the hearings imagined in great detail the benefits of professional recognition. For ex-ample, Elizabeth Smith noted:

The advantages will be that we will be more accessible, and we will be able to be professional—to enjoy the benefits of working in the professional sector. I can look at this in a couple of different ways, but for me, ever since I have been doing midwifery I have always kept records; I do my taxes and take all my deductions. I always spend a lot more on midwifery than I make. I just want to get other benefits that other businesses get. I don't know ex-actly what those are but I know there are some. Like I would like to set up a decent office and . . . I would like to be able to have a birth center where we can work and we can function parallel to all the other alternatives or options for families. Other specific kinds of benefits—the psychological part of it, having credibility and I am not always having to fight to defend who we are and the fear factor and things like that that are more subtle but just as real—confidence.[11]

Connie Baker desired a clear sense of professional boundaries:

Women who work in the informal section have no social security . . . and this is something I saw through all of Latin America. The midwives always lived in the crummiest houses. Everyone in town adored the women and would say, "Oh, she delivered six of my kids and four of my nieces and two of my grandchildren," and then you would go over and her front door would be falling off the hinges and she'd have a dirt floor in her house, and every time I asked someone, "Would you bring me the midwife?" they wouldn't go without some tortillas or flowers. They brought her something every time but obviously it's not a lucrative profession. I just think that working in the informal sector is oppressive. There are just certain rights that workers have that people who work outside of the formal section are deprived of.

It's always been unclear in the past about how to report or whether to report [our taxes]. Are we leaving a paper trail? Is what we are doing illegal, is it gray, who is really responsible? Is this something that we want to test in court? There weren't really too many people who were willing to go to court to find out what our rights were . . . It's been real unclear as to how much we want to say about what we do or how incriminating it would be to say what we do. So as a legal profession we can hang a shingle and have a business.[12]

With the ability to advertise and to be recognized by other medical professionals, the direct-entry midwives felt that their practices would become not only more lucrative but also less legally ambiguous.

Yet these advantages of professional standing were countered by a potential loss of autonomy, so some of the direct-entry midwives worried their community would experience further division after professionalization. As midwife Greta Godwin said:

And the people [who] are working on the state level . . . feel comfortable that they are doing something by incorporating this licensing and they feel that that's in the best interest of the parents. But once licensing is in place, then you have different types of parents looking for home birth. Some of those parents would be appropriate for a licensed provider, and some for an unlicensed provider. Because we have to realize that just because there is licensing doesn't mean that there will not be unlicensed providers. In fact, it will be the unlicensed providers who keep the skills of midwifery in the future: breeches, twins, VBACs [vaginal birth after cesarean], even natural birth. The licensed midwives will refer these mothers to their unlicensed colleagues.[13]

The direct-entry midwives realized that if they succeeded in gaining professional standing, if their practices were defined within the licensing genre along clear jurisdictional lines, then some members of the midwifery community would embrace licensing to gain clarity and visibility, but others would wish to retain their autonomy. The direct-entry midwifery community would split into the licensed and the unlicensed, the legal and the illegal, the normal and the deviant.

Attitudes About Midwifery Professionalization Across the United States

The Minnesota direct-entry midwives involved in the midwifery hearings were not unusual in their mixed feelings about professionalization. In a 1996 listserv discussion, nurse-midwives and direct-entry midwives debated the many meanings of licensure.[14] This thread on the listserv contrasted midwifery and medical systems of knowledge and debated whether medical care providers would recognize a midwife's experiential knowledge and intuition once she achieved professional standing. The participants did agree that professional standing could free a midwife from legal prosecution. Finally, although some listserv participants felt that licensing ensured safe care and that formal education proved that midwives could deliver that care, others felt that only individual protocols reflected quality of care. For example, Sally started this listserv thread by questioning the significance of formal schooling and whether it ensured safe care:

> A crucial element for me here is what is anybody's definition of "schooling"? If schooling is to mean only formal education that has come thru a classroom, I highly disagree . . . There are many-a-midwife who have been self-taught who I would not hesitate to match skills with school-trained midwives. . . . a license does not show a person's skill or capabilities at applying testing knowledge in a real-life situation . . . licenses will not PROVE safety for any profession, no more than all licensed drivers are safe & use sound judgement.
>
> (listserv communication, August 11, 1996, and August 15, 1996)

Although Jane agreed that self-taught midwives can be as capable as those with formal training, she cautioned that examination and licensing can keep a direct-entry midwife free from state harassment as she can "prove" her knowledge and skills. Jane mentions the legal prosecution that New York direct-entry midwives have experienced:

> I totally agree . . . that self taught midwives can have skills that match school trained midwives. The only difference in many states, that I know of is that the school trained midwife is tested on her skills and has proven that she has attained a body of knowledge. This (supposedly) protects the public from hiring someone who may or may not know basic midwifery material . . . Isn't the point that one have the knowledge and someway to prove it, not where (or at what school) the knowledge was attained? . . . One can have a legitimate reason for not being licensed, but in that choice it is imperitive [sic] ethically to also be realisitic [sic] about the legality of that choice. Having come from a two year legal battle in New York (which is still ongoing) and not being licensed (yet) I personally feel that while I did not consider licensure an advantage (especially in the homebirth arena) I was not always realistic about the consequences of not being licensed. In this state, being unlicensed may mean arrest, handcuffs, possible jail time, cease and desist orders, restraining orders, huge fines (we are talking many thousands) AND YOU DON'T HAVE TO HAVE A BAD OUTCOME, just for doing an unlicensed prenatal or unlicensed labor support . . .
>
> (listserv communication, August 12, 1996)

However, other listserv participants, such as Minnie, asserted that licensing ensured safe care and assumed that the licensed direct-entry midwife had the status to interact with medical care providers. Moreover, licensing is the only way that those medical care providers might accept the knowledge system of midwives:

If one is licensed then one has shown proficiency, PERIOD. Whether one is schooled or trained in a particular way should make no difference . . . While I certainly agree that far too much esteem is attached to certain avenues of education—the birthing world, and world in general, needs midwives who are also willing to face the established authorites in their own sphere of influence—academia (that MD behind a name is a very powerful tool) . . . In addition, as midwives begin to produce midwifery based literature, statistics and research materials to bolster the many truths that are now seen as "anecdotal" evidence [in] the world of academia (and hopefully those with other letters behind their names) will ultimately be obliged, however reluctantly and slowly, to accept the incontrovertible evidence of safe and sane midwifery care when presented by midwives credentialed in "their own" world . . .   (listserv communication, August 12, 1996)

To other listserv participants, such as Leah, professional benefits were distinct from professional competence:

Having a licence [sic] is simply a quick and easy means for your clients to see that other professionals feel that you have met the minimum standard for your profession in whatever year it was that you obtained it . . . It does not indicate your competance in dealing with any one specific problem, nor does it replace experience. It is a piece of paper to hang on the wall which may serve to ally clients fears if you are, in fact, inexperienced and it may yield certain professional perks such as hospital priviledges [sic], cool letters after your name, discounts on journals and newsletters, etc. (listserv communication, August 14, 1996)

Finally, Tallia proposed that midwifery knowledge is best reflected in the midwife's individual protocols, not in licensing rules:

Actually licensing, et al, is neutral. . . . Licenses and certification make a statement to the public and to our colleagues, it gives us a shared base of training and knowledge and a place to begin to work together. I think where we need to focus is: what are the protocols we operate under, what are our policies and procedures—do we have them written down and available to the public so they can decide about our practice, do we share them with physicians so they can know what they can count on us for in an emergency, do we use and follow our own protocols??
      (listserv communication, August 16, 1996)

The observations offered by the Minnesota direct-entry midwives about the advantages and disadvantages of professionalization, supported by the comments made on the midwifery listserv, suggest that when a practice gains professional standing, some of its members may regret their loss of autonomy. As the knowledge system and practices of the emerging profession become normalized, diversity might be devalued, if not impossible. In eighteenth-century England, Elizabeth Nihell argued for the value of the midwives' experiential knowledge. Historical and current definitions of the "good midwife" call upon her to know when to consult with practitioners more formally trained. When a practice becomes normalized, jurisdictions are clearly delineated, knowledge is abstractly defined and categorized, and individual practices either conform or are branded as deviant, even unsafe. As seen in the next section of this chapter, in the genre of licensing rules and regulations, language represents and reinforces the reification and normalization of the practice. Moreover, the practice is often defined by dominant professions, including supervision by practitioners in these dominant professions, who use discourse to maintain their jurisdictional boundaries.

The Genre of Licensing Rules and Regulations

In the first hearing of the Licensing Rule Writing Group (LRWG) on December 1, 1993, Leonard Boche, executive director of the Board of Medical Practice, explained that, although board staff member Jessica Ramsey would help write the rules, she would not define direct-entry midwifery practice. LRWG participants had the responsibility to do that. Boche reassured the LRWG that, although the writing process would be "arduous," there were boilerplate materials available, and, even though the language of the law had to "stay" and the format of the board's licensing rules was set, there was a lot that the LRWG could "put its teeth into." So when Jessica Ramsey passed out a draft of the licensing rules, various sections were already complete, while others were left blank. However, as Ramsey, who held both a nursing and a law degree, explained, genre conventions determined the nature of these sections—from Definitions to Fees, from Licensure Requirements to Forms of Disciplinary Action. Although other forms of communication became important during the public hearings, including legislative statutes, policy and procedure manuals from such organizations as the Minnesota Midwives' Guild, and informed consent agreements between midwives and home birth parents, the genre of licensing rules and regulations became the discursive mode used to maintain or challenge professional jurisdictional boundaries. Again, through this genre, we see how midwifery practice was to be normalized through professionalization.

Boilerplate language within the genre provided to the Licensing Rule Writing Group participants consisted of procedural requirements, including requirements for license application and renewal, and definitions of the surveillance and disciplinary powers of the board, including prohibition of sexual contact with clients. Also addressed were lists of obligations to report information to the board, including the results of malpractice suits against insured midwives; definitions of cooperation between the midwife and the board, including the obligation to testify during board investigations; and categories of disciplinary action, such as suspension of the right to practice. To demonstrate the conventions of the genre, the Board of Medical Practice gave LRWG participants the scope of practice sections for other Board-regulated practitioners: physician assistants, respiratory care practitioners, and athletic trainers. Thus, the LRWG members understood that they would have to describe quite specifically midwifery practice when they read that respiratory care practitioners' services included such tasks as "obtaining physiological specimens and interpreting physiological data including . . . analyzing arterial blood gas" (Minnesota Department of Health, "Respiratory Care" 5). Moreover, LRWG participants read about supervisory relationships between practitioners and physicians, such as the section noting that physician assistants prescribed and administered drugs and used "medical devices" but only "if this function has been delegated to the physician assistant by the supervising physician and approved by the board . . ." (Minnesota Board of Medical Examiners, "Physician Assistant" 7). These practitioners had to refer certain cases to supervising medical authorities; for example, respiratory care practitioners' services "whether delivered in a health care facility or the patient's place of residence, must not be provided except upon referral from a physician" (5). Also, "to ensure the supervising physician assumes full medical responsibility for patient services provided by the physician assistant, the supervising physician . . . shall review and evaluate patient services provided by the physician assistant on a daily basis from information in patient charts or records" (6). Thus, regardless of what tasks and tools were sanctioned within the practices, what jurisdictions were determined, these examples of genre conventions dictated state surveillance and medical supervision.

For this first LRWG hearing on December 1, 1993, board staff member Ramsey drafted an extensive list of prohibited practices, practices labeled "unsafe," for the section on "Grounds for Disciplinary Action." For example, direct-entry midwives were not to attend births of women "who have been diagnosed with a medical condition which requires medical supervision" (Licensing Rule Draft 30 November 1993, 10).[15] Thirteen conditions, from cardiac arrest to congenital anomalies in the newborn, required referral or transport to "appropriate medical care." LRWG members were invited to review and revise these grounds or contraindications, and their responses to these sections later sparked substantive conflict in the hearings. However, the genre determined that these contraindications—grounds for losing one's license—must be included. Thus, in this first draft, the LRWG inherited specifications of the licensed direct-entry midwife's relationship to a supervising agency, the Board of Medical Practice, and the limitations on her practice, including when medical care providers must approve her choices.

As seen in chapter 3, midwives have long struggled to avoid supervision by medical caregivers and have resisted a place in the hierarchical structure of medical institutions. Although Elizabeth Cellier was willing to enter into this hierarchy to achieve professional status, as were British midwives in 1902, Elizabeth Nihell and others feared medical supervision of their practices. During the time of the Minnesota hearings, the midwives on the midwifery listserv voiced definite opinions about the disadvantages of medical supervision. For example, Ida, a nurse-midwife in Michigan, responded to one participant's comments on how health care providers may discourage home birth:

> Oh I WISH it was just that "providers pass on a less that optimistic view" [about home birth]. IMNSHO [in my not so humble opinion] the providers pass on the cultural view, and that surrounds women everywhere everyday. The American view of birth in general is that it's a terrible ordeal, best man-

aged by LOTS of "Experts" IN the hospital with drugs. Why put yourself at risk and suffer to be some kind of hero? Women who don't get overwhelmed by that view are the minority . . .

(listserv communication, September 13, 1996)

For Ida, suspicion of home birth seemed inherent in the supervisory comments offered by medical care providers. Laura, a practicing midwife in Las Vegas, agreed that these differences were irreconcilable when the two systems of care collided:

> I can only speak from the experiences of midwives in my area, but, we seem to get the same reactions from hospital staffs whether we get the mom there at the first sign of a problem or after things have gotten fairly complicated. I have heard many a hospital staff say "Well, that's what you get when you try a home birth!" no matter what the problem!!!
>
> Not only are the parents treated like they have had no previous care (yes, I always accompany the mother and bring all records), but the second we leave they are told many lies about how serious their condition really was, how close to death they and their baby came and how many home birth tragedies they see. Our relationship with the parents is seldom the same afterward.   (listserv communication, September 17, 1996)

Moreover, the very language that medical health care providers used seemed to the midwives on the listserv to denigrate their practices and have differing effects on their clients. For example, Ida cautioned another midwife that the words doctors used had linguistic capital:

> You said words communications etc cannot disempower anyone—they do it to themselves [women disempower themselves]. I can't go along with that. At all. Words are powerful and can wound , stop, wither—or they can nourish, open, soothe. Witness any labor. See the difference in a newly pregnant Mom who's told about her pelvic "I don't know, you're kind of small there, but we'll see." versus "Wow, great bones—made for babies, feels wonderful." Witness "Shut up and stop screaming" versus "Let it out, let it be low in your throat, you're so strong." Witness "Mother and baby" versus "Maternal-fetal unit."
>
> Listen. Look. See what happens. Your words scare me.
>
> (listserv communication, August 30, 1996)

Finally, one nurse-midwife working in a rural health clinic, shared a birth story with the midwifery listserv in which she suggested that her laboring client's needs were disregarded in the hierarchical structure of the hospital. Also, she saw her only alternative was to avoid the situation again, even though she had to find another way to practice:

> Don [pseudonym for the physician with whom she works] and his resident want me to check the patient who is understandably reluctant since when Don did his last vag exam, he stayed in for awhile stretching her cervix and she was in tears when the exam was complete. I promise I will be quick

and easy and not do that. Well I can't even reach her cervix. 5 cm? [Don's last assessment] Hmmm . . .

I let mom go and walk. I see Don and tell him that her cervix is too posterior for me to reach without causing quite a lot of pain. Nothing has changed much with the intensity of her contractions so I can't imagine there has been any big change. I am really trying to be diplomatic. I have short fingers but I can feel a dilating cervix, thank you.

A few hours they are bugging me to check her again . . . I can reach her cervix now (though it is still posterior) and she is 4 cm and 70 to 80% effaced. I have to explain to the couple that measurements can vary between examiners and that I feel that progress has definately [sic] been made because her cervix has come forward, contractions are stronger, etc. But when I report to Don, he decides he wants to check her. According to him, she is 6 cm. I trust my own assessment.

She walks more and hangs out in the shower a lot. Around 6:30 p.m., the quality of the contractions change and knowing that the good doctors will be bugging me, I ask to check her again, but she doesn't want to be checked which I respect and [she] wants to hang out in the shower which is helping her cope. In the next half hour, things seem to be picking up nicely . . . So at 7:00 p.m., the resident decides she is 6 cm, and this means she has made "no progress" . . .

The resident is pushing to rupture her membranes and to "do something." He starts talking about pain medicine although this woman has been doing quite well, especially when she is in the shower which seems to help her cope and stimulates stronger labor. He leaves to talk to Don who decides to check her now and pronounces her 7 cm. He does rupture her membranes and the head comes down a bit more, and encourages her to walk if she wants to. However, in a few minutes they are back in wanting her to have a hep lock and for me to give her some pain medicine (which she has never requested). Now contractions are really strong. She is up on the toilet. I put the hep lock in and ask her if she really wants the pain medication, indicating that she does have a choice. But I think all the suggesting from the resident that she might need pain medicine along with the slow progress has unnerved her and she wants pain meds now . . .

(listserv communication, July 28, 1996)

This nurse-midwife described how her medical care supervisor disregarded both her own knowledge of cervical dilation and her client's intuition to labor without medication. To the midwife, the care provided by Don and his resident so intervened in the birth process that she decided to disregard their instructions and her client lost track of her own needs. The midwife's perception was that she could not give quality care under the supervision of this team of medical care providers.[16]

Moreover, the direct-entry midwives in the Licensing Rule Writing Group in Minnesota found that not only medical supervision but also state surveillance, as expressed in generic licensing rules and regulations, seemed to disregard their knowledge and intuition as well as the particular circumstances of their practices. For example, standard language added to the licensing rules by Jessica Ramsey, a board staffer, stated that direct-entry midwives would be prevented from "revealing a communication from, or relating to, a client except when otherwise required or permitted by law." This stipulation was designed to protect the privacy of clients, in this case home birth parents, and to enable the board to gather information about any practitioner's actions that it wished to investigate (February 14, 1994 draft).[17] However, the direct-entry midwives found that the rule would eliminate one of their main sources of knowledge and emotional support—birth stories presented for peer review. In the small, close home birth community in Minnesota, it would be impossible to continue to tell birth stories and maintain the privacy of clients. For example, as Connie Baker, a guild midwife, argued before LRWG: "This is a real issue. [If a midwife asks me for advice,] I know who her mother [due] in June is. She hasn't told me, but it's a little community. And I was at the last home birth gathering [of the guild] and I could tell who was due in June. This is real. This is real" (LRWG hearing, February 15, 1994).[18] Here the direct-entry midwives within LRWG resisted the conventions of the genre that would have excluded an important source of their knowledge.

Thus, although the Minnesota Board of Medical Practice considered the language of the licensing rule genre standard or even neutral, the direct-entry midwives tested the language against their realities and found it vague, too restrictive, or, at times, not up to their own community standards for safe practice. For example, the board rules called for disciplinary action when a practitioner was found "engaging in sexual conduct with a client." The direct-entry midwives wanted to know when the practitioner-client relationship would end. Phillip McAfee asked, "What's the matter with 'never'?" He suggested that the rules for direct-entry midwives could mirror those for psychotherapists. But the direct-entry midwives often helped members of their large extended families give birth at home; they worked not just with clients but with a couple and their family; and some cared for second and third generations of home birth families. Thus, they found it problematic to take "a hard line on these things" as they resisted the conventions of the genre that did not reflect the actual nature of their relationships with their clients.

The licensing rule genre also included statements pertaining to prohibited conduct, such as the following:

> Conduct likely to deceive, defraud, or harm the public; or demonstrating a willful or careless disregard for the health, welfare, or safety of a client; or any other practice that may create unnecessary danger to any client's life, health, or safety, in any of which cases, proof of actual injury need not be established. Prohibited conduct includes, but is not limited to, the following practices which have been identified as unsafe . . .

The direct-entry midwives proposed a positive statement about their practices as an alternative to language that specified what they could not do. As one midwife stated, the language of the genre was "loaded"; the guild version was "more like our language." Thus, they suggested in their version of the licensing rules that this section opened as follows:

> A midwife's conduct will be honest with highest regard for the health, welfare and safety of the mother and baby. The midwife willfully and openly inspires confidence in the birth process. The midwife's care includes screening for conditions or situations that have been identified as unsafe which include the following . . .

Although the content of the list that followed was not remarkably different in either version, the language was. The language provided by the direct-entry midwives, however, was alien to the conventions of the genre. The licensing rules had "to be negative," Jessica Ramsey stated, as the language had been established by case law. The midwives were told that they would have the opportunity to describe their positive relationships with their clients in the scope of practice section of the rules. However, the direct-entry midwives, in particular those who had been involved in writing the Minnesota Midwives' Guild's own *Standards of Care and Certification Guide*, wished to emphasize the supportive relationship between the midwife and the mother in both sections, resisting again the conventions of the genre.

For example, the guild members recommended changing the first prohibited item, "Attending birth as the primary caregiver in which the woman has obtained no prenatal care, except in an emergency," to "Attending birth as the primary caregiver in which the midwife has not provided thorough and complete course of prenatal care, except in an emergency." Much as her relationship with Don and his resident was described by the nurse-midwife to the listserv, direct-midwife Connie Baker commented to LRWG participants:

> One of the major differences between home birth and hospital birth is the relationship. In the hospital if the mother gets to a point where she cannot give birth, there are drugs and devices that will help her. In a home birth situation, we really rely so much on our relationship with women to help them through the hard stages of their labor . . . Because [of] the relationship building—those are the tools that we use in a home birth.

In suggesting the language for this section, the direct-entry midwives were in fact articulating a higher standard of thorough and careful care. Thus, the direct-entry midwives participating in the licensing rule writing process wished to place in the foreground the benefits of the midwife forming a relationship with her home birth parents rather than the aspects of practice that would be prohibited by the state and overseen by medical caregivers.

In subsequent hearings of the Licensing Rule Writing Group, the direct-entry midwives continued to resist the conventions of the licensing rule genre that narrowed their practices and challenged their autonomy by requiring medical consultation on certain conditions. Although the 1995 version of the Minnesota Midwives' Guild's *Standards of Care and Certification Guide* specified thirty-eight conditions "requiring documented medical consultation"—from "suspected multiple gestation" to "marked decrease or cessation of fetal movement," from "mother over age 45" to "failure of laceration/episiotomy site to heal properly with signs of infection or breakdown" (appendix C), during the June 21, 1994, LRWG hearing the guild midwives protested the notion of required medical consultation:

> [The need to consult] doesn't make sense. It doesn't seem really workable.
> From a midwife's perspective . . . the difference between the midwife and
> physician in terms of status and belief system is so great . . . that a need to
> consult sets up a situation where there is no coherence, no communication,
> no understanding from one belief system to the other. And this is hard on
> the autonomy of the profession, on the midwife. From the physician's per-
> spective, it seems to make even less sense in that it puts the physician in the
> position of saying "Yes, it's OK for the woman with serious psychological
> problems or whatever to stay home" and then if she does and anything hap-
> pens . . . it's the doc who has the liability insurance . . . who would be in
> slightly hotter water than the midwife. It's just not going to work on either
> side.   (LRWG hearing, June 21,1994).[19]

Mary Emerson, a lobbyist for the guild, confirmed this resistance on the part of the guild: "My bottom line is that if we or the Board of Medical Practice say this fall that Connie [Baker, for example] has to get Dr. Miller's [one of the physicians attending the hearings] approval to do such and such that we had just as well quit right now . . . You made it impossible to function under the conditions of the license." Instead, the direct-entry midwives proposed that individual midwifery protocols and informed consent agreements between the direct-entry midwife and her client substitute for required medical consultation as called for by the conventions of the genre. "These boundaries belong in protocols but not in these rules," Emerson said.

The conventions of the genre, however, supported the medical systems of knowledge of birth and therefore supervisory relationships between medical ex-perts and other practitioners. Judy Miller, representing both the American College of Obstetrics and Gynecology and the Minnesota Ob/Gyn Society, proposed to LRWG that midwives would more easily work with medical caregivers if, in the future, the midwives could speak with a more united and seemingly professional voice: "Perhaps in the future as traditional midwives become more cohesive and up front and respected by the medical community, then there will be potential for co-operation, interaction and consultation." Also, seemingly forgetting the long his-tory of midwifery and the current direct-entry midwives' knowledge systems, one nurse offered LRWG members examples of how midwives might misdiagnose con-ditions, conditions that should not be "left to standards of what might be in the [mid-wifery] community. Because we are not talking about a broad spectrum of medical practice in the system that has grown up over the years." Finally, nurse-midwife Henrietta Kramer, president of Region 5, Chapter 11, of the American College of Nurse-Midwives, questioned whether, after professionalization, direct-entry mid-wives could be truly autonomous: "You are part of the system [e.g., using the med-ical labs] even though you are autonomous." The conventions of the licensing rule genre, then, supported the notion that professionalism normalizes a practice so that practitioners and practices are uniform and cohesive. These conventions also in-corporate supervision by practitioners of dominant professions who are culturally and professionally granted expertise and oversight by representatives of the state who depend on these experts' systems of knowledge.

Other states that licensed direct-entry midwives at the time of the Minnesota hearings (1991–1995) required various degrees of either supervision or consultation. Most restrictive of the midwives' autonomy was Wyoming, where direct-entry mid-wives could attend births, but only supervising physicians could offer prenatal or postnatal care (Becker et al. 55; Wyoming Board of Medicine). Some states, such as Montana and Alaska, required a midwifery client to undergo a physician exam-ination by a physician, physician assistant, advanced nurse practitioner, or certified nurse-midwife before committing to a home birth. Arkansas "encouraged" each midwife to "develop a close working relationship" with a physician who served as her "referral physician," who "supported" her when "potentially serious conditions" arose. Other states, such as South Carolina, held that it was the direct-entry midwife's duty to recognize "the warning signs of abnormal or potentially abnormal conditions necessitating referral to a physician." However, South Carolina's Health and Hu-man Services department promised to review the requirement "that each midwife have her own backup physician as it continues to be a problem for everyone" (Gaskin, "Regional Reports").[20]

In fact, at the time of the Minnesota hearings, direct-entry midwives across the country were expressing via the listserv a concern that required medical consultation not only threatened the autonomy of their practice but also could be used as a tool to eliminate their practices, giving medical care providers full jurisdiction over birth. For example, Hope, a community midwife, described her suspicions as follows:

> The same states that are mis-using Roe v. Wade/Bowland are the ones that make all licensed midwifery (CNMs & direct-entry) dependent on "physi-cian-supervision". These laws were purposefully constructed by the med-ical establishment to make the doctor culpable for the midwife's practice (as a "disincentive to home birth") and thus virtually eliminate the LEGAL practice of domiciliary midwifery (including free-standing birth centers) by midwives of all educational background.
>
> (listserv communication, July 25, 1996)[21]

One way that the direct-entry midwives testifying before the Licensing Rule Writing Group proposed to avoid required medical consultation was to include in the licensing rules a Midwife Client Statement of Rights and an informed consent agreement form that all midwives must use. Rather than simply resisting the con-ventions of the genre by deleting or protesting certain sections, the direct-entry mid-wives suggested instead sections describing their practices in ways that were unique or alien to the licensing rules and regulations genre. They proposed that the State-ment of Rights section be based on the previous work of the Midwifery Study Ad-visory Group and contain stipulations such as "a brief summary, in plain language, of the approach used by the midwife in providing services to clients" and the mid-wife's degrees, training, and experience. Although informed consent agreements are required of physicians and other health care professionals and were included in the Minnesota Midwives' Guild's *Standards of Care and Certification Guide*, they were not a convention of the licensing rules and regulations genre in Minnesota. In essence, informed consent agreements were created to protect the practitioner, in this case the direct-entry midwife, by limiting her liability, and the client, in this case the home birth parent, by offering enough information about risks and benefits so that she could make a safe choice.

At the June 1994 hearing two examples of informed consent forms were distributed to LRWG participants. The guild submitted a very simple form, including a definition of the direct-entry midwife and a disclosure of the midwife's background, education, training, professional affiliations, malpractice insurance (or lack thereof), association with a physician, and a statement "that clearly outlines the expectations the midwife has of the parents." On the other hand, Judy Miller shared the informed consent form of the hospital in which she practiced in Minneapolis, which gave the patient's consent to the physician to perform all necessary procedures related to treatment and contained such statements as "I am aware that the practice of medicine is not an exact science and I acknowledge that no guarantees have been made to me concerning the results of the operation or procedure(s)." The guild's version appeared to confirm the midwife's decision-making relationship in consultation with her client, whereas the hospital's form authorized the physician to treat the patient unilaterally.

The guild's version of the informed consent agreement was similar to that of direct-entry midwifery organizations in other states and therefore seemed a common part of midwifery practice. For example, the New Mexico Midwives' Association includes a statement of "parental responsibility" in its *Policies and Procedures*: "Most parents seeking a birth at home or in a birth center accept responsibility for their health, sharing information about changes in their pregnancy and matters that may affect their pregnancy and birth"(7). However, in fact, the informed consent agreement was a strategy that other direct-entry midwives had used to get around some of the strict parameters of their licensing rules. Licensed direct-entry midwives in Arkansas, for example, alarmed that families were electing "do it yourself (DIY)" home births when a condition was on the contraindications list, believed an informed consent waiver was the solution, as the Licensed Direct-Entry Midwife chair of the Arkansas Department of Health Midwifery Advisory Board told the midwifery listserv:

> Here in Arkansas we are working on rewriting our rules and regulations. This does not require new legislation, but does require a public hearing and a presentation to the Board of Health for their vote. We are trying to get a waiver approved so that if a family wants to have a home birth with a licensed midwife and yet do not want all of the procedures or fall outside the regulations, they may still have a licensed midwife in attendance. There are many families who have DIY home births because they do not meet the criteria for low risk: vbacs, 8th timers, etc. This is unsafe and we are trying to change that. We also have woman in monogamous relationships who do not want a repeat GC culture and the midwife can lose her license over allowing that. So we hope to have a waiver that the parents can sign and thus still have us in attendance.   (listserv communication, July 25, 1996)

Nurse-midwives and direct-entry midwives in other states had developed specific informed consent releases for some of the conditions that the medical caregivers attending the Minnesota hearings wanted to see contraindicated for home birth. For example, nurse-midwives and direct-entry midwives in other states developed their own informed consent releases for specific conditions, such as vaginal birth after cesarean or VBAC at home.[22] States, such as Texas and Montana, allowed home birth VBACs if parents signed an informed consent form. Finally, New Hampshire had set a precedent for the Minnesota direct-entry midwives by including the agreement itself, in this case for VBAC, within the licensing rules. However, the New Hampshire agreement was more similar in language to those offered by Judy Miller than that offered to LRWG by the Minnesota Midwives' Guild. The New Hampshire informed consent agreement outlined the risks for the condition in some detail and specified that the midwife had explained what additional medical care might be provided should these risks be realized:

> I appreciate that there are certain risks associated with this procedure including uterine rupture and its potential consequences of fetal distress, fetal death, maternal hemorrhage, hysterectomy and maternal death and I freely assume these risks. I also understand that there are possible benefits associated with this procedure including less chance of surgical intervention, birth in the familiar surroundings of my own home, with the support of the certified lay midwife. However, I appreciate that there is no certainty that I will achieve these benefits and no guarantee has been made to me regarding the outcome of this procedure . . .
>
> The reasonable alternatives to this procedure have been explained to me including attendance of VBAC within the hospital setting where there is more immediate access to surgical intervention, should a significant rupture occur intrapartally, and more intensive care facilities such as blood transfusions and neonatal resuscitation equipment and personnel.

The conventions of the licensing rule genre confronted by the direct-entry Minnesota midwives confirmed their concerns about the normalization of their practice leading to a loss of autonomy by requiring medical consultation and by dictating conditions they could not treat at home. They resisted these conventions by proposing alternative language that cast their relationship with home birth parents in a positive light and alternative content that substituted informed consent agreements for required medical consultation and supervision. Given the professional status of the dominant medical profession, whose knowledge about birth was already sanctioned by state recognition, the direct-entry midwives' resistance to the licensing rule genre might seem doomed to fail. However, as they began the process of writing the licensing rules, the LRWG participants decided to grant equal voice to the emerging profession—the direct-entry midwives—and to use the shared-document collaborative process to respond to the genre. This decision was supported by the Board of Medical Practice. The decision enabled the direct-entry midwives to resist to conventions of the genre—but spelled the eventual failure of the rule writing effort, as medical caregivers responded forcefully when their knowledge systems and jurisdictional claims were challenged.

The LRWG Drafting Process: Resisting the Conventions of the Genre

Again, the shared-document collaborative process assumes intellectual negotiation, with all collaborators having equal rhetorical status. Thus, conflicting knowledge systems and the direct-entry midwives' resistance to the genre of licensing rules and regulations were publicly articulated as were the discursive attempts by the nurses, nurse-midwives, and physicians in the group to normalize midwifery practice. Regardless of the impulse of the collaborative writing process, however, the medical care providers participating in the Licensing Rule Writing Group hearings represented the incumbent profession; they had established professional status, wide cultural regard, and legal standing. Outside the hearings, some members of LRWG predicted the problems that the shared-document collaborative process would generate. For example, Emma Davidson, who represented the Minnesota Nurses' Association, described the potential impact of these problems: "The Board should have been honest . . . and said, 'listen, we are not going to approve this [early drafts that maintained direct-entry midwives' autonomy] but within these edges here is where you can go'—I just think that this thing is doomed."[23]

The process of granting equal authority to all LRWG voices began when the participants collaborated on the scope of practice section of the licensing rules. Here, although the genre conventions did not provide boilerplate language for the group, Minnesota Statute 148.30 served as the starting point according to the agenda set by the board for the January 13, 1994 hearing: "The Scope of Practice should answer the question: What does 'attend women in childbirth' encompass or mean?'" because that phrase formed the essence of the statutory definition of direct-entry midwifery. However, LRWG participants had to spell out in great detail direct-entry midwives' approved tasks, services, and tools. Jessica Ramsey initiated the shared-document collaborative process by asking individuals or representatives from various discourse communities to work outside the LRWG hearings to produce text and then to present their drafts for open discussion. Ramsey's suggested process proved to be so challenging that the Minnesota Midwives' Guild hired a conflict resolution expert to guide their discussions and to resolve the differences among guild and non-Guild members. The guild was expected to return to the LRWG hearings with a united voice, in essence to contribute willingly to the normalization of their practices.

Upon Ramsey's recommendation, three members of LRWG submitted drafts of the scope of practice for direct-entry midwifery: the co-chairs of the Minnesota Midwives' Guild; a family practice physician who also participated in the MSAG hearings; and Judy Miller, who represented both the American College of Obstetrics and Gynecology and the Minnesota Ob/Gyn Society. The three groups responded in distinct ways, which signaled not only the midwives' resistance to the genre but also the negotiations that would have to take place between the emerging and the incumbent professions. The guild's draft of the scope of practice was quite specific, detailing prenatal, intrapartum, and postpartum physical and emotional care, referring to the midwife as "the primary care provider," and leveling the relationship between the home birth and medical communities. For example, the guild's draft stated: "If the required repair [of a perineal or vaginal laceration] does not fall within the expertise of the primary care giver, arrangements should immediately be made for transfer and proper attendance." The direct-entry midwife was to be the judge of what kind of repair was required and what kind of attendance necessary. The guild's draft was based on its own *Standards of Care and Certification Guide* and its interpretation of the licensing documents of other states (LRWG hearing, January 13, 1994).[24]

The family practice physician's draft was a two-paragraph statement stressing that direct-entry midwives attended women with "normal, low-risk pregnancies" and "normal term newborns." Any condition that was not normal must be referred. For example, the second and longest paragraph of this draft focused on the limits of direct-entry midwifery and the surveillance of medical authority:

> Midwives do not diagnose or treat disease, but ascertain risk factors and recognize deviations from the normal course of pregnancy, labor, birth, and the post-partum/neonatal period. Any significant risk factors or deviations from normal should lead to appropriate consultation and/or referral. Midwives should quickly recognize and provide initial stabilization for obstetric and neonatal complications which may arise emergently and/or unexpectedly. In the case of home birth, adequate plans and procedures must be in place to assure timely transport to an appropriate medical facility when necessary.

The third draft came from the representative of the American College of Obstetrics and Gynecology and the Minnesota Ob/Gyn Society, Judy Miller. Her draft also stated that direct-entry midwives "support the natural process" of pregnancy with "alertness to the parameters of normality." However, in her draft, "contraindications requiring medical referral" were not listed but instead were to be referenced in some other document, such as MANA Core Competencies or Minnesota Midwives' Guild's *Standards of Care and Certification Guide*. She admitted that she was not sure about the adequacy of these references. Therefore, she prefaced her draft with a list of questions and comments about the guild's *Standards of Care*: "Do traditional midwives perform vaginal birth after cesarean section?" "I think a patient who truly has a diagnosis of incompetent cervix is very high risk, and I am surprised that traditional midwives would consider caring for a patient under these circumstances."

However, despite these initial differences between the three drafts presented to the LRWG, Judy Miller's questions seemed to confirm that LRWG participants could collaborate not only to write the scope of practice section but also to modify the licensing genre to suit their purposes. Working from the drafts submitted by the guild, by the family practice physician, and by Miller, LRWG decided to create a scope of practice section that contained essential definitions of midwifery that would satisfy the majority of voices. Their first effort focused on the direct-entry midwife herself and what services she provided: "Midwives provide prenatal, intrapartum, and postpartum care for women with initial and continuing assessment for feasibility of midwifery care. Midwives also provide neonatal care for normal term newborns."

The guild midwives then proposed instead that midwives be called "primary health care providers"so they could be included in the health plan that President Clinton had proposed that year. Although the family care physician warned that this was "hot language," as primary health care providers "assess and diagnose and serve as gatekeepers for others," LRWG reached a modest and uneasy compromise: "The midwife is a health care professional who provides primary health care services during pregnancy, birth, and the postpartum period for women and newborns." Then the guild recommended that LRWG add "autonomous" to "health care professional." Thus, the very definition of the direct-entry midwife seemed to offer both professional standing and autonomy to the midwives, problematic language in light of the purpose of the genre itself and the normalization of practices that usually came with professional status.

LRWG then used the draft that was prepared by Judy Miller to list midwifery services as follows:

A. Initial and ongoing assessment for suitability for midwifery care.
B. Comprehensive prenatal care with attention to the physical, nutritional, emotional and social needs of the woman and her family.
C. Attending and supporting the natural process of labor and birth with alertness to the parameters of normality.
D. Postpartum care of the mother and newborn including physical and emotional assessment.
E. Information and/or referrals to community resources on childbirth preparation, breast-feeding, exercise, nutrition, parenting and care of the newborn.

One sentence, initially contained in C, "Emphasis is on insuring the well-being of the mother and baby throughout labor, delivery, and the postpartum period via the art and practice of midwifery" became a concluding statement: "The art and practice of midwifery care emphasizes the safety and well-being of the mother and baby throughout pregnancy, labor, birth, and the postpartum period." And the sentence that followed— "The midwife has a mechanism for consultation and referral with continuing involvement, when appropriate"—came from MANA Core Competencies and the guild's *Standards of Care and Certification Guide*.

Thus, through the shared-document process, a process which gave the direct-entry midwives the ability to shape their own licensing rules, the midwife herself— as an autonomous health care professional, well versed in her art and practice—remained prominent in the scope of practice section. She was to be "alert" to what is normal and decide when and with whom to consult or refer. This definition of the direct-entry midwife—couched in words that in the first versions of the Minnesota licensing rules preserved the autonomy of the direct-entry midwife and resisted normalization of the practice—was atypical of licensing rules in other states.[25] In their initial definitions of midwifery, other states limited rather than empowered the practitioner.

For example, in the scope of practice section in Louisiana's licensing rules, both state and medical authority were stressed:

> The licensed midwife may provide care to low risk patients *determined by*
> *physician evaluation and examination* to be essentially normal for preg-
> nancy and childbirth. Such care includes prenatal supervision and coun-
> seling; preparation for childbirth; and supervision and care during labor
> and delivery and care of the mother and the newborn in the immediate post-
> partum period if progress meets criteria generally accepted as normal as
> defined by the board. (2, emphasis added)

South Carolina as well stressed this authority and assigned to the midwife low-risk care only: "The licensed midwife may provide care to low-risk women and neonates *determined by medical evaluation* to be prospectively normal for pregnancy and childbirth . . . and may deliver only women who have completed between 37 to 42 weeks of gestation, except under emergency circumstances" (8–9). Some states, such as Alaska, referred to the midwife's knowledge and responsibility but included medical consultation in that responsibility. States such as Texas acknowledged the right to choose where to birth but still limited direct-entry midwives to low-risk births: "Midwifery care supports individual rights and self-determination within the boundaries of safety" but the midwife "will not knowingly accept nor thereafter maintain responsibility for the prenatal, intrapartum, or postpartum care of a woman or neonatal care of an infant who has or develops a high risk condition or compli-cation" (19, 21).

Only New Mexico's licensing rules contained language similar to that in Min-nesota's first draft of the scope of practice. Using the strategy suggested by Judy Miller in the Minnesota hearings, New Mexico's rule writers directly referred read-ers to the state's midwifery guild for "management" standards of pregnant women and newborns. Also, in the New Mexico Midwives' Association's *Policies and Pro-cedures*, midwives' autonomy was confirmed: "All midwives will be able to inde-pendently assume responsibility for the management and care of the healthy, low-risk woman and her infant during pregnancy, labor, birth and puerperium" (New Mex-ico Midwives 2). However, the New Mexico rules also directed readers searching for more specific direction to the *Standards of Care* of the American College of Ob-stetricians and Gynecologists and procedures and policies of the Department of Health (New Mexico Department of Health 102). Thus, in the scope of practice sec-tion, the first part of the licensing rules upon which the Minnesota LRWG collab-orated, the group departed from the conventions of the genre by attempting to balance the autonomy and professional standing of the direct-entry midwife.

Outside of the public hearings, LRWG participants expressed concerns about the definition of midwifery that the group had produced. Henrietta Kramer, repre-senting the Minnesota nurse-midwives, worried that the definition invited direct-entry midwives to "take anyone."[26] Emma Davidson from the Minnesota Nurses' Association believed that the medical community would "have a hard time with 'autonomous' health care professional,"as the medical community "doesn't even like nurse-midwives having an autonomous practice. They will want all sorts of supervisory language." However, Davidson predicted that if such supervisory language were added, the direct-entry midwives "might find that insulting in the same way that many nurse-midwives find some of the relationships they are forced into insulting. There is no way under these rules that all midwives would be pulled in [become licensed]."[27]

Even the guild midwives who contributed to this definition of midwifery worried about how it would be received outside of LRWG. For example, Rita Ortiz said that although "in essence the midwife has to be an autonomous health care provider . . . putting it in here in such language is like saying, 'kill me, kill me' . . . This is politically suicidal language."[28] The direct-entry midwives were aware that, outside the LRWG discourse community, they had no control over how others would interpret their words. As Elizabeth Smith said, "The word 'normality' gets me . . . I just think it's such a loaded and judgmental word. But I think it works. If everyone who uses it comes from a certain kind of consciousness, it can be OK. It depends. Most of the midwives would probably agree on what it means, but an Ob might not."[29] Finally, both guild and non-Guild midwives believed that the definition still did not represent adequately the relationship between the midwife and her client and the special nature of this gendered practice. For example, Gloria Olson, a guild midwife, found the definition "uneven, like the midwife is more powerful. But in actuality, in my experience, it's a very equal relationship."[30] Kris House also feared that the definition implied that the midwife had more authority than the home birth parents:

> Midwife means with women—I feel like we are with women in the sense that they have a sense of their own health . . . and well-being and even their own babies, and they want to bounce it off someone, and what better person than another woman who has birthed previously . . . This definition of midwifery, it puts the burden on the midwife and not on the families. . . . When I read that I provide primary health care—no, this couple is doing primary health care.[31]

Finally, Elizabeth Smith was aware that in the very act of writing the licensing rules, midwifery would lose what she considered its female nature, that it would be "masculinized":

> But again, it's [the definition within the scope of practice section] talking about a health care professional, and licensing is creating another tier. Now you have nurse midwifery on the most medical level, licensing [of direct-entry midwives] on the next medical level. Creating a tiered level of midwifery further masculinizes midwifery because you are taking a feminine tradition, an art, and pushing it into a male model of definitions. Certainly female models have had control issues and power issues, but we are putting this into a more linear model—labeling, defining, editing the art, putting it into the male model of health care. Modern medicine is the cut and

dry version of health care, whereas midwifery, by nature, is much more holistic.[32]

Although the LRWG members collaborated on this definition, one that would seem
to retain the autonomy of direct-entry midwifery even after licensing, they suspected that after licensing the practice would be normalized through professionalization. They feared that the direct-entry midwives would find themselves in a
hierarchy, that the midwives' knowledge systems would be devalued, and that the
relationship between the midwife and her female client would be compromised.

The final comments Judy Miller offered at the end of the February 1994
LRWG hearing foreshadowed the jurisdictional problems that this definition, created through shared-document collaboration, would raise. In this section of the draft,
omitted from the list of conditions that required referral or transport to medical care,
were certain conditions that she predicted physicians would expect to see, such as
malpresentations, multiple gestation, and history of postpartum hemorrhage:

> But I understand that it's a person's right to choose, and as long as there is
> informed consent, I personally don't have a lot of trouble with it. Though
> I know that a lot of my colleagues would feel that that's neglecting the well-
> being of the baby. Sometimes I think a lot of those particular issues, it's
> the mother taking responsibility for the baby, and it's the baby who loses
> eventually when things go wrong.

Up to this point, she did not engage in substantive conflict over these conditions
nor did she propose a different collaborative process, for example, one in which she
would represent her medical colleagues more directly or one in which medical and
state authority would have a greater voice than the direct-entry midwives. At this
point, however, she wondered whether LRWG would create a set of rules that would
be unacceptable to the professional medical associations that she represented.

Resolving Issues of Professionalization
for Direct-Entry Midwives

Most studies of interprofessional conflict focus on the advantages of professionalization to the emerging profession. However, the Minnesota direct-entry midwives entered into the rule writing process with mixed feelings—looking forward
to the advantages of professional standing while fearing a potential loss of autonomy through the normalization of their practices. Their feelings were similar to
those expressed by their sisters across the nation, as they tried to balance the
advantages of becoming more visible to a broader community and having state-
sanctioned protocols against potential disadvantages of the normalization of their
practices and the imposition of state surveillance and required medical consultation. The conventions of the licensing rules and regulations genre seemed to dictate
that surveillance and consultation and a narrowing of the midwifery scope of
practice.

However, the direct-entry midwives continued to resist conventions of the genre, conventions that could devalue their knowledge systems and place them in a hierarchy relationship with the medical community that midwives had resisted for centuries. Resistance revolves around the question of "Who are we?" says Foucault, much as the direct-entry midwives resisted the conventions of the licensing rule genre that did not accommodate their identities in telling home birth stories, in their caring for generations of families, and in their relating to home birth parents on a case-by-case basis rather than according to prohibited conduct. Their struggles represent what Foucault would call "a refusal of these abstractions, of economic and ideological state violence which ignore who we are individually, and also a refusal of a scientific or administrative inquisition which determines who one is" ("Subject" 212). The shared-document collaborative process, and inclusion of informed consent agreements in the licensing rules, seemed to offer a way to resist the conventions of the genre, balance autonomy with professionalization, maintain midwifery knowledge systems, and leave room for some diversity in practice.

Within LRWG, the direct-entry midwives were granted equal rhetorical status with participants representing more medical discourse communities, and they helped produce a definition of the direct-entry midwife as an "autonomous health care provider." However, the LRWG participants predicted that this definition and other changes to the genre would be received negatively outside of the LRWG discourse community. In particular, the broader incumbent medical profession had jurisdictional authority over birth that would not allow the midwives to be granted state sanction to perform tasks and solve problems that were considered part of medical practice. As Andrew Abbott maintains, the medical profession has "a very narrow and particular object of work, the body, but a deep and formally rich body of knowledge about it. Medicine's jurisdiction is thus compact, although surrounded by imperialistic abstractions" (104). The worries expressed outside the hearings by LRWG participants would soon emerge in more open and public conflict within the hearings.

Thus, through a study of the genre of licensing rules and regulations, in this chapter, we gained a greater understanding of how, through recurrent discursive forms and strategies, jurisdictional boundaries of an incumbent profession may be maintained legally and publicly. The direct-entry midwives' resistance to these genre conventions exposes the assumed hierarchical relationship that practitioners must have with the dominant medical experts and the reification of medical knowledge systems. The midwives' attempts to define their practice in their own "positive" language, to focus on relationships with individual clients in their informed consent forms, and to maintain autonomy in practice contrast with the genre conventions that support the hegemonic, technologically based knowledge systems of the medical community. The next chapter analyzes how the Minnesota direct-entry midwives' attempt to write into the licensing rules and regulations the state-sanctioned right to carry certain drugs and perform specific procedures pushes them further into the jurisdictional territory of the medical community, escalating conflict with medical authority and, at the same time, producing a seemingly irreconcilable division within the midwifery community.

CHAPTER 6

Jurisdictional Boundaries:

CLAIMING AUTHORITY OVER SCIENTIFIC DISCOURSE AND KNOWLEDGE

*From a medical standpoint, I felt quite strongly that twins and breech
birth were contraindications . . . I am personally uncomfortable with
. . . relying on the individual traditional midwife to judge her own skills
in this regard as well as relying on the patient to inherently understand
the risk and thus choose medical care rather than home birth with a
traditional midwife . . . Again, the medical community felt strongly
about this and these [breeches and twins were] left out of the
contraindications. I personally think this risks losing the licensure
possibility completely once it reaches the medical board.*
—*(Judy Miller)*

*The newer midwives wanted to keep breeches and twins in there . . . but
the people who had experience doing breeches said that they could
give them up . . . As a group we sat down and agreed not to put that
[breeches and twins] in there—it was a political strategy to make it
work. If the option is for all to be illegal, we would rather make
some compromises in order to keep on practicing.*
—*(Julia Dylan)[1]*

$\mathcal{A}$s seen in chapter 5, the conventions of li-
censing rules and regulations dictated that not only would the Board of Medical
Practice monitor Minnesota direct-entry midwives but also the incumbent and dominant medical profession would maintain its jurisdictional authority by supervising
the midwives when it came to certain conditions of pregnancy and birth. Many Minnesota direct-entry midwives, particularly members of the Minnesota Midwives'
Guild, desired increased visibility through state sanction to advertise their practices
and clarification about which procedures they might perform legally during home
births, but, with the conventions of the licensing rules and regulations, they also encountered normalization of their practices and risked potential loss of autonomy.
However, the collaborative writing process employed by the Licensing Rule Writing Group (LRWG) to draft the licensing rules and regulations seemed to offer the
midwives a way to resist those conventions of the genre that threatened the autonomy and diversity of their practices. Unlike the situation that Rita Ortiz and Mary

Emerson encountered before the Midwifery Study Advisory Group (MSAG) hearings, all LRWG participants were granted equal rhetorical status. Therefore, the direct-entry midwives employed their own language to describe their practices and ideologies as they defined themselves as autonomous health care providers. They focused on their relationships with the clients through informed consent and avoided strict categories for transfer or transport into the medical system. Their choices give us a close look at the relationship between the midwifery and medical knowledge systems and the effect of jurisdictional boundaries on that relationship.

This chapter focuses on the next stage of the Minnesota licensing rule writing efforts, beginning with the fourth LRWG hearing (April 21, 1994), when the representatives from the Minnesota Midwives' Guild requested legal sanction to use the technologies of birth claimed exclusively by medicine. This request once again seemed to be accommodated by the collaborative process that granted all voices equal rhetorical status within LRWG, but this stage of writing the licensing rules revealed additional divisions within the direct-entry midwifery community. In part, these divisions, made public within the hearings, defeated the guild's planned strategies about the most convincing way to argue for legal access to these technologies of birth. Before the LRWG deliberations, guild members, such as Julia Dylan, had decided that they were willing to give up attending multiple and breech births at home to gain legal permission to carry pitocin, perform emergency episiotomies, suture, and perform other procedures that fell within medical jurisdiction. However, this decision alienated a portion of the direct-entry midwifery community who still wanted to include such conditions as twins and breeches in their practices. The decision also alarmed LRWG representatives from nurses', nurse-midwives', and physicians' organizations that considered these conditions strictly within the boundaries of medical practice and therefore unsafe practice in home births.

Thus, the direct-entry midwives' continued resistance to the conventions of the licensing rules and regulations, and the ways in which the guild's planned rhetorical strategies to trade breeches and twins for legal access to technologies of birth claimed exclusively by medicine played out in the LRWG public hearings, add to our understanding of the role of discourse in interprofessional competition. Moreover, we continue to see the uneasy relationship between medical and midwifery systems of knowledge, as the dominant medical profession sought to maintain its jurisdictional boundaries and the emerging direct-entry midwifery profession challenged these jurisdictional boundaries. In this chapter, in particular, we witness the problematic relationship between women's experiential knowledge, on the one hand, which is informed by intuition and embodied knowledge about birth, and medical knowledge systems, on the other hand, which have appropriated scientific discourse and claimed exclusive authority over scientific knowledge. Finally, we see the power of the medical community's claim to scientific discourse and knowledge when the midwives' challenge fails.

Feminist studies of science and technology further our understanding of the context and significance of the Minnesota direct-entry midwives' bid for legal access to tools and procedures claimed by the medical community. The Minnesota midwives, as did their sisters throughout history, identified their knowledge systems as women-centered, based on their experiential and embodied knowledge combined with intuition. But, for many, midwifery knowledge was also supported by whatever scientific and technological knowledge they found appropriate for home birth. This knowledge is, in essence, knowledge of the body. However, when modern direct-entry midwives petitioned for legal access to the technologies of birth, they confronted powerful fields whose knowledge systems have historically negated the experiential and embodied knowledge of women. In effect, medical science has the capacity to do gender work by organizing the worlds it describes, by including only certain knowledge systems, and by defining what is normal or abnormal. As Evelyn Fox Keller has defined the gender work of science, gender is "the basis of a sexual division of cognitive and emotional labor that brackets women, their work, and the values associated with that work from culturally normative delineations of categories intended as 'human.' . . . From this perspective, gender and gender norms come to be seen as silent organizers of the mental and discursive maps of the social and natural worlds we simultaneously inhabit and construct—*even of those worlds that women never enter*" (*Secrets* 16–17; original emphasis). Practices supported by women's knowledge systems—for example, the midwifery practice of version or manually turning the breech baby to avoid cesarean section or Ina May Gaskin's celebrated method of maneuvering a baby with shoulder dystocia (the baby's anterior shoulder is stuck behind the mother's pubic bone)—may then be negated within medical communities.[2]

However, many modern direct-entry midwives would assert that they are indeed practicing science, as they develop their experiential knowledge, finish their apprenticeships, educate themselves about anatomy, physiology, and pharmacology, and refine such practices as version and manually correcting shoulder dystocia.[3] Therefore, these midwives would insist that they have a knowledge basis to seek legal sanction to use the technologies of birth. Some scholars speculate that only by rethinking our cultural definitions of science would alternative knowledge systems such as midwifery gain a legally sanctioned claim to scientific knowledge, while others propose that first we must expose cultural assumptions about male and female nature or gender ideology before such practices as midwifery can gain this access.[4] However, important to the Minnesota story is the realization that many of the direct-entry midwives were already employing birth techniques claimed by medical science—they were carrying pitocin, performing emergency episiotomies and versions, suturing, and so on without legal standing to do so. At the same time, they were also using the midwifery tools and techniques handed down to them by their sisters throughout history, such as using comfrey root and shepherd's purse to control postpartum hemorrhage, lubricating the perineal tissue to avoid tearing, and changing the position of the mother to deliver breech births. Finally, they had developed their own midwifery practices, which they felt would inform birth no matter what the setting; for example, they were successfully delivering VBACs (vaginal births after cesarean) at home before many physicians adopted the practice in the hospital. When the Minnesota direct-entry midwives asked that licensing rules and regulations grant them legal access to the technologies of birth claimed by medicine, however, they confronted a discourse community that was accustomed to excluding their midwifery knowledge, perpetuating certain beliefs about women and their bodies, and remaining suspicious or unaware of midwifery practices that combined touch and herbs with modern drugs and procedures.

As we saw in chapter 5 and will see again in this chapter, the gender work of medicine in its claim of authority over scientific knowledge is done through language and discourse. As Keller explains, the association of science with objectivity and masculinity reveals "a set of beliefs given existence by language rather than by bodies, and by that language, granted the force to shape what individual men and women might (or might not) do" (*Secrets* 25). Within that discourse, we can see the conceptual universe that scientists might share—their knowledge systems. The world that science studies, the nature that science names, is rather mediated by language, such as metaphor, and scientific arguments express these shared conventions (Keller, *Secrets* 27–28). For example, scientific language and its metaphorical base often define pregnancy as a medical event to be controlled by technology:

> From the beginnings of the medicalization of childbirth in the nineteenth century, we are now faced in the 1980s with a situation in which all aspects of reproduction have come under the command of science. Viewed as medical events, pregnancy and childbirth can be monitored and controlled by the latest technology, while in the laboratory, women's role in reproduction is increasingly open to question; IVF [in vitro fertilization] and the burgeoning of genetic engineering offer to fulfill, with undreamt of specificity, earlier versions of science as the virile domination of the female body of nature.
>
> (Jacobus, Keller, and Shuttleworth 3)

Within this metaphorical base, the body might be depicted as a machine itself and the fetus as an entirely separate entity from the mother; therefore, intervention into birth by technology often seems appropriate.[5] As Emily Martin finds, the metaphor of the body as machine "continues to dominate medical practice in the twentieth century and both underlies and accounts for our willingness to apply technology to birth and to intervene in the process" (*Woman and the Body* 54). Therefore, the technologies of birth are generally important tools used by medical science to diagnose, classify, and treat a condition, activities associated with a profession's ability to abstract and apply knowledge (Andrew Abbott 40–46). Technology itself is not only a human activity and set of physical objects but is also a system of knowledge. Human or professional activities evolve around and support technologies, such as the reproductive technologies that some scholars believe serve women but others suspect are used to control women.[6] For example, Judy Wajcman has proposed that ultrasound technology "serves to discredit and then displace women's own experience of the progress of the foetus in favour of scientific data on the monitor" (71). Moreover, those who control birth technologies also can claim the cultural and professional right to extend existing technologies or invent new ones: "New technology typically emerges not from sudden flashes of inspiration but from existing technology, by a process of gradual modification to, and new combinations of, that existing technology" (Wajcman 21–22).[7] The Minnesota public hearings afford another opportunity to see how, through discourse, the female body and its reproductive functions might be defined by the medical and midwifery communities and to what extent women might be knowers of their own bodies.[8] But more important, the Minnesota hearings give us a unique opportunity to see the results of an alternative and gendered practice making a bid for legal access to the technologies of birth already claimed by medicine, a bid that, ironically, given the leveling of rhetorical status among LRWG participants, was expressed within the words and language of a genre created to support the dominant profession of medicine.

Finally, if we accept that the metaphorically based language of medical science may represent women's bodies as machinelike, and pregnancy as a process that can be aided when necessary by technological intervention, we must also consider the metaphorical base of midwifery language. For example, one Minnesota direct-entry midwife, Connie Baker, contrasted how she viewed birth to how a surgeon might, organizing her thinking around the metaphor of sewing:

> I had a really interesting flash one time when I was sewing. I was making some pants for my mother for a Christmas present, and I was having the hardest time getting the pockets into them. And finally I did it, and then I decided I would make her another pair, and the second pair I just zip-zip, I got the pockets in; it was so cool. And I was sitting there feeling really proud of myself and I thought, Gad, it's like a cesarean—if you look at it as just a mechanical process, once you know how to put the pockets in, it's no big deal, you don't have to look at who the person is, *the fabric of her life, the belief system.* That's what midwifery is all about; it's not at all technical; it's really understanding a woman and helping to guide her through the process. And you can get totally around that if you do it surgically. It [surgery] doesn't matter what you believe; what you think; what your past experiences are; what your future aspirations are. I can just get in there, knock you out, cut you open. . . . It's really an efficient, economically more feasible process than caring about the person. (emphasis added)[9]

To Baker, surgery was like sewing that second pair of pants, mechanically operating on the body, whereas midwifery considered the unique needs and experiences in each woman's life. Thus, Baker and other midwives participate in what Davis-Floyd and Davis call the normalization of uniqueness:

> The midwifery normalization of uniqueness must be understood in the context of the technomedical pathologization of uniqueness. The technomedical model of birth defines as "normal" only those births that fall within specific parameters— twelve hours of labor, cervical dilation of one centimeter per hour, steady fetal tones, and so on. Labors that take too little or too much time, cervixes that remain "stuck" at four centimeters for hours on end, heart tones that speed up or slow down, meconium in the amniotic fluid, all are defined as dysfunctional "deviations from the norm." Aware of technomedical parameters, midwives must constantly weigh their trust

in and acceptance of women's individual rhythms against the consequences of straying too far outside of the medical protocols that are regarded as authoritative in the courts. (336)

One system assumes that a universal procedure serves women's bodies best under certain conditions, while the other relies on an intuitive relationship with each woman to determine how to guide her through her birth experience.

Thus, the language that direct-entry midwives use to represent their ideologies seems to conflict with those of medical science and to underlie a suspicion of technological intervention. In another example, the participants in the midwifery listserv noted that although they requested legal access to the birth technologies to determine when to transfer their patients to medical health care practitioners and when to transport an at-risk mother or infant to the hospital, they remained suspicious of technological intervention in the birthing process and discouraged complete reliance on technology's diagnostic capabilities. In one thread, Gail commented on the unreliability of ultrasound:

> Well, I think I can top this for misread ultrasounds. I once assisted on a labor which we brought to the hospital for FTP [failure to progress] (about 7 cm I think). She was 41 weeks. An ultrasound showed she had twins! A second ultrasound showed two hearts/two chests, but one head. She was taken to cesarean for this suspected severely deformed cojoined twin. She had ONE perfectly normal baby boy!
>
> (listserv communication, July 12, 1996)

Other midwives, such as Ellie, proposed that technology should empower rather than limit choice but that, even then, technology provided no guarantee for a healthy baby or even a fully informed parent:

> I guess that I just want them [parents] to be fully informed about what these tests could do for them. I also stress that these are screening tests, and there could still be a problem with a baby that was never diagnosed prenatally in spite of having these tests. The second home birth I ever attended (as a friend) was the birth of a child with very severe spina bifida. His home birth was a precious event to his mother, because from that time on, his life was a series of surgeries and medical problems. The mother told me that parents of other spina bifida babies she had talked to had their babies whisked away from them before they even knew what the sex was.
>
> (listserv communication, July 12, 1996)

Not only would medical technology detect the presence of a birth defect, such as the spina bifida of the infant born to Ellie's friend, but also the system interpreting technology would rule out home birth for her, therefore limiting her choices, according to Ellie. Moreover, the listserv participants found that the diagnostic procedures themselves involved risks. For example, Grace wrote back to Ellie:

If, in fact, a fetus is found to have spina bifida, it may be good to know so that the birth can be planned for a tertiary care center where corrective surgery can be done ASAP. If a child has Downs and a significant heart defect, it might again be appropriate to change birth site in order to protect the child's health.

I do point this out to my clients, but also remind them that the risk of their child having these problems may be less than the risk of the procedures to detect them, so the decision may still be a difficult one.

(listserv communication, July 12, 1996)

To Ellie and Grace, technological knowledge and innovation should provide the tools to enable choice, but these midwives' experiences with birth revealed to them that these tools were not infallible diagnostic devices.

When considering the value and use of birth technologies on the simplest level, then, the knowledge systems of midwifery and of medicine, and the language used to represent these systems, seem in direct contrast. However, the Minnesota direct-entry midwives' request for legal access to the birth technologies claimed and controlled by medicine reveals a more complicated relationship. Some of the direct-entry midwives involved in the Minnesota hearings already used birth technologies in their practices to diagnose and screen for certain conditions, to control emergencies, and to prevent a mother or infant from having to go into the hospital for care the midwife felt they could receive at home. Other midwives felt that birth technologies created more problems than they solved and had no place in home birth. Certainly, during the Minnesota midwifery hearings, the direct-entry midwives argued that they would contribute to the overall body of authoritative knowledge about birth in American culture, and that their experiential knowledge might be more valid in understanding the female body than was the knowledge system of medicine. The medical representatives to the LRWG hearings came from communities that claimed exclusive control of scientific knowledge and some thought that if direct-entry midwives had legal access to these technologies, the midwives' practices would expand to such an extent that midwifery would compete with medical practice and make home birth unsafe. After all, the jurisdictional boundaries claimed by the modern medical profession were distinguished by this claim to birth technologies that medical professionals used to diagnose and treat mothers and infants. This chapter first explains this complexity by tracing the public discourse that emerged when the LRWG participants debated multiple births and malpresentations, the tradeoff that some guild midwives were willing to make to get legal access to birth technologies. The chapter next analyzes the discourse that evolved around the midwives' potential legal use of certain drugs and devices—suturing, episiotomies, pitocin, needles, and oxygen tanks and masks—and the issue of how midwives would be educated to use these drugs and devices. Finally, the chapter describes the medical community's reaction to these discussions, inside and outside the hearings, and the rhetorical strategies used by the Board of Medical Practice to suspend the writing process of the LRWG.

Challenging the Authority of Medical Knowledge About Birth: Breeches and Twins

As represented by the quotations that open this chapter, the direct-entry midwives of the Minnesota Midwives' Guild, such as Julia Dylan, and the medical care providers, such as Judy Miller, seemed to agree that the licensing rules should stipulate that certain conditions of pregnancy, such as malpresentations and multiple gestation, were contraindicated for home birth. However, the reasons why they thought the direct-entry midwives should not be permitted to attend these conditions at home differed. The guild midwives considered this move a compromise in their practices and a rhetorical strategy in the LRWG hearings: They would stop attending breeches and twins at home if they could gain legal access to pitocin and other drugs, if they could get legal permission to perform emergency episiotomies and to suture those episiotomies and minor perineal tears. For example, Rita Ortiz described her personal decision to support this rhetorical strategy, a decision similar to Julia Dylan's:

> I thought I was trying to be manipulative. I have done most breech births in the state of Minnesota, and I was the person most against breech births [in the hearings] because I knew politically that it could not be defended . . . it could not be won politically, not because I believed that home breech shouldn't happen, not because I didn't think that people couldn't have the skills to do it, after all I had done tons of breeches at home. . . . I just knew that we don't have the power base to be able to defend that and in order to have traditional midwifery accepted at all you had to start building a very broad, simple, innocuous power base. And then you had to refine it as you go along; you cannot start with 100 percent.[10]

These Minnesota Midwives' Guild members decided to give up the right to attend breeches and twins at home, to suppress their experiential knowledge of and skills in attending such conditions, in order to establish what Ortiz called a strong enough power base to argue for other home birth options in the licensing rules.

On the other hand, Judy Miller, representing the American College of Obstetrics and Gynecology and the Minnesota Ob/Gyn Society, proposed that, because medical knowledge systems considered these conditions high risk, obviously they must be ruled out for home birth—this was not a compromise or a rhetorical strategy. Other medical practitioners agreed. For example, nurse Emma Davidson commented:

> The way I have always been able to "get ahold" of lay midwifery is—it's a normal labor and delivery. It's not unusual—it's not likely to have any problems. It's a statistically safe delivery. It's being attended by somebody who's got a lot of experience but not a lot of formal training. It's their experience which carried them through that normal delivery. So, when you begin thinking about breeches and twins, or complicated deliveries, it falls outside how I imagine lay midwifery to work. And, it starts in my mind to not be an average labor and delivery any more. That's where I am having trouble seeing lay midwives delivering breeches and twins.[11]

The diagnostic and treatment capabilities of medical technology, found within the hospital setting, according to Miller and Davidson, were needed to deliver breeches and twins safely.

However, the fate of these contraindications to be listed in the licensing rules rested not only on the opinions and rhetorical strategies described by Julia Dylan and Emma Davidson but also on the collaborative process employed by LRWG. When discussing these contraindications, LRWG continued to employ the shared-document collaborative process, granting each participant an equal voice. During the process of collaboratively writing the contraindications for home birth, it became clear that not all direct-entry midwives were willing to accept the compromise described by Dylan and Ortiz. The collaborative process not only allowed the midwives to resist the conventions of the licensing rules, as in the early hearings of LRWG, but also encouraged some midwives to articulate their disagreements with Ortiz, Dylan, and others within the midwifery community. To a great extent, these disagreements centered on the worth of midwifery experiential knowledge and the opportunity to contribute to the authoritative knowledge about birth within American culture.

Between February and April 1994, LRWG had taken a two-month break so that smaller groups, such as the guild midwives, could meet on their own to prepare preliminary texts for the contraindications and scope of practice sections of the licensing rules. As they did with the definition of direct-entry midwifery, the LRWG representatives of various discourse communities submitted these preliminary versions of approved midwifery services and contraindications for home birth for LRWG's consideration. Judy Miller, representing the American College of Obstetrics and Gynecology and the Minnesota Ob/Gyn Society, had reflected on her role as representative of the medical community during this two-month hiatus. She prefaced her draft of contraindications for home birth, presented at the April 1994 hearing, with the following statement:

> I would be remiss in my responsibility to the obstetricians and gynecologists whom I represent, if I did not bring to this group a list of obstetrical circumstances for which we have strong reservations about midwifery care and home birth. These conditions are open to discussion, and I would hope that the midwife community would see the risk inherent in these circumstances and would agree that medical referral is appropriate. I would also hope that recognition of these circumstances and subsequent willful continuance of midwifery care or attempted home birth would result in disciplinary action by the Board of Medical Practice.
>
> (LRWG hearing, April 14, 1994)[12]

Miller made clear that she represented a powerful medical organization, which asked the LRWG participants, and, in essence, the Board of Medical Practice, to recognize medical authority in these matters.

Miller then presented a list of eleven contraindications for home birth, including "previous classical cesarean section," an incision seldom used in the 1990s but one that can more easily rupture during labor, "known or suspected multiple pregnancy," "primipara [first-time mother] with breech presentation, non-frank breech presentation at term, or malpresentation [in this case meaning transverse lie or when baby lies horizontally to the birth canal] at term," and "history of difficulty controlling hemorrhage."[13] Miller also noted fifteen conditions that required medical consultation or transport, including "uncontrolled maternal hemorrhage." In contrast to the other lists submitted, Miller's version was brief, although it contained the two conditions that became the focus of debate within this stage of the rule writing process—breeches and twins.

Henrietta Kramer, who represented the Twin Cities chapter of the American College of Nurse Midwives, submitted a more extensive list of twenty-one contraindications for home birth. She also listed sixteen conditions that required consultation, including breech births and "multifetal gestations [such as twins]," and "persistent transverse lie." Finally, she presented nineteen conditions that required transport, including "vaginal and perineal laceration" and "uncontrolled maternal hemorrhage."

The Minnesota Midwives' Guild's list was more detailed and complex than those submitted by the two LRWG members representing physicians and nurse-midwives. The guild's list included forty-nine contraindications for home birth, including breech birth, transverse lie at term, and multiple gestation; thirty-four conditions requiring consultation; and thirty-nine conditions requiring transport, including "laceration requiring medical attention." Stricter than their *Standards of Care and Certification Guide*, the guild's list seemed a narrowing of current direct-entry midwifery practices, an acknowledgment of the concerns about home birth expressed by medical practitioners in previous LRWG hearings, and a rhetorical strategy to demonstrate the midwives' willingness to compromise their practices in order to achieve professional standing.

In preparation for its members taking the NARM exam and becoming Certified Professional Midwives, and in contemplating eventual professional standing in Minnesota, the guild had revised its *Standards of Care and Certification Guide* and placed even more restrictions on contraindications for home births. For example, although "persistent transverse presentation" and "breech baby on a first time mother" were contraindicated for home birth in both the 1989 and 1995 versions of the *Standards of Care*, the guild added "multiple gestation with one or more baby presenting other than vertex [or head down]" to the 1995 version (appendix B). The 1995 version listed "suspected multiple gestation" and "suspected malpresentation or abnormal presentation" as requiring "documented medical consultation," whereas in the 1989 version the midwife had to consult but not necessarily with a medical caregiver (appendix C). In both versions, "known multiple gestation and mother wants a home birth" and "breech presentation at term" also required consultation with other midwives. If the multiple births or breech presentations were unforeseen, both versions of the Guide advised midwives to transport to the hospital unless birth time was shorter than transport time (appendix E). However, the guild did continue to recognize that home births should be assessed on a case-by-case basis:

Common sense and intuition play an important role in the traditional mid-wife's assessment and response to each specific situation. Midwives are by nature innovative, creative and flexible. In acknowledging the exception to the rule, we set forth the following conditions and situations to be assessed and determined by consultation with at least two other certified traditional midwives.   (1995, appendix D)

Overall, though, the guild's revision of its *Standards of Care and Certification Guide* contained contraindications for home birth more acceptable to medical care providers.

Faced with differences in the length and content of the three lists, Jessica Ramsey, the medical board staff member who coordinated LRWG, recommended that the lists be merged according to the following process: Any item on all three lists should be considered noncontroversial and should remain on the merged list of contraindications for home birth, and then groups and individuals could lobby to include or exclude other items. This process continued the conventions of the shared-document collaborative writing process—each person or organization submitting a list of contraindications for home birth would have equal authority. Therefore, even though Judy Miller alerted LRWG to the considerable medical authority that informed her list, her voice was again treated as no more important than others. Because the three lists were quite similar, at the time it did seem that the collaborative process would ensure that Miller's concerns would most likely appear on the final contraindications list.

However, during the open lobbying that followed the merger of the three lists at the April hearing, it soon became clear that not all direct-entry midwives were willing to concede delivering breeches and twins at home. The concessions seemed not only to negate their experiential knowledge but also their opportunity to contribute to authoritative knowledge about birth within American culture. Individual midwives again resisted the narrowing of their practices and loss of autonomy. In earlier LRWG hearings, the direct-entry midwives had resisted medical supervision as required by the conventions of the licensing rules and regulations genre. Now some resisted abandoning their own protocols for handling particular conditions of pregnancy and birth; they refused to assume that these conditions were high risk or pathological. Specifically, they were not willing to abandon the techniques they had developed to treat such conditions, such as their ability to diagnose through touch and to turn the breech baby through version or manual manipulation. For example, Gloria Olson argued that midwives had developed unique knowledge about breech and twin birth:

Almost the only people in this country who know how to deliver breeches [vaginally] are traditional midwives. They do a lot of them. And they do know how to deliver them. A lot of twins are born at home, very safely. And midwives are better at that too, because they come at it with an attitude that the woman can do it and the babies are meant to be born; whereas in the hospital, a twin birth is done in the delivery room, with stirrups, and ready to do a cesarean in a second.[14]

Greta Godwin agreed that the midwives' experiential knowledge in dealing with breech birth would be lost by such concessions:

> This is one of the areas in which you are talking about giving up one of the long standing traditions in midwifery in order to make a political appearance and to make midwifery fit the medical model who is in charge of the legislative and legal processes. . . . Traditionally frank breech in some midwifery books in the past was not considered an abnormal presentation. I think that the skills for breech births are among the few remaining midwives, and we are talking about giving up these skills for several centuries.[15]

This compromise within the licensing rules would actually decrease knowledge about birth, proposed Olson, an opinion shared by other midwives across the nation. For example, direct-entry midwife Valerie El Halta admits that during her twenty-year career she has "often come under harsh criticism for continuing to attend what many consider to be 'high-risk' deliveries," but she has "caught" more than 100 breech babies and more than 20 sets of twins (22). These births, "while demanding greater respect, do not necessarily portend greater risk to either mother or her baby," says El Halta. In fact, although expressing her gratitude for the technological advances that have benefited mothers and babies, El Halta is also "appalled by the amount of empirical knowledge which has been cast aside for the sake of technical advancement" (22). Ina May Gaskin's videotape on breech birth and external version has been used by direct-entry midwives for over a decade; in fact, some women seek help at the Farm specifically to have a vaginal breech birth.[16] Thus, Norma, a nurse-midwife working at a hospital in California, proposed to the midwifery listserv that, because of this loss of experiential knowledge, vaginal breeches were ceasing to become an option in the hospital:

> In my current practice none of the physicians feel comfortable doing vaginal breeches . . . Because it is an HMO, with all the docs taking turns at call, they feel it is unfair to offer vaginal breech delivery, as not all of the doctors feel comfortable doing that type of birth and there's no telling who will be on at the time of delivery . . . The only vaginal breeches I've seen at my current hospital have been second twins . . . There was a recent discussion about the availability of vaginal breech delivery as an option on the OB/GYN list a couple of months ago. Generally speaking, teaching institutions do them and a few rare private OB's do them (more in the Midwest, it seems), but most private OB's won't consider it. Such a shame.
>
> (listserv communication, July 31, 1996)

To Olson, El Halta, and Norma, in the face of scientific and technological diagnosis and treatment of birth conditions such as breeches and twins, midwives had difficulty contributing their techniques and protocols to authoritative knowledge about birth. Licensing would increase that difficulty, believed Olson and a number of direct-entry midwives participating in the Minnesota hearings.

Thus, the collaborative process of merger and then debate as suggested by Jessica Ramsey exposed the divisions within the midwifery community. The merged version of the contraindications list yielded only eleven contraindications and eleven conditions requiring transport, a considerably shorter list than those presented by the three groups. At the top of the list of contraindications appeared breeches and twins but to remain on the list, according to Jessica Ramsey's definition, conditions should be noncontroversial. Because the appearance of breeches and twins on the merged list dictated the exclusion of all such cases from direct-entry midwifery practice—regardless of an individual midwife's experiential knowledge and her personal protocols—to some direct-entry midwives the list represented the first tangible sign of loss of autonomy through professionalization. Kris House argued before LRWG, "We should write who we are and what we feel . . . The reality is that there are breeches being done [at home]." To House, breeches and twins were a matter of informed consent, parental decision making, and midwifery experience—matters to be settled on a case-by-case basis. They did not represent an acceptable compromise made to gain advantages through professionalization. House's and others' objections meant that breeches and twins must be removed from the contraindications list—they were too controversial to remain, according to the process recommended by Ramsey.

In the Midwifery Study Advisory Group hearings, the recognition of the "other" midwife—the direct-entry midwife who did not represent the image of the thorough and discerning practitioner—advanced the midwives' rhetorical status. By contrast, the midwives were expected to present a united front in the LRWG hearings. For example, physician Judy Miller reflected upon the debate over breeches and twins: "I was disappointed and actually somewhat surprised at the lack of consensus among the group."[17] According to Miller, only if the direct-entry midwives were able to present a united front did they deserve the rhetorical status accorded to each discourse community in LRWG.

Some of the direct-entry midwives attributed their lack of consensus to the independent nature of midwifery, to some midwives' unwillingness to compromise individual values and protocols, and to the exclusion from the guild of those other midwives, Kris House, Karen Mist, and now Greta Godwin. Therefore, lack of consensus among the direct-entry midwives participating in LRWG represented not only a breakdown of a rhetorical strategy but also an ideological issue that went to the very core of the independent midwife. For example, Connie Baker noted that the guild meetings might have presented a false sense of agreement, as those who disagreed stopped attending the meetings:

> I suppose that we were a group of very independent women trying to figure out a way to appear in solidarity. . . . For the most part, the majority of midwives in the state came together . . . There was some concern regarding what should be said and what should not be said. We have practiced underground and are used to protecting ourselves. . . . At the time I believe that decisions were reached by consensus. However, there is a matriarchy in the home birth community and some women simply did not return to meetings when they felt they were not in agreement with the "consensus."[18]

To midwives such as Elizabeth Smith, the consensus that the guild attempted to reach in order to bring back a united face to the LRWG hearings failed because some midwives clung to their individual protocols and felt their voices were excluded:

> This image was perpetuated from the past that there were the in's and there were the out's, and I think that's not so because in the past I would have been considered on the "out." I think it had a lot to do with people's commitment to hang in there and work shit out and to be willing to do the work . . . But there were people it seemed who wanted to get hung up on personal behavior patterns rather than the bigger picture. So, I think, a lot of people left feeling like they were being excluded, or they weren't being heard but a lot of time it had more to do with people isolating themselves. In some ways, there is a hierarchy of power in the midwifery community, but it is not insurmountable.

To Smith, those who felt they were excluded had to take partial responsibility for that position. However, Kris House described her dilemma of choosing between going along with the rhetorical strategy and continuing to attend these breech and twin births openly:

> When we started to talk about breeches and twins, I realized that I was supporting what they wanted, but I didn't feel supported or that they were really hearing what I was saying. So how could I belong to a group where I didn't feel represented where I am at? There was one midwife meeting, where we sat around the table, and I verbalized to myself, "How can I live with that? . . . "And someone turned to me and said, "Just don't tell anyone." And I have heard that kind of comment in the past. Now it certainly isn't written anywhere. But I though, un't-uh [no] . . . I just feel that [the] only way to be me is to share the truth that I understand.

Finally, to Gloria Olson, a guild midwife, such compromises ultimately would not have increased the midwives' rhetorical status and credibility. They would simply have diminished their personal choices. Olson attributed this willingness to compromise to the midwives' internalized sense of oppression, to their marginalization as women in society and as practitioners suppressed by dominant professions:

> Nothing you do is politically wise. I don't think there is anything. I have never seen any way in which we have won any political battle no matter what we do. I am beginning to realize that compromising or trying to get around or trying to avoid certain things is not a powerful position. If someone has good self-esteem and really believes in what they are doing, why would they bother to do that? They won't do it. It wouldn't even seem responsible. So it's just the nature of our oppression that would make us even think of doing stuff like that.

While some of the midwives, such as Olson, doubted that they would really increase their rhetorical standing by narrowing their practices, others, such as House, refused to remain publicly silent about conditions they intended to continue to treat at home regardless of legal rules and regulations. At this stage, the direct-entry midwifery community divided about whether to compromise on breeches and twins or to include them in their practices regardless of the cost to their professional and legal standing.

Permitting Minnesota direct-entry midwives to attend breeches and twins at home would have made the state laws somewhat exceptional in the national context. At the time of the Minnesota hearings (1991–1995), the states that licensed direct-entry midwives considered multiple births and babies in other than vertex or head down positions to be at high risk. Only Alaska authorized midwives to deliver breeches and twins. The majority of states required that both conditions be handled by a physician unless the midwife found herself in an emergency situation. The New Mexico Midwives' Association, with official recognition in state licensing rules, was cautious in its approach to breeches and twins, and in November 1994 direct-entry midwives in Texas openly admitted that they "did give up the right to do breeches and twins in a compromise for less restrictive protocols" (Penn 15).

However, the personal conflicts faced by the Minnesota midwives who fought to retain twins and breeches in their practices were not unusual, despite the licensing rules in other states. The birth stories shared on the midwifery listserv during this time indicated the numbers of direct-entry midwives who attended home births for babies in breech or transverse lie position. For example, Grace asked for advice about her transverse lie case:

> Hi List—I have a multip at 34+ weeks who has a fetus in a transverse lie. This kid must like this position because it hasn't changed in the last few visits or so since I've started intentionally palpating position. This mom really wants a home birth—it will be her first. Last baby was to be at home, but had PROM [prolonged rupture of membranes] at 35 weeks and chose to go to the hospital. I'm concerned that this kid isn't varying the position any and am wondering how best to encourage it into a head down position . . . Do people use the same things (i.e., slant board, anything else?) as they do to encourage a breech to turn around?
>
> (listserv communication, August 6, 1996)

Moreover, in October 1995, one direct-entry midwife urged MANA to include twins, breeches, and other conditions in home birth protocols. To do otherwise would divide the midwifery community and isolate those who continued to treat such conditions at home. She warned:

> Currently, twins are considered high risk. This label itself is what creates much of the risk for mother and babies. The medical assumption that twins will birth prematurely is self-perpetuating. Many obstetricians know little about fostering the wellness and empowerment that would help twin mothers carry their babies to term. Most twin mothers seeing doctors are exposed to an extreme amount of intervention . . . The birth is conducted as

if the presence of two babies makes it a medical emergency. Midwives offer superior care for healthy twin mothers during their pregnancy, birth and postpartum . . . As MANA moves toward certifying midwives, I hope we can remain inclusive and supportive of variations in practice. Rigid standards of practice for Certified Professional Midwives (CPM) would create more separation and isolation among midwives. I hope MANA will support midwives who attend twins and other variations of normal [birth], creating an attitude of mutual respect. Rather than restrict the practices of CPMs, I think it would be appropriate for midwives to use informed consent— outlining information and consideration for twins, breeches, and other special circumstances. It is essential for midwives to continue to support women's right to choose.   (Sawyer 16–17)

She argued that home birth parents should be allowed to choose to stay at home with their twins or breech babies, as long as they are well informed and supported by their midwives.

Again, the issues at this stage in the Minnesota hearings centered on the authority that midwives impute to experiential knowledge versus the authority the wider culture imputes to biomedical ways of knowing. Therefore, in arguing to include breeches and twins on the contraindications list for home birth, some LRWG rhetors distinguished between the professional status and knowledge of the incumbent profession and that of the direct-entry midwives. For example, chair Joan Montgomery stated at the April 1994 hearing that the physicians' medical practice act contained specific protocols and practices, which were debated within recognized professional organizations. Therefore, the licensing rules for physicians could be less specific: "The medical practice act changes as stuff happens but they have years and years and years of having gotten together as a practice . . . officially at the MMA [Minnesota Medical Association] . . . they already come with a whole set of understood and accepted knowledge and standards." Jessica Ramsey agreed: "Traditional midwifery is not as organized or above board . . . does not have the history." Therefore, the long history of midwifery and its knowledge systems were negated in contrast to the authority of the medical community. Moreover, physician Judy Miller reminded the direct-entry midwives that without some contraindications for home birth, this powerful and legally recognized medical community would oppose the licensing of direct-entry midwives:

> From the standpoint of general acceptance to the public and maybe the medical community . . . you would go a long way to have at least some basic, spelled-out contraindications for midwifery care and home birth . . . Fighting for the privilege of delivering a handful of breeches or multiple pregnancies at home over a lifetime of practice, I think you risk some respect of . . . the medical profession . . . a list of the bare minimums done there says you have given some thoughtful consideration to your practice . . . that's the privilege of continuing your profession at home under licensure standards.

Guild lobbyist Mary Emerson reminded the direct-entry midwives of the necessity to compromise midwifery practice and knowledge in order to become licensed:

> We have one community that says multiple births and breeches are fine at home. And yet we are not out here by ourselves. We have another community standard which has years of legal basis and the law and malpractice cases. Are we risking the entire profession for the sake of this one issue?

Even Jessica Ramsey, who invited LRWG members to lobby openly for or against any contraindications for midwifery care they felt strongly about, reminded those advocating delivering twins and breeches at home that they were risking the licensing process:

> Keep in mind what we are doing here. The state is saying we recognize you as professional people, and we are saying that you are licensed. You hold yourself out to the public as having a certain amount of competence and skill. And furthermore you have the right to charge for that . . . Even though parents have rights . . . the state as a governing agent has an obligation to protect the public . . . because the general public does not have the knowledge to choose who is competent.

However, despite the urging of these rhetors, the collaborative process recommended by Ramsey determined that only those items that represented agreement remained on the list. Individual midwives and home birth parents remained adamant that breeches and twins should be possible in home birth: "I was doing breeches in the 1960s until the academics ruled it out"; "It's a sellout"; "What we end up with here is not going to help the public," they said. At the end of the April 1994 LRWG hearing, physician Judy Miller issued a final warning that the group may indeed list only the contraindications about which there was no controversy but, "Believe me," she said, "I will get my list in one way or the other." For the moment, however, breeches and twins remained within the scope of practice for direct-entry midwifery and home birth.

To the direct-entry midwives who protested the possible exclusion of breeches and twins from their practices, it appeared that this concession would negate their experiential knowledge. They would have to accept as authoritative, medical knowledge about birth that excludes these conditions from the definition of normal birth. Finally, as midwives—and to a great extent as women—they could not contribute to authoritative knowledge about birth; they would not be viewed as "knowers" by the larger society. They would have to rely on the incumbent profession to handle these cases in ways that some midwives felt displayed less knowledge and experience than the midwives themselves had. Such feelings so deeply divided the direct-entry midwifery community that they could not provide a united front before LRWG, despite how rhetorically effective Ortiz, Dylan, and others felt that united-front strategy might be. Some of the midwives resisted this concession despite the expectation that, as an emerging profession, they must normalize their own practices and include in their newly defined jurisdictions only those conditions determined by the dominant profession to be safe for home birth.

Again, this resistance came from the Minnesota direct-entry midwives' belief that their midwifery knowledge did constitute authoritative knowledge about birth. In fact, as revealed in the midwifery listserv, those celebrating such experiential knowledge often argue that all authoritative knowledge is not "truth" but is socially constructed. For example, when Audrey suggested to the midwifery listserv that "all forms of health care, even biomedicine . . . are 'cultural constructs' rather than unshakable truths," Peg responded, "I like to say that they [lay] claim to the Science of Obstetrics while we know we practice the Art of Midwifery" (listserv communications, September 6, 1996). In responding to Peg's distinction, the listserv midwives asserted that midwifery was as valid as what the medical discourse communities call a "science":

> Ah yes Peg, but even science is a "cultural construct." Would Linnaeus have come up with the animal classificatory system in which Homo sapiens, particularly white european [sic] Homo ss were at the level of most evolved if he'd been from East Asia? And science still bases many of it's assumptions on ideas of white European males from the 17th century. Would those assumptions still be true today . . . or even at that time in other places?
>
> (Audrey, listserv communication, September 6, 1996).

The listserv midwives are aware of how much medical knowledge about birth changes from year to year:

> I think we were saying the same thing. Most of us understand that there is no exact science of birthing. Wait two years and you will see that what we thought was a fact has now become fiction. Take the old "once a cesarean, always a cesarean." Think of how just a short time ago, that was considered a fact. Think about how short a period of time ago we thought that there was nothing to do about the fact that some mothers carried beta strep. Prophylaxis didn't work so we ignored it. And that was just weeks ago. Now they want us to treat everyone in labor. Etc. Etc. Etc.
>
> (Peg, listserv communication, September 6, 1996)

However, regardless of how astute these direct-entry midwives might be about the social construction of knowledge, what government agencies, legislatures, and the broader culture consider to be authoritative knowledge is used to legitimize professional jurisdictions. In the next LRWG hearings, those professional jurisdictions played an important part in discussions of whether, as emerging professionals, direct-entry midwives would gain legal access to drugs and state permission to perform certain procedures at home. The next section of this chapter analyzes the debates about legal access to birth technologies and the role of formal education in this access. The section ends with a description of how these issues contributed to the failure of the Licensing Rule Writing Group to draft licensing rules and regulations for direct-entry midwifery in Minnesota.

Asking for Legal Access to Science and Technology: Drugs and Devices

The next two hearings of the Licensing Rule Writing Group (June 21, 1994 and July 28, 1994) focused on several direct-entry midwives' requests that their scope of practice, as described within the Minnesota licensing rules and regulations, include permission to obtain and administer pitocin, a drug effective in stopping postpartum hemorrhage, to perform emergency episiotomies at home, and to suture first- and second-degree perineal lacerations.[19] Such practices would make home birth safer and more comfortable, the midwives proposed, as they could handle excessive bleeding, deliver babies quickly if they were distressed, and suture what they considered minor tearing rather than disrupt the new mother by transporting her to the hospital. In essence, they asked for legal access to the drugs and devices of science and technology and recognition that their apprenticeships and self-education were sufficient training in how to use these drugs and devices. Again, the direct-entry midwives were resisting the supervisory and surveillance activities of the state and medical experts as dictated by the conventions of the licensing rule genre—the midwives wanted to suture, administer drugs, and perform episiotomies independently and outside the hospital setting. They were also asking to expand their practices by entering the boundaries of the dominant profession's jurisdiction, because the medical profession had historically distinguished its practice by maintaining exclusive claim to birth technologies. In a way, the direct-entry midwives had to argue much as Jane Sharp did in her 1671 *The Midwives Book* when she claimed that midwives could and should learn anatomy and physiology. The LRWG medical practitioners argued against the midwives' requests by doing boundary work—they argued that such practices would be outside the realm of midwifery and were only within the scope of medical practice. In order to do this boundary work, they distinguished between formal education and training on the one hand, and apprenticeship on the other, between medical and midwifery knowledge, and they proposed that all diagnostic procedures and pharmaceutical tools pertaining to birth were within the sole jurisdiction and purview of medical science.

For example, one nurse participating in the LRWG hearings responded to the midwives' requests by saying, "Nurses cannot perform injections without medical direction."[20] The only nurses who have the option of administering pitocin are "in advanced practice and have been legislatively given the right" to prescribe such drugs. Henrietta Kramer, representing the nurse-midwives, confirmed that, if granted their request to legally administer pitocin, direct-entry midwives "are into medicine." Up until this time, nurses and nurse-midwives participating in LRWG were relatively quiet. To a great extent, Emma Davidson, representing the Minnesota Nurses' Association; Kramer, representing the Twin Cities chapter of the American College of Nurse Midwives; and Elaine English, representing the Board of Nursing, had merely audited the public hearings. Davidson and Kramer had offered some comments and helped develop lists of contraindications for the licensing rules and regulations. They had kept in touch with each other and their organizations outside the hearings, but, with the discussion about legal access to birth technologies, they became more outspoken. They wanted to ensure safe home birth, they generally believed that the direct-entry midwives should be regulated or licensed, but they drew the line at granting the direct-entry midwives legal permission to carry drugs and perform certain procedures.

However, the direct-entry midwives believed that their request was an essential one—after all, many were willing to give up breeches and twins to more effectively argue for legal access to these birth technologies. Moreover, the midwives were already performing such procedures and using such tools, even though they did not have legal sanction and access, because they believed that they had the knowledge and experience to do so. As Julia Dylan said: "If pitocin is going to save a life . . . that's such an easy [emergency measure] to have. People don't want to carry a lot of technology, but if people are doing it, like suturing, to say now you can't do it . . . it's really unfair to the consumer. There are many moms who won't go into suturing; if their midwife doesn't know how to suture . . . they won't go in [but stay at home and heal without suturing]. If a midwife can do it and save a lot of money compared to going into the emergency room and having it done . . ."[21] Elizabeth Smith agreed: "We absolutely have to be able to suture. Emergency episiotomies—I cannot speak to that one because I have never seen the need for it. That's not to say that it wouldn't come up, and if it did I would want to be able to do it. Although my focus is much more on preventing the need for it so it's kind of a funny one to fight for because we really work to make sure that women don't have one." Moreover, Gloria Olson believed that excluding suturing in the scope of practice section would represent not only a loss of midwifery knowledge but also the deliberate narrowing of midwifery practice:

> If you are going to deliver babies at home, you have to know how to suture. It's ridiculous to bring every woman in who has a little tear. It's part of the practice of midwifery. Women did it with needle and thread long before doctors ever learned how to do it, [before doctors] got their cat gut and forceps and needle holders and all that stuff. It's part of the whole thing. Some women just tear and they deserve to be stitched.

For Olson, the practice of midwifery had always included suturing, long before medical practitioners determined their own professional boundaries and claimed exclusive ownership of birth technology.

However, if the scope of practice for direct-entry midwifery in Minnesota included these procedures and access to these tools, the licensing rules would authorize these skills for all direct-entry midwives. If all direct-entry midwives were authorized to suture and carry drugs, then all licensed direct-entry midwives would have to demonstrate formally before the board their skills and knowledge to do so. The conventions of the licensing rule genre dictated exclusive categories and definitions. Moreover, if the direct-entry midwives argued successfully to expand their scope of practice, then they would be given more authority and autonomy in their practices than nurses and nurse-midwives but would not have the same required formal education. Yet, if no direct-entry midwives were authorized, then, as Rita

Ortiz, said, all midwives would be faced with "bringing into the metropolitan hospitals everyone who needs three or four stitches," a fair number according to Ortiz. The midwives who continued to suture at home could be charged with practicing medicine without a license.

Arguing for this expanded scope of midwifery practice was risky. The direct-entry midwives had carefully defined their practices as supportive of their clients' needs and choices. Some midwives resisted giving up the ability to deliver breeches and twins at home to strengthen the midwives' credibility before LRWG. Some of these same midwives would resist what they would consider a "medicalization" of their practices—and their home birth parents would join this resistance. Thus, those midwives arguing for the expanded practice were in danger of losing their close identification with some of their clients. One aspect of social and professional prestige can come from treating clients on their own terms, as Andrew Abbott suggests: "A profession clearly derives general social prestige from meeting clients on *its* own, rather than on *their* own, grounds just as it derives prestige from strictly enforced rules of relevance. But a profession that forces clients to take treatment completely on its own terms risks heavy competition from those who talk to the clients in their own language" (47, original emphasis).[22] Certain home birth parents chose midwifery care to avoid dependence on medical science and technology. The argument was made even more difficult because, without the formal education of nurses, nurse-midwives, and physicians, the direct-entry midwives were asking for legal sanction to diagnose and treat. For example, in identifying and repairing first- and second-degree perineal tears or lacerations, the direct-entry midwives would be classifying the degree of tearing. In performing an episiotomy, the midwives would be diagnosing fetal distress and deciding upon a treatment. Finally, the direct-entry midwives arguing for expanded practice were challenging the professional boundaries of modern medicine that were defined by formal educational routes.

Suturing and Episiotomies

In anticipation of the July 1994 LRWG hearing, Jessica Ramsey drafted the list of specific services within the scope of midwifery practice. These services reflected the most expansive scope—those services that, in Ramsey's estimation, could be construed as practicing medicine or nursing and therefore subject the midwives to felony arrests if not included in their scope of practice.

These special services included the following:

A. Artificial rupture of membranes, during the second stage of labor, just prior to crowning of the baby's head.

B. Episiotomy, in emergency situations.

C. Repair of perineal lacerations and/or episiotomy.

D. Administration of oxytocin by intramuscular injection, for emergency control of postpartum hemorrhage.

E. Administration of RhoGam, by intramuscular injection.

F. Administration of eye prophylaxis to the newborn.

G. Administration of vitamin K to the newborn by injection.

H. Emergency cardio-pulmonary resuscitation by the mother and/or the newborn.

Items E, F, and G involved drugs that could be obtained by the client herself and so they were quickly struck from the list. Considered by some an acceptable "low tech, low invasive procedure," the direct-entry midwives decided to strike item A because of the difficulty of defining "prior" to the LRWG nurses and nurse-midwives who immediately requested a definition. However, the guild's *Standards of Care and Certification Guild* contained a similar statement: "The artificial rupture of membranes is not to be done at any point in labor except if the membranes bulge at the vaginal opening, just prior to the crowning of the baby's head" (20). Finally, item H was revised to read "Use of deelee suction and oxygen during emergency cardio-pulmonary resuscitation of the mother and/or the newborn" and seemed acceptable to the group. Four items (B, C, D, and H) then provided the focus for intense debate.

Direct-entry midwives generally take great care to avoid having to perform episiotomies. For example, the Minnesota Midwives' Guild's *Standards of Care and Certification Guide* states: "The midwife should make every attempt to help the woman keep her perineum intact. Hot compresses, perineal massage with oil, controlled pushing and attempting to birth the baby's head as gently as possible [are very helpful—from first version] for avoiding perineal lacerations." However, the *Guide* also includes the following stipulation: "In rare occasions where it may be necessary to protect the health of the baby, an emergency episiotomy may be done" (22, both 1989 and 1995 versions). Birth stories posted on the midwifery listserv attest that direct-entry midwives across the country, regardless of their legal status, perform emergency episiotomies at home if other means of delivering babies in distress quickly fail. For example, a direct-entry midwife practicing in Indiana, where midwifery is illegal, posted this birth story to the listserv:

> Her labor was hard, with almost no time between contractions . . . I told her to follow her body urges, and within an hour she was pushing some. I finally checked her again, to find the lip still swollen . . . We iced it, and put her on her side . . . We started getting bright red blood running down her legs. Heart tones were excellent, at about 120–125 throughout. We perservered. The head had come down, so that we could see a lot of it. We had her doing everything that we could think of, but we couldn't get it any farther . . . Finally, the baby started slowly moving. Slowly, slowly, slowly, we got to some sort of small crown. She had a hymenal band like steel. And now the baby won't move past that. At that point we started getting bright red blood coming out around the baby's head . . . I cut a small medline episiotomy, into the hymenal band, and we hauled out the baby.
>
> (listserv communication, August 4, 1996)

During the time of the LRWG hearings (1993–1995) states that licensed direct-entry midwives, such as Delaware, Montana, Alaska, Florida, and Arizona, permitted midwives to perform this procedure in an emergency. In Arkansas, licensed direct-entry midwives could perform an episiotomy in certain conditions such as "the mother pushing more than one hour in prolonged labor" after they consulted a physician by phone and followed his or her instructions (Section 407.02). States such as South Carolina and New Hampshire required midwives to obtain the necessary training or education for performing emergency episiotomies but did not specify where they must do so.

Finally, the texts that direct-entry midwives use in their self-education contain information on episiotomies. For example, Gaskin's *Spiritual Midwifery*, in its third edition in 1990, suggests that if the baby's heartbeat drops below 100 beats per minute, and "[i]f the mother is late in the second stage, give her oxygen, do an episiotomy if necessary and deliver quickly"(432). Moreover, Gaskin gives instructions for how to perform a small midline episiotomy and includes such comments as: "If the cut is made at the height of a rush when the skin is blanched white, the mother won't feel it" (356). However, the LRWG nurses and nurse-midwives continued through the July LRWG hearing to object that the direct-entry midwives did not have the formal education and training to perform emergency episiotomies— an episiotomy was a form of surgery and therefore a medical procedure.

To support their objections, the LRWG nurses and nurse-midwives challenged the validity and reliability of the version of the NARM exam available at the time. This version of the NARM exam did not yet contain a mechanism for testing clinical skills such as suturing and administering injections, the nurses and nurse-midwives pointed out. The direct-entry midwives countered by stating that other states included not only a licensing exam but also educational components that allowed direct-entry midwives to administer pitocin, suture, and perform episiotomies. Some of these educational components were formal. For example, Colorado specified that only "verified graduates from approved Colorado direct-entry midwifery programs" could take the state licensing exam (chapter 1, section 1.5). The program, which had to be offered by a university, college, or vocational-technical school, had to be accredited by a regional or national accrediting agency or hold a certificate of approval from the private occupational school division of the Colorado Department of Higher Education. However, as of May 1995, the Colorado Midwives' Association's certifying program was not approved because it was not administered by a school as defined by the private schools act (Carrie Abbott). Other states such as Oregon allowed licensed direct-entry midwives who had completed board-approved continuing education courses in prescriptive medications to "administer local anesthetic as indicated at the direction of a state licensed health care provider who is authorized to administer local anesthetic" in an emergency—anesthetics that could be used to numb the site of an episiotomy (section 8). Finally, some states allowed midwives to gain these skills through an apprenticeship experience or specified that the midwives must have skills such as suturing but did not regulate their route to gaining these skills. By 1997 the majority of states licensing direct-entry midwifery would accept NARM certification as their state licensing procedure.

However, in the face of the nurses' and nurse-midwives' criticism of direct-entry midwifery education and their suspicions about the NARM exam available at the time, seasoned Minnesota midwives such as Gloria Olson still resisted any educational requirements that would limit the paths to direct-entry midwifery:

> This is an area that I personally have a lot of feelings about. Partially because we are all women, and all white, and probably predominantly middle class. And I have a deep concern that whatever we regulate won't alienate the Native American community, the Hmong community, the African American community, the poor people . . . All of our pathways into midwifery were so diverse and I want to respect a wide variety of pathways and also preserve a high quality of care.

However, the LRWG nurses and nurse-midwives argued against alternative routes to midwifery. A well-defined educational component is a "basic philosophy" of licensing, said nurse Emma Davidson:

> The wider the scope, the more educational preparation you need; the more educational preparation you need, the more you've got to prove. If we cannot get an education preparation we can agree upon, then we are going to have to narrow the scope. Because if you're going to be doing suturing and whatever, you are going to have to have training on that . . . If this gets way too controversial to the point where it's going to throw up lots of red flags to the rest of the medical community, and for the BMP [Board of Medical Practice] . . . all this effort . . . is going to go right down the tubes . . . Save something [rather] than end up with nothing. . . . The nursing community would find much of it quite controversial.

Davidson predicted that the midwives could not convince the LRWG and the review bodies that would follow the LRWG hearings that their educational routes were sufficient to expand the practice of direct-entry midwifery to include legal access to birth technologies.

Moreover, the nurses and nurse-midwives objected to the direct-entry midwives suturing those emergency episiotomies and to repairing perineal lacerations (item C of the specific services section) for the same reasons. Although the direct-entry midwives agreed to limit this repair to first- and second-degree tears, nurse-midwife Henrietta Kramer argued that before the direct-entry midwife could repair first- and second-degree perineal tears, they had to distinguish between these tears and third- or fourth-degree tears:

> I think that in treating lacerations it's difficult to recognize tissue damage. And if you only do ten to twelve births a year and only see several bad ones a year, are you going to miss a third degree [tear] that required suturing? You are saying that everyone can do it [suture], if you put it in the law.

To Kramer, distinguishing between degrees of tearing constituted diagnosis, a medical skill.

Indeed, the participants of the midwifery listserv agree about the difficulty of making these distinctions. For example, a nurse-midwife shares a birth story in which she has difficulty spotting a tear:

> Midwives, I have an interesting case to share with you. A tall, healthy mom having her second baby, first a c/s [cesarean section] for breech. She had a three hour labor, yelped when she went complete and slowly pushed out a 8 pound baby over an intact perineum. When I checked for vaginal lacerations, I found a BIG hole in her vagina. She had torn her rectal sphincter. After pondering this for a very long time (like a half hour) and asking an OB out in the hall what he'd do, I CUT an epis(!) to be able to visualize the layers. I still couldn't visualize well and didn't feel comfortable doing the repair and called in my back-up to do it.
>
> (listserv communication, August 13, 1996)

In response to her story about repairing this tear, other listserv participants discussed the difficulty in determining the degrees of tearing. For example, a childbirth educator and doula in Oklahoma asked a question about her own birth:

> Along all these lines, I have a personal story to relate to you all: When birthing my last child (2 years ago—Successful VBAC I might add :-)), the doctor stated that as my son was coming out, his elbow caught my perineum right in the back and tore me pretty good (no episiotomy) . . . Now, my question is, my doctor recorded the tear as being a 4th degree tear. However, from everything I have read a 4th degree tear tears INTO the rectum and when my doctor described my tear it tore just up to the opening of my anus and just *slightly* over the lip. It did not tear into the rectal barrel at all, so how can this be termed a 4th degree?   (listserv communication, August 28, 1996)

The listserv participants then shared a list of characteristics to use in making these distinctions:

> The definitions of the different degrees of perineal lacerations as I learned them are:
> 1st—Skin, mucuous membrane, and subcuticular or submucosal layers only.
> 2nd—Muscle
> 3rd—Anal sphincter muscle (may be partially or completely torn)
> 4th—Rectal mucosa [the tissue of the rectum] (listserv communication, August 30, 1996)

Despite the difficulties in determining the degree of tearing, licensed direct-entry midwives in other states at this time were able to suture first- and second-degree tears. For example, Montana's law stated: "A licensed direct-entry midwife may not perform any operative or surgical procedures except for an episiotomy or simple surgical repair of an episiotomy or simple second-degree lacerations" (Section 37-27-303). Such texts as Gaskin's assumed that "[t]he midwife can repair first and second degree tears if she knows how to suture"(377; Davis 149–52). However, to the LRWG nurse and nurse-midwives, direct-entry midwives did not have the education and training to make such diagnoses and therefore they should not have legal sanction to perform these procedures.

Drugs, Needles, Tanks, and Masks

The final two items (D and H) on the specific services list provoked similar discussion among Licensing Rule Writing Group participants. Although suturing and performing episiotomies seemed to depend on the direct-entry midwives' ability to diagnose and treat, their ability to administer oxytocin to stop hemorrhage and oxygen rested upon their legal access to these drugs and the tools to use them—hypodermic needles, IVs, oxygen tanks, and masks. Inherent in any approval of repair of lacerations and emergency episiotomies was the question of anesthesia, an option that the group decided to add to item C ("with or without local anesthesia"). To obtain these drugs and tools legally, the direct-entry midwives would have to deal directly with the medical community, pharmacists or physicians who would supply and prescribe, or state agencies such as Departments of Health, which would supply the drugs and tools and monitor the frequency and amount of their use. Some direct-entry midwives obtained pitocin from "friendly docs" even though to administer such drugs was clearly practicing medicine without a license, a practice not unusual across the country for unlicensed midwives (Rooks 271). However, in the previous LRWG hearings, the direct-entry midwives had resisted required supervision by medical practitioners—and they continued to do so in the June and July 1994 hearings.

The direct-entry midwives who asked for access to pitocin made their case on the warrant of safety—the common good that would appeal to all LRWG participants. As a guild lobbyist Mary Emerson stated:

> Postpartum hemorrhage is not easily predictable . . . [I]n a low-risk home birth mom there is still a possibility of a postpartum hemorrhage. I would like to speak very strongly for permitting midwives to carry oxytocic agents [such as pitocin] for use in emergencies only. It is one very appropriate use of technology. We cannot have midwives operating as if the death rate is the same as in 1900s. It's not OK. We are covered by the standard of care that exists in the community as a whole. We need to keep moms alive when it's a simple matter of you have to stop bleeding, and I have a tool. There is a tool that is low-tech, easily carried.

The representatives from the medical communities immediately questioned this request. "I see this as something that you are doing while you are calling 911. You aren't going to keep her there [at home], are you?" asked Judy Miller. Also for Miller, doing deelee suction at home meant that direct-entry midwives were not transporting to the hospital infants who have aspirated meconium fluids, which come from the baby's first bowel movement. Therefore, the infants might experience respiratory problems in the first few days of their lives: "What oxygen implies goes right to the guts about the fears about home birth," Miller cautioned. Nurse Emma Davidson challenged the request to carry pitocin by stating that, again, the direct-entry midwives would be engaging in diagnosis: "But what does 'uncontrolled' [hemorrhage] mean?" Finally, nurse-midwife Henrietta Kramer asked again about the education and training required for such drug administration: "How many hours of pharmacology are you going to require each year? You have to know how to give them [the drugs] and how to assess the patients."

Again, the Minnesota direct-entry midwifery community divided over expanding midwifery practice to include such drugs as pitocin and oxygen. For example, Kris House shied away from such technical tools in general: "This is a home birth situation! If you think you're going to need oxygen, an IV, then I think you should be in the hospital. That to me is part of my screening. I just say 'Whoa.'" Herbal remedies and, in extreme cases, bimanual compression or pressure directly on the womb were alternatives to administering pitocin. However, Gloria Olson believed that direct-entry midwives had as much right as physicians to use such drugs:

> I think that pitocin is a safe and simple thing. I don't know why it has to be monitored. I don't know who would overuse it. It would be tough to overuse it unless someone was starting to induce labor at home. I don't know who would do that, but I suppose someone could do that too. Carrying drugs is a medical privilege in this country. I think that they [physicians] are continually surprised that we even exist. [They think that] birth is just fraught with danger [and that] you have to have a medical degree and a few more years to deliver a baby.[23]

Not all direct-entry midwives agreed with Olson that they were capable of making these decisions, assessing these conditions, and administering these drugs. For example, Rita Ortiz questioned whether, given the different educational paths to midwifery, carrying substances such as oxygen and drugs such as pitocin, and performing such procedures as emergency episiotomies and suturing, really were safe:

> You are going to cut, which is surgery, and you are going to repair, which is surgery, and you've never even taken anatomy and physiology, you don't know anything about sterile technique. How did you get these supplies . . . these are controlled substances? Some people were going to restrict these things [the special services] in ways that are dangerous. You could have oxytocin but no methergine. If you are going to have people control postpartum hemorrhage at home, you need methergine because you don't have intravenous fluids and without fluids oxytocin is not as effective. But methergine is a dangerous drug. Without an education, these things wouldn't provide a safety net that was desired.[24]

Ortiz felt that without formal and universal training, such substances would not provide the desired safe practice, and her own experience warned her that the special services section of the licensing rules might not address all complications. Direct-entry midwives would be allowed to carry only pitocin, not the more powerful methergine, but without intravenous fluids pitocin was less effective in controlling postpartum hemorrhages. Whereas Ortiz, Dylan, and other direct-entry midwives agreed that they would relinquish the right to deliver breeches and twins at home to gain legal access to these birth technologies, in the LRWG hearings the direct-entry midwifery community publicly debated ideological differences about whether these drugs and devices were appropriate and safe in home birth.

The debate within the Minnesota LRWG about pitocin, oxygen, IVs, and other drugs and devices reflected national concerns about direct-entry midwifery during the mid-1990s. Although other states that licensed direct-entry midwives at this time varied in granting legal access to drugs, oxygen, local anesthetics, and other tools and devices, those that granted access usually required that the midwives have formal education in using such tools and techniques and that a physician or state agency office prescribe their use. For example, some states such as Alaska extended to their licensed direct-entry midwives even more special services than did the third draft of the Minnesota rules, but only after "training in administration" and on condition of continuing education in pharmacology were Alaskan midwives permitted to use xylocaine hydrochloride and cetacaine to numb tissue for suturing, rhogam to prevent Rh disease, eye prophylaxis to prevent infection, pitocin and methergine, and to give injections or set up IVs (section 14.570). Direct-entry midwives in Montana had access to all these drugs except methergine, but the drugs had to be prescribed by a physician, requiring midwives to establish a link with the medical community and potentially subject themselves to its control. Moreover, many midwives found it extremely difficult to find a physician who was willing to work with them. Oregon midwives had access to "antihemorrhagical agents" as well as needles, IV tubing, and scalpel blades. The state health officer in Oregon assisted with access to the mandated prescription medications if a licensed direct-entry midwife was unable to locate an appropriate state licensed health care provider to prescribe medications, but Oregon midwives had to take continuing education classes in prescription medications (section 8, subsection 4). Florida, Washington, South Carolina, and Texas had similar rules, but Colorado prohibited its midwives from administering any drugs except for required eye prophylactics.

States in which midwives were not licensed might aggressively prosecute midwives if they used such drugs and devices. For example, in 1994, midwife Lori Albrecht of Bismark, North Dakota, was issued an injunction against her practice by the state attorney for allegedly administering pitocin to control a third-stage of labor hemorrhage (Tulip 9). The Minnesota Midwives' Guild's *Standards of Care and Certification Guide*, in both the 1989 and 1995 versions, dealt with this dilemma by discouraging the use of "medical technology" at home but required the midwife to have the knowledge to use it if she must. The *Guide* stated:

> Parents ultimately make the decision concerning the use of birth-related technology while the midwives determine whether they can ethically help them at home under such conditions. In keeping with their values, traditional midwives accept that a birth that seems to require the use of medical technology should occur in the setting of a hospital facility. (8)

However, the *Guide* also declared: "The midwife shall have the knowledge and ability to recognize and control postpartum hemorrhage and perform emergency resuscitation of the mother and/or newborn" (20). The *Guide* did not specify how that hemorrhage should be controlled or how resuscitation should be performed or where the midwife was to access the tools or learn the techniques to use them.

At the time of the Minnesota hearings, discussions on the midwifery listserv were just as divided, depending on the midwives' legal status and their individual protocols. For example, Renee, in Michigan, related her experience with carrying pitocin illegally:

> In Michigan, as most of you know, there is no licensing for non-nurse midwives. I was arrested in 1983 for practicing medicine w/o a license for giving pitocin to a woman who was hemorrhaging. Complaint was filed by the doc who took over care when we transported; charges filed by the state. In my (and our) naivete with the legal system, I honestly and forthrightly told the investigating detective (who said first thing about my home "This is nice. I didn't know whether to expect dead birds, feathers and voodoo-type stuff"), after Miranda rights were read, "Of course I gave her pitocin!"
> (listserv communication, July 26, 1996).

Bonnie, in Ohio, related a similar experience about starting an IV at home without standing orders from a physician:

> Standing orders from an MD? Hee Hee! Ha Ha! Forgive me while I ROT-FLOL [roll on the floor laughing out loud]!!! You will find Ohio colored in all black on the state legal status charts (meaning "clearly illegal" for DEMs), so no, I have no standing orders from anybody for anything. *I am legally at risk for everything I do.* My philosophy is that if I'm going to do it at all, I'm going to do it right, and if doing it right increases my legal risk, so be it. The only time this has come up in regards to IVs, was with a client with pph [postpartum hemorrhage] and a convulsion (the only 911 transport I've ever made), and I had my apprentice call 911 while I was setting up the IV. The ambulance got there quickly and I had the bag and tubing hung, but hadn't got the needle in yet (I had tried twice, but her BP [blood pressure] was pretty much nonexistent, as were her veins). So they stuck her (took them 3 tries) and they ended up using my bag of LR and tubing.   (listserv communication, August 5, 1996).

Finally, the direct-entry midwives themselves reflected on how pitocin might save a mother's life but also on the traumatic experience of having to use it:

> I recently had a horrendous home birth experience and feel the need to exorcise it by sharing . . . Mom had some bleeding, so I tried cord traction—no placenta . . . Had mom squat over a bedpan, and she proceeded to dump 500cc blood (yes, I measured it) but no placenta. Called paramedics into the room. Started two IV lines. Called our back-up hospital to tell them we were on our way. Gave mom 20 IV pitocin and rushed to the hospital via ambulance with mom bleeding the whole way there . . . I am having a hard

time regaining my trust in the birth process. Had we been further away
from the hospital, our client most likely would have died.

(listserv communication, August 2, 1996)

Despite the trauma this midwife experienced with this case, she and many other
direct-entry midwives contributing to the listserv made it clear that, regardless of
their legal status, they continued to administer pitocin, oxygen, and intravenous fluids to their home birth clients. The Minnesota direct-entry midwives who also carried pitocin and other drugs and tools were not exceptional in making these choices
and asking that they be legally sanctioned to do so.

However, at this point in the LRWG hearings, home birth parents attended
by Kris House and other midwives who had departed from the Minnesota Midwives' Guild also opposed including these special services in the scope of licensed
direct-entry midwifery. For example, one home birth parent said, "I don't want to
just have the hospital to roll into my bedroom when I am wanting a home birth." In
phone calls to Jessica Ramsey, these parents expressed their concern that, if their
direct-entry midwives carried such drugs and devices, as parents they would no
longer be "in charge of birthing their babies":

> They [the parents] call on a midwife because they want the midwife there
> for assistance, but they don't want to turn over any power, if you will, to
> the midwife. It's a power thing. They were concerned about the content of
> the rules because they feel the rules are giving a lot of power to the mid-
> wives . . . that the midwives wouldn't be any kind of alternative to the doc-
> tors and the nurse-midwives.[25]

These parents felt in conflict with the midwives over who should decide how much
technology should be used in home birth and who actually accepted the risks of
home birth. To these parents, their desire to determine how "medical" their birthing
experiences would be conflicted with the midwives' need to define their own practice and gain legal sanction to perform certain procedures. Despite an emerging difference between the direct-entry midwives and the home birth parents attending the
LRWG hearings, the guild midwives decided to challenge the medical care
providers' negative assessment of their education. Before the August 1994 LRWG
hearings, the guild met to create an educational series to cover the special services
within the scope of licensing midwifery practice. This series would confirm to the
Board of Medical Practice that experienced midwives had the ability to assess perineal tears and suture, administer oxytocic drugs and oxygen, and perform emergency episiotomies—"to assure the Board of Medical Practice that midwives are
adequately trained to do so" ("Midwifery Licensing Series"). The educational series was to further the education of practicing midwives who "already meet the criteria for numbers of births, prenatal and postpartum exams, etc." Later the guild
intended to design a second series for midwives just beginning their apprenticeship. This educational program—the Midwifery Licensing Series—was to include
sessions on "Anatomy and Physiology for Midwives," "Physical Assessment of
Mothers and Babies," "Pharmacology for Midwives" (including oxytocic drugs),

"Practical Medical Skills for Midwives" (including use of O_2 and injections), and "Suturing for Midwives" (including assessment of vaginal and perineal tears, repair of first- and second-degree tears, and emergency episiotomies). Five sessions would extend over a period of nine months and would be taught by the guild midwives and family practice physicians.

Suspending the LRWG Process and Reaffirming Jurisdictional Boundaries

In the late summer of 1994, the Minnesota Board of Medical Practice became increasingly concerned that the latest version of the licensing rules and regulations would not pass the scrutiny of the larger medical community, particularly because of the special services section that granted direct-entry midwives legal access to birth technologies. The dissemination of licensing rules and regulations in Minnesota includes publication of a notice of intent and a complete copy of the rules in the state register and then submission of the rules to the state attorney general and to the secretary of state, and publication of a notice of adoption in the state register. If any objections are submitted within twenty-five days, a public hearing is held to air those objections. Licensing rules and regulations that draw objections are then reviewed by an administrative law judge. If the warnings expressed within LRWG by Emma Davidson and Henrietta Kramer about granting direct-entry midwives legal access to birth technologies exclusively claimed by the medical community were any indication of the potential reaction of the larger medical community, then the rules would certainly provoke objection and subsequent legal review.

The Board of Medical Practice began to hear complaints about the licensing rules emerging from the LRWG hearings from physicians or their organizations, some participating in the hearings and others monitoring the hearings from the sidelines. For example, one physician clipped an article from his local newspaper in which one of the direct-entry midwives attending the LRWG hearings asserted that many births were safe at home. Before sending the clipping to the board, he annotated the article, highlighting it with question marks and expressing his professional opinion that attending to the delivery of a child was something to be handled by licensed medical doctors.

More specifically, a letter from the Minnesota Medical Association (MMA) formally requested that certain sections of the rules be changed to restrict the direct-entry midwives' practices and to strengthen surveillance by the board and the medical community as expressed within the third draft of the licensing rules discussed in the June and July 1994 hearings. For example, the MMA asked that the words "autonomous and primary care services" be deleted because they implied that direct-entry midwives could provide a range of health care services. The introductory language of the scope of practices section—"midwifery services include, but are not limited to"—was problematic to the MMA which felt the words implied that the midwives had unlimited scope of practice. The MMA recommended that the licensing rules specify what the risks of home birth were, which midwifery educational programs were accepted as requirements for licensing, and what a qualifying score on the NARM exam must be. The MMA also requested that an additional physician representative from the MMA, the Minnesota Ob/Gyn Association, or the Minnesota Academy of Family Physicians be added to the proposed Midwifery Advisory Council. Finally, phone calls from various MMA members suggested that the board limit the number of midwives who could be licensed—a request that would control the "market share" of home birth practitioners.

Nurses and nurse-midwives also called the board to say they would not support the rules unless certain conditions, such as twins and breeches, were contraindicated for home birth and unless the midwives had to meet formal educational requirements before they could legally practice. They were concerned that the public would confuse their nurse-midwifery practices with those of the direct-entry midwives who might treat at home what the nurse-midwives considered high-risk conditions. Nurse-midwife Henrietta Kramer hoped that strict licensing would clear up this confusion, narrow the scope of direct-entry midwifery practice, and ensure contact with the medical community:

> Somewhere in the last twelve months I had gotten two phone calls . . . [from people] who had talked about this nurse-midwife doing these really poor practices and shouldn't we do something about this . . . and I looked into it and discovered it was a traditional midwife . . . Unfortunately a good share of the public assumes it's nurse midwives [when they hear the word "midwife"] . . . In response to some of the negative stuff, it seemed like a good idea if there were some sort of regulation . . . used to upgrade some of the practice and perhaps put teeth into some sort of law that would get rid of the real egregious practitioners . . . really high risk stuff, twins, breech, premature, and you decide to deliver them at home, that person could be nailed for that. There is no accountability now . . . we have never had a problem with them practicing out there. Because it's apparent when they talk that they can do a really nice job. I think that they could have some lovely births . . . if there was some licensure and accountability then perhaps . . . they would not be quite so shunned, there would be a little more open flow into the health care system . . . if you do say this was going to be a home birth there is gnashing of teeth. [With clear regulation, the direct-entry midwife is] going to be more comfortable in talking to the health care system . . . and maybe make a difference so the mother and the baby would have a safer chance.[26]

Nurse Elaine English raised the issue of jurisdictional boundaries and formal education as she maintained that the tasks "performed in the area of delivery and medication administration and treatments" are "delegated medical functions," for which the direct-entry midwife had "very little preparation." English opposed the third draft of the rules because it allowed midwives to use drugs such as pitocin "in a [home birth] setting where there are additional dangers such as infection." Moreover, English began to doubt that licensing was indeed the best approach for recognizing direct-entry midwives. To her, "licensing should be retained by the group that had the total scope of practice in an area. . . . So, it's appropriate for the physicians and nurses to be licensed" but direct-entry midwives could not claim jurisdictional authority over birth.[27] Thus, the nurses and nurse-midwives within LRWG joined the physicians in their uneasiness with an extension of the boundaries of direct-entry midwifery, encompassed in the latest draft of the licensing rules.

At the same time, at the request of some medical representatives to the LRWG hearings, the Minnesota Board of Medical Practice completed a survey of the educational background of direct-entry midwives in the state and disseminated the results before the August 1994 hearing. Judy Miller was "surprised" by the "obvious disparity in education amongst members of the group which was not apparent by just their speaking." Upon reflection, Miller was "sorry that we did not tackle the education issues first."[28] The survey revealed that some of the direct-entry midwives within LRWG had only a high school education, but, perhaps as a testimony to the boundary spanning they were able to achieve or the rhetorical status given to them by the shared-document collaborative process, their lack of formal training was not obvious to Miller and others before the results of the survey were made available. Only formal education within an institution of higher learning was acceptable training, according to Miller, Kramer, Davidson, and English and the physicians', nurses', and nurse-midwifery organizations they represented. Connie Baker's education at the Farm in Summertown, Tennessee, Rita Ortiz's education at the Santa Cruz Birth Center, and others' self-education and apprenticeship would not meet the medical care providers' requirements for formal, uniform training in order for any practitioner to have legal access to medical tools and procedures and to handle conditions they considered high risk.

In general, even though they sensed that other voices were being heard by the Board of Medical Practice, the direct-entry midwives were not privy to these lobbying efforts before the August LRWG hearing. For example, Julia Dylan commented:

> I do think that there are some people involved in the BMP who are supportive of traditional midwifery, but I think there's a lot that goes on in between those [LRWG] hearings that we just don't know about. I am not a paranoid person, but I just have a real strong feeling . . . that decisions are made . . . I wish I knew. I have heard through the years that the BMP [Board of Medical Practice] had complaints about midwives, and I wish that those were public. So we can find out if it's legit.[29]

Dylan was correct in suspecting that important discussions were taking place outside the LRWG hearings.

Before the August hearing, Mary Emerson, the lobbyist for the guild; Joan Montgomery, who chaired the majority of the LRWG hearings; Jessica Ramsey, who had drafted each version of the rules thus far; and Leonard Boche, who, as executive director of the board, anticipated widespread negative reaction to the licensing rules and regulations in their current form, discussed the necessity of suspending the LRWG hearings. The direct-entry midwives' requests for legal access to the technologies of birth, exclusively claimed by medical practice, so alienated the Minnesota medical community that the board felt that the licensing rules and regulations would invite too many objections to survive the scrutiny of an administrative law judge. The objections to the direct-entry midwives' bid for legal access to birth technologies would only be compounded by the exclusion of breeches and twins from the list of contraindications for home birth. Even Emerson, who strongly supported the efforts of direct-entry midwives to become licensed, knew that those efforts were doomed to failure for two key reasons: first, because the Minnesota Midwives' Guild's planned compromise to exclude breeches and twins from their practices had been publicly rejected by others in the home birth community, and second, because their bid for legal sanction to carry and administer pitocin, to suture, and to perform episiotomies would be rejected by the majority of medical representatives on the board and by medical practitioners who were following the hearings carefully. The guild's proposed education series did little to counter these objections. Granting all LRWG participants equal authority in creating the licensing rules and regulations seemed only to result in public disagreement among the direct-entry midwives and in a set of licensing rules and regulations that granted the midwives such extensive scope of practice that they clearly intruded into the jurisdictional boundaries of the medical community. The licensing rules and regulations for direct-entry midwives in other states suggested that the only way the midwives would gain professional standing would be to accept normalization and narrowing of their practices. Even with such professional standing granted through licensing, they would have legal access to birth technologies only under the supervision of physicians, which constituted a loss of autonomy in the eyes of many direct-entry midwives. However, the August 1994 draft of the licensing rules and regulations for Minnesota direct-entry midwives also contained no requirement for medical consultation. Thus, the fourth and latest draft of the rules and regulations allowed the midwives to continue to treat conditions considered high risk by medical authority, to have legal access to the birth technologies exclusively claimed by that medical authority, and required little or no supervision by that medical authority.

Regardless of the rhetorical status gained or granted to the direct-entry midwives participating in the MSAG and certainly the LRWG hearings, medical authority over birth—an authority meant to be supported by the conventions of the licensing rules and regulations genre—finally asserted its voice before the Board of Medical Practice in the summer of 1994; as a consequence, the direct-entry midwives of Minnesota lost their bid for professional status. That voice was articulated by physician Judy Miller, nurses Emma Davidson and Elaine English, and nurse-midwife Henrietta Kramer. But perhaps the most powerful articulation came from outside the hearings: The phone calls and letters from the Minnesota Medical Association and individual physicians were enough to eventually silence the direct-entry midwives.

Thus, the Board of Medical Practice, again a group dominated by physicians, suspended the LRWG hearings. Leonard Boche and Jessica Ramsey were well aware that the voices lobbying to suspend LRWG would carry credibility in the larger public, legislative, and juridical spheres that would hear the licensing rules next. Given her experience with the Pappas-Flynn-Brown legislation, Emerson, the guild's lobbyist, felt that the nurses', nurse-midwives', and physicians' concern over the expanding boundaries of direct-entry midwifery doomed the licensing rules but that the midwives needed to be carefully led to such a conclusion:

> I felt that the . . . midwives . . . were up against the wall . . . That's what happened to us with the Legislature [with the Pappas-Flynn-Brown bill]—we thought that we would be able to stand up and make a great case and our best debate team members would be up there and in fact all of the lobbying had been done back behind closed doors.[30]

Montgomery and Emerson, who were to co-chair the August LRWG hearing, needed a rhetorical strategy to persuade the direct-entry midwifery community that their licensing efforts had failed.

The purpose of the August hearing was to have been a final discussion of each section of the fourth draft of the licensing rules. Given the rhetorical challenge of shutting down the rule writing process without betraying the direct-entry midwives who had worked so hard on the effort, Montgomery, Ramsey, and Emerson interjected the notion that licensing no longer matched the interests of direct-entry midwifery, and, to gain credibility for this argument, they revealed the medical profession's objections to the current licensing drafts and reminded the midwives of their own divisions. Thus, Joan Montgomery opened with a "philosophical question" about the specific services in the fourth draft: "On one hand, we hear about home birth being non-invasive, not hospital like . . . [but] these kinds of things [pitocin, episiotomies, suturing, etc.] appear to be medicine-stuff . . . [I]s this what we want to talk about when we talk about the home birth option . . . from a consumer point of view?"[31] Jessica Ramsey hinted that the fourth draft represented the needs of only a portion of the direct-entry midwives:

> I wonder if people who have been speaking in favor of these services represent the group of people who are practicing lay midwifery in the state . . . I know that there is other literature out there that says midwifery is an art; it doesn't include these invasive services—this kind of active participation; it's more of a passive-assistive service. Is there anyone here today that feels these services should not be considered part of the midwife's tools?

Ramsey and Montgomery then argued for a definition of midwifery that excluded medical procedures and tools—midwifery was an art, not a science, they asserted. This distinction offered rhetorical authority to anyone who wished to dispute the fourth draft of the rules.

The medical representatives to LRWG, having made their concerns known publicly at the last hearing, and privately to the board, were noticeably absent. The home birth parents, who had already communicated their reactions in private to the board, remained silent. The direct-entry midwives began to argue among themselves and with Montgomery. Greta Godwin asked whether individual midwives could write their own protocols, which might not include the specific services; it was "unfair" to ask the midwives not interested in learning how to suture or to administer pitocin to spend the time and money to do so. Rita Ortiz snapped back:

> The bottom line is that people practicing midwifery are going to be held accountable to case law and community standards of practice . . . [which] do not permit a midwife to write a protocol that says that she will not use oxytocic drugs and therefore she can transport a woman to the hospital who has lost an incredible volume of blood . . . Community standard of practice does not permit us to bleed to death in the later years of the twentieth century.

Montgomery then suggested that the licensing rules might include these services but still avoid any specific references to medical tools and procedures: "Is there a way we can say this [use of oxytocic drugs, suturing, performing episiotomies] in a way that isn't medical? Can we say 'use of acceptable community interventions . . . [to] ease the birth . . . '?" Some direct-entry midwives protested that vague language could land the midwives in legal trouble— for example, "ease the birth" could mean vacuum extraction, a method that would never be accepted for home birth by direct-entry midwives or by medical caregivers.

When the guild midwives seemed unwilling to back away from a detailed specific services section in the rules, Jessica Ramsey revealed more about the nature of the comments that the board had received over the summer:

> One of the things that I need to point out is that I have gotten a number of calls since the last hearing, and I just want to *put you all on notice* that there are some very concerned groups out there . . . [who think] that the Board of Medical Practice is going to *sanction a bunch* . . . some people who are not properly trained to do these activities. There is this concern about the lack of training, about the lack of ways to measure competence. There is a concern about the validity of the NARM exam. You heard Emma Davidson from the Nurses' Association talk about . . . the need to measure competence. (emphasis added)

Ramsey cast the midwives in a no-win situation with the fourth draft. She described the unflattering image that these "concerned groups" had of the midwives, even though she doesn't finish her phrase—"a bunch . . ."

Moreover, Montgomery proposed that, if the direct-entry midwives found themselves resisting the conventions of the rules and regulations genre, they should reconsider licensing because the rules did not represent the true spirit of midwifery:

> If we are saying that this is a body that is going to be licensed, then why should we treat ourselves as different than any other licensed body? But on the other hand, if we are saying that we don't think we should be licensed, then we would [want to have the statement of rights and informed consent forms required within the practice] . . . [A]re we saying in the final analysis we don't really want licensure? . . . Think about it. It's a good question.

But, again, many direct-entry midwives were not ready to give up on licensure. Some guild midwives, among them Rita Ortiz, said that the midwives wanted licensing and were optimistic about changing these conventions of the genre: "I think that a lot of the other health-related occupations would benefit if they provided their clientele with this kind of information. There would be a lot less misunderstanding and legal problems . . . It's definitely nonharmful and possibility helpful." However, by now others were beginning to believe that Montgomery and Ramsey had information that they needed to hear. One midwife asked Ramsey directly: "One thing I heard through the grapevine, and maybe you can set me straight, is that the powers that be have already decided the outcome of traditional midwifery, and this is just like going through the required motions . . . Do you have any idea at all how close to this or how extremely far from these rules it will actually end?"

Upon this invitation, Ramsey revealed more about what had gone on outside the LRWG hearings:

> I can tell you that there are some big groups out there who have a very keen interest and are watching this project as it evolves and those groups obviously include the physicians, whether they are represented by the Minnesota Medical Association or not . . . and nurses, in particular nurse-midwives, are very interested. If you consider those groups "the powers that be," I think it is fair to say that they have something in their minds that they want and that they have some limits that they will not be allowed to be crossed . . . Those groups believe that, by and large, breeches are not appropriate for home delivery . . . There are also groups out there who are very concerned about getting formal educational programs, something comparable to what they have to go through.

In the confines of LRWG, all voices were equally empowered and the fourth draft appeared to represent a consensus of opinion. Now, however, voices outside the hearings asserted their right to rein in the boundaries of the midwives' practices. At this news, the midwives' determination wavered.

Given the direct-entry midwives' reaction to this news, Montgomery asked again: "Is licensing what we really want?" and framed the words that LRWG participants could use to stop the licensing process. In August 1994, the version of the NARM exam that the Minnesota Board of Medical Practice intended to use to license direct-entry midwives was not yet in final form. The first two versions of the exam were taken as a pilot project by experienced midwives, all of whom passed. Later versions of the NARM exam, deemed to be psychometrically valid, contained a rigorous hands-on skills component, and many midwives taking these later versions failed to pass. Moreover, NARM certification was designed to demonstrate knowledge, skills, and experience of midwives regardless of their educational route, and the candidate for certification had to document her attendance as a primary caregiver at twenty births and seventy-five prenatal sessions. However, in referring to the version of the NARM exam that existed in August 1994, Montgomery suggested that the LRWG suspend the hearings on the warrant that the NARM exam was inadequate for demonstrating the midwives' knowledge and abilities:

> You guys, this was a practical thing when you thought you had an exam.
> We don't have an exam; we don't have an exam that you are going to ac-
> cept because we have no validation studies and [because] everyone has
> passed it [the exam]. And I have never heard of an exam that everyone has
> passed. . . . I just need to tell you that validation-testing psychologists . . .
> generally will not accept the fact that 100 percent will pass. . . . We all came
> here because it was the only way that was open right now. But let's assume
> that this is not the only way because right now the way has been chopped
> off because the vehicles don't exist. What would be our recommendation
> to the board based on this information? Do we say licensure or die?

Montgomery's pronoun choices reveal her rhetorical strategies: She cast herself as
part of the "we," the group she defined as having believed that writing licensing
rules for direct-entry midwifery would be successful, and now she was entertain-
ing doubts that the process would work. However, as the "I," she also had special
knowledge of testing validity; thus, she had authority but not necessarily allegiance
to the board or the medical community. Moreover, anyone in LRWG who still supported licensing was to be viewed as going against common sense and as being too
extreme—willing to "die" for an unattainable goal. In Emerson and Montgomery's
view, meanwhile, as long as the discussion remained open—as long as the direct-
entry midwives were working on their educational component—the midwives would
avoid the kind of legal prosecution that New York direct-entry midwives faced.

Without any way to document their own authoritative knowledge about birth,
the direct-entry midwives could not challenge the jurisdictional boundaries of the
medical profession. The minutes for the August LRWG hearing contained the following statement:

> Several members of the group expressed concern about the current draft of
> the rules. The reliability of the NARM exam is still in question and there
> is no approved program of study. Some members still believe that VBAC,
> breech and twin births are contraindications for home birth. Nurses will
> not support the rules in their current state. Perhaps it is time to rethink the
> issue of registration versus licensing . . . Licensing would help define and
> legitimize the practice of midwifery. The group also agreed, however, that
> the rules as written are problematic and additional work needs to be done.

In the MSAG public hearings about direct-entry midwifery in Minnesota, the
Minnesota Midwives' Guild midwives convinced the group that they were "good
midwives," who acknowledged the limits of their practices and carefully screened
out high-risk mothers. The recommendations of the Midwifery Study Advisory
Group would have increased the visibility and rights of direct-entry midwives within
the state. However, when the Board of Medical Practice charged the Licensing Rule
Writing Group with writing the rules and regulations for direct-entry midwifery
in Minnesota, the midwives expressed mixed feelings about becoming state-
recognized professionals. Direct-entry midwifery would be normalized and no
longer autonomous, as the midwives would be expected to follow clearly defined

protocols. Therefore, the direct-entry midwives involved in LRWG resisted the conventions of the licensing rules and regulations genre by defining themselves as autonomous primary health care providers, providers who were not required to be supervised by the medical community. The shared-document collaborative process granting all LRWG members equal rhetorical status further enabled this resistance. However, those midwives unwilling to sacrifice delivering breeches and twins at home were soon pitted against those willing to compromise these practices to gain legal access to administer antihemorrhagic and other drugs and permission to suture and perform episiotomies at home. Home birth parents appearing before LRWG sided with one faction of the midwifery community as they resisted what they considered the medicalization of midwifery. The genre of licensing rules and regulations contained exclusive categories and definitions—for example, if direct-entry midwives were granted permission to suture, then all must offer this service and prove that their training and education were sufficient to do so. The direct-entry midwives wanted to continue to obtain their education through a number of routes, including apprenticeships, self-study, and a variety of formal programs, and to validate this education through NARM certification. Finally, those asking to expand the jurisdiction of direct-entry midwifery were confronted by the boundary work that medical communities used to confirm their own jurisdictions. Episiotomies were defined as requiring surgical procedures, suturing as involving medical diagnostic skills, and drug administration as demanding pharmaceutical education.

As seen in the LRWG hearings, the conventions of the licensing rules and regulations were one discursive means by which the authority of a dominant profession—the medical community—maintained its jurisdictional boundaries. The midwives resisted these conventions, at times simply recasting phrases into their own language but at other times including new sections, such as the special services section, to include practices for which the genre typically left no room. The medical community seemed to have assumed that its jurisdictional boundaries and authority would be upheld by the genre—after all, the conventions of the genre were designed to do just that. However, the scope of practices and special services sections, as represented by the August 1994 draft, granted the midwives legal access to birth technologies without medical supervision. These sections also affirmed the midwives' ability to deliver twins and breeches at home. As a result, they created a discourse that directly challenged medical authority over scientific knowledge, a challenge to which the medical community responded forcefully. The response mounted by the medical community ensured that physicians would maintain their exclusive claim over scientific knowledge and their appropriation of scientific discourse as it pertained to pregnancy and birth.[32]

CHAPTER 7

Issues of Gender and Power:

THE RHETORIC OF DIRECT-ENTRY MIDWIFERY

*I think that traditional medicine is pretty strong and feels that they
should control how health care should be delivered. It's difficult to see
how the traditional midwives will get through that.*
—Henrietta Kramer

*A lot of it has to do with the oppression of women—that women are
competitive with each other, and that they are unable to support each
other. And we are just this tiny little group that is seen as this big
threat. Because, for one thing, we are not under the domination of the
system. We have somehow, in some little way, escaped it, although we
certainly have our own oppression. So in that way we are a threat.*
—Gloria Olson[1]

        *T*his book has focused on four rhetorical
sites within the history of midwifery and on the public hearings about direct-entry
midwifery in the state of Minnesota held between 1991 and 1995. Within the historical sites, we saw how the early midwifery texts and proposals written by Jane
Sharp in 1671, by Elizabeth Cellier in 1687, and by Elizabeth Nihell in 1760 taught
midwives basic aspects of anatomy and physiology and promoted an independent
midwifery corporation. These early texts also acknowledged that professional standing for midwives would mean that they would have to consult with male medical
practitioners, and the texts argued against the expanding use of birth technologies
by celebrating the midwives' traditional remedies such as herbs and touch. We saw
how the obstetrical forceps and other birth technologies increased the practice of the
male practitioner, who could now claim to deliver, under adverse conditions, a living child from a living mother. We also read the arguments in *JAMA* at the end of
the nineteenth century both for and against the forceps, debates that also considered whether any birth was natural and therefore safe. We realized that the issue of
whether birth was natural and safe continued into the beginning of the twentieth
century, as many officials sought to outlaw the U.S. midwife while others proposed
to educate her by using the funding available through the Sheppard-Towner Act.
Finally, we saw a resurgence of interest in midwifery during the natural and home
birth movements at the Farm and the Santa Cruz Birth Center in the 1960s and 1970.
These movements celebrated the birth story as a means of sharing experiential

170

knowledge, but suffered prosecution for practicing medicine without a license when the state successfully argued that its right to protect its citizens outweighed parents' right to privacy.

Within the Minnesota midwifery hearings, we realized how, through discourse, a dominant profession can maintain its jurisdictional boundaries. Within the Midwifery Study Advisory Group meetings, the direct-entry midwives of Minnesota gained the rhetorical status to help draft recommendations to increase their visibility and their place in attending home births. Key rhetors, such as Rita Ortiz and Mary Emerson, challenged the professional boundary work of pathologist Rachel Waters by promoting the image of the good midwife who carefully screens her clients for high-risk conditions. However, in the Licensing Rule Writing Group hearings, we saw how the midwives' authoritative knowledge about birth, supported by their experiential and embodied knowledge, challenged the medical authoritative knowledge about birth. But we also learned how the genre of licensing rules and regulations helped a dominant profession assert supremacy over an emerging profession. Thus, we saw the results of the midwives' drive to obtain legal access to birth technologies and for legal sanction to attend conditions such as breech birth and twins, conditions considered high risk by medical knowledge systems. The medical community successfully lobbied the Board of Medical Practice to suspend the hearings. Finally, the statutory definitions and regulation of direct-entry midwifery in other states, and the conversations among midwives and medical practitioners on a midwifery listserv, set the Minnesota hearings within a broader context. Thus, the Minnesota hearings reveal some issues central to understanding the rhetoric of midwifery. These issues include the uneasy relationship between the hegemonic, technologically based knowledge system of medicine and the marginalized, experientially based knowledge system of midwifery. They include the conflict between normalization and autonomy of practice and the maintenance of medical jurisdiction through exclusive claims to scientific knowledge and control of scientific discourse. This chapter concludes the study of the rhetoric of midwifery by further speculating on the relationship between gender and power, a relationship that informs the central issues raised throughout the book. These final speculations are supported by the reflections offered and arguments made by the principal rhetors who participated in the Minnesota story and by the midwifery listserv participants who discussed similar issues during the Minnesota public hearings.

In understanding the relationship between gender and power in modern and historical debates over midwifery, one confronts the problem of defining direct-entry midwives by their sex and their involvement in birth, while acknowledging that gender is a social concept constructed through discourse. Like the body, gender is a "boundary concept," Anne Balsamo notes (9). Even if the "body has been recoded within discourses of biotechnology and medicine as belonging to an order of culture rather than nature," Balsamo contends that "gender remains a naturalized marker of human identity" (9). Gender, then, is an organizing feature of power relations, "a determining cultural condition and a social consequence of technological determination" (Balsamo 9). In the words of Lois McNay, "On a fundamental level, a notion of the body is central to the feminist analysis of the oppression of women because it is upon the biological difference between the male and female bodies that the edifice of gender inequality is built and legitimized" (*Feminism* 17).[2] New reproductive technologies and current medical models of the body might be used to cast it as a cyborg, a creature for whom the boundaries of machine and nature are blurred, to identify the fetus as a separate and primary patient, or to divide the mother into body parts—womb, breast, limb. However, these impulses are also marked by cultural constructs of gender, the ways in which a community organizes and assigns roles and status to its members.

Therefore, any study of direct-entry midwifery is complicated by the midwives' own sense of what they learn from being female and from birthing and mothering their own children, from engaging in a practice that ministers to women during pregnancy and birth, and from experiencing how, as women, their knowledge and experience may be devalued. As Emily Martin says, "The overall picture assumed in the present day is that knowledge of the natural world is produced by scientists doing proper science. This knowledge is concentrated in its purest form in the scientists who produce it; then, to a limited extent, it filters out or trickles down to other professional groups and the general public" (*Flexible* 5). In creating their own knowledge system about birth, direct-entry midwives celebrate their unique and personal involvement in reproduction. Their experiential knowledge is gained through helping others deliver their babies or "catching" for other women. This experiential knowledge is often supported by the midwives' embodied knowledge, the ways in which they understood the processes of their own bodies as they labored to deliver their own children. Finally, the laboring woman's own instincts and the midwife's intuition contribute to midwifery knowledge about birth. Therefore, the midwives themselves often point to their roles as mothers and women—the unique processes of their own bodies because they are women and they give birth to children. Rather than receiving knowledge as "trickling" down from the medical community, the midwives create knowledge through experience and instinct, and they inherit knowledge from their sister midwives who are practicing now or who practiced centuries ago. However, they also recognize the challenge presented by their socially assigned places as women and as "knowers" in society. They recognize, as does Gloria Olson in the opening quote to the chapter, that because they are women, they face a society that may discount their experiential and embodied knowledge, and they confront dominant professions that claim authoritative knowledge about women's bodies and, through discourse, successfully maintain that claim.

Within the Minnesota hearings on direct-entry midwifery, the medical community asserted the authority of its knowledge system to define normal and abnormal birth, to categorize high-risk birth, and to support its use of birth technologies to ensure safety. As Foucault says, through discourse, power is exercised as it creates knowledge and identifies what it considers as truth (*Discipline* 26–27).[3] Topics become appropriate for discussion, statements become elevated to facts or evidence, experience is valued, and knowledge is created when power relations establish them as such. Individuals may resist those impulses and definitions, and they may also be normalized by them. Women may consider hospital birth, expert management of their bodies, and visualization of their fetuses through technologies as the norm, but they may also resist these constructions of their bodies. For example, the direct-entry midwives resisted the conventions of the licensing rules and regulations genre that supported medical knowledge about birth. In this resistance, we understand how gender, or women's assigned social roles, affects their ability to assert their experiences and knowledge.

Additionally, to understand how, in the end, the Minnesota hearings supported medical authority over women's bodies through an exclusive claim to scientific knowledge and discourse, we must consider discourse on the body as an aspect of what Foucualt called biopower. Biopower takes two forms—disciplinary practices and regulatory power. Disciplinary practices represent the body within institutions and in everyday activities by "creating desires, attaching individuals to specific identities, and establishing norms against which individuals and their behaviors and bodies are judged and against which they police themselves"(Sawicki 67). Establishing the definition of normal birth or the good midwife would be a function of disciplinary power. Such disciplinary power would specify the particulars of midwifery practice and establish hospital birth under the supervision of a medical caregiver as the norm for birth. On the other hand, regulatory power is inscribed in the policies and interventions governing a population in which the body "serves as the basis of biological processes affecting birth, death, the level of health and longevity" and is the target of state agencies (Sawicki 68). Declaring that only licensed medical caregivers could administer pitocin or suture would be a function of the regulatory power of the Minnesota Board of Medical Practice. Biopower, constituted by disciplinary and regulatory power, then, supports social and professional justifications of birth technologies. However, once we understand how biopower supports disciplinary and regulatory functions, we can propose alternative stories about gender and power. These stories add to our understanding of how power and subsequent gender relations negate women's voices, experiences, and knowledge, and how these relations may be maintained or resisted through discourse. For example, Jana Sawicki proposes an alternative story of the development of birth technologies. This story has been told as "the entrance of the enlightened male physician with scientific knowledge into the birth room and the dismissal of female ignorance and superstition" or as "the medicalization of childbirth, the identification of pregnancy as a disease, takeover of a female-centered natural process attended by skilled and caring midwives by a group of male physicians interested in establishing and expanding their practices, their occupational status and authority, and their control over women" (75). However, Sawicki asserts that the history of reproduction is actually a story of both power and resistance. This story is reflected in the discourse of the dominant medical profession and the moments of resistance to medical practices (81). In these moments of resistance, we can see how birth technologies, such as ultrasound, fetal monitors, amniocentesis, and antenatal testing procedures create new norms of motherhood, "attach" women to their "identities as mothers," and normalize birth (83–85). By assessing biopower, we better understand how systems of thinking and regulating are able to establish bodily norms and to examine and survey bodily functions, and how individuals and groups cooperate in or resist those systems.

Therefore, to understand the relationship between gender and power, we must further study oppression from the point of view of the oppressed and within moments of resistance to or participation in that oppression. To do so will help us capture the voices of those who know their worlds in different ways—know different worlds—than those expressed by dominant discourse. Bodies and their reproductive roles are both material and discursively constructed through disciplinary practice and through regulatory policies. Thus, important to understanding the relationship between gender and power in the Minnesota story are midwifery's authoritative systems of knowledge, informed by women's embodied knowledge and midwives' experiential knowledge. Also important are medical authoritative systems of knowledge, which engage in biopower to produce new norms of motherhood and offer women technological solutions to the birth problems they face.

Finally, we must also resist simply labeling the medical community in the United States as powerful and the direct-entry midwifery community as powerless. To do so would negate the relationship, however uneasy, between the two systems of knowledge and would fail to acknowledge the achievements of such organizations as the Minnesota Midwives' Guild, the Midwives' Alliance of North American (MANA), and the North American Registry of Midwives (NARM). Certainly the Minnesota direct-entry midwives failed to achieve professional standing during the time of the hearings (1991–1995). Moreover, as Paul Starr has said in his study of medicine, "Modern medicine is one of those extraordinary works of reason: an elaborate system of specialized knowledge, technical procedures, and rules of behavior. . . . In America, no one group has held so dominant a position in this new world of rationality and power as has the medical profession" (3–4). Nurse-midwife Henrietta Kramer's statement, which opens this chapter, reflects this belief that the medical profession controls health care in this country. However, although the medical systems might claim exclusive control of birth technologies, many midwives use birth technologies to screen their home birth clients and to manage difficult births, regardless of whether or not they have legal access to these technologies. Home birth parents manage to find midwives in the underground networks, and midwives find "friendly docs" who will provide them with pitocin and other drugs to deal with emergencies during home birth. At the end of the twentieth century, more and more direct-entry midwives are achieving the status of Certified Professional Midwife through NARM. In Minnesota, a consumer group, Minnesotans for Midwifery, sprang up after the hearings to support direct-entry midwives in their practices. As reported in the September 1998 MANA newsletter, "Midwives are quietly helping babies be born" in Minnesota (Dixon 9). In states such Florida, California, Alaska, and Oregon, midwives appear to flourish.

However, direct-entry midwives continue to confront the normalization of birth that so negates their experiential and embodied knowledge and the ways in which parents have become dependent on medical expertise to determine how and with whom they will birth. As Paul Starr says,

> Power, at the most rudimentary personal level, originates in dependence, and
> the power of the professions primarily originates in dependence upon their

> knowledge and competence . . . Indeed, what makes dependence on the
> professions so distinctive today is that their interpretations often govern
> our understanding of the world and our own experience. To most of us, this
> power seems legitimate: When professionals claim to be authoritative about
> the nature of reality . . . we generally defer to their judgment. (4)

The vast majority of women in the United States give birth in the hospital because
that is where they feel safe. Indeed, as we saw in the history of midwifery, women
often deferred to medical judgment when they sought relief from pain and death
during childbirth. However, the history of midwifery tells the story of resisting this
normalization with varying degrees of success. The establishment of the Farm and
the Santa Cruz Birth Center constituted moments of resistance. Direct-entry midwife Gloria Olson's assessment as to why the nurses rejected the Minnesota Midwives' Guild's education plan, in the quote offered at the beginning of this chapter,
reflects this resistance. The nurses have accepted their oppression within the medical profession, Olson said, but direct-entry midwives have resisted the system.
Rhetors Mary Emerson and Rita Ortiz successfully resisted images of direct-entry
midwifery that aligned the practice with a modern form of witchcraft, and they resisted Rachel Waters's assertion that their clients were poor and uninformed. At
least through the fourth draft of the Minnesota licensing rules and regulations, created in 1994, direct-entry midwives resisted the conventions of the licensing genre
that dictated supervision by medical caregivers. The rest of this chapter attempts to
once more capture the perceptions of the direct-entry midwives as they reflected
on gender and power during the time of the Minnesota public hearings. Allowing
the midwives to speak for themselves further clarifies the Minnesota hearings and
their eventual failure. This chapter, then, concludes by summarizing the essential issues raised in this study of the rhetoric of midwifery.

Direct-Entry Midwives' Reflections on Gender and Power

The direct-entry midwives involved in the Minnesota public hearings articulated the sense of personal freedom they realized in operating outside the dominant
medical profession's jurisdictional boundaries and knowledge systems, while they
sought the professional power to be gained through licensing. In a sense, then, they
felt themselves freer than nurse-midwives, who functioned within the medical system and were under the supervision of physicians. For example, Elizabeth Smith,
in considering the special services of direct-entry midwifery, questioned uniform
protocols for every midwife: "One way to get around it would be to mandate something for everyone, but that goes against every cell in my body. It's like a censor-
ship of free speech or any of the fundamental rights we have."[4] Mary Emerson
confirmed that practicing midwifery "takes sort of a renegade and anarchist": "So
that's the personality that's drawn to this—the combination of nurturing, mothering, rescuing, and renegade. So a lot of people come to it with some very, very high
purpose and high calling . . . a certain kind of rebel—I am above the law. And there
is a certain amount of personal power in that."[5] Therefore, practicing outside the

system of the professions—outside the surveillance of state agencies—seemed to give the direct-entry midwives personal freedom and choice—and, in fact, motivated some to enter midwifery in the first place. However, midwives such as Smith also accepted that in joining the system of the professions, direct-entry midwifery might gain another sort of power. To Smith, the guild's educational plan "is a great thing": "And I am really excited that the guild is doing it, and that we are becoming a powerful force and that as an organization, I think, that whenever you have that unity, you have a lot more power." To Smith, operating as a formal organization meant professional and discursive power, even though it might also mean loss of personal freedom.

Moreover, the direct-entry midwives' perceptions of power were often directly linked to their gender identity and their experiences with birth. Often, after giving birth for the first time, they saw the world quite differently and felt empowered by the experience. As direct-entry midwives, they might be attracted to the unregulated practice, in part, *because* it afforded them the opportunity to live beyond legal and state surveillance. As new mothers, they might have experienced their ability to resist discursively constructed limitations, particularly if they gave birth outside the hospital setting. To be women meant to be powerful. For example, Connie Baker reflected on her experience of giving birth at the Farm:

> It was really my first time of thinking how choosing a home birth really resonates throughout your life. I started thinking of how I have started to take control of my reproduction, what I am going to do about raising and educating my children. It really brought up a lot of questions. Also there is something about once you question that funnel of women into the hospital, when you step out of that, I wondered how many funnels am I in here? . . . It [giving birth] was such a powerful experience. When it was over, I just felt like I could probably do anything I wanted to.[6]

Elizabeth Smith used similar words to describe the birth of her first child:

> I was completely blown away by how powerful birth was and how empowering it was to become a mother. The amazing changes that I went through in becoming a mother were a pivotal turning point—it was a time I knew that I could take on the world.

Both Baker and Smith felt they could do anything—take on the world. Reflecting on the alternative of hospital birth, the midwives often felt that giving birth in this institutionalized setting decreased a woman's self-worth. Smith said, "It's just stressful to be in an environment [like the hospital] when you know you have to be on the defensive . . . When you are at home, it's just giving. The woman is in her power." To Smith, that empowerment is possible only in a women-controlled setting, in a different world than that experienced in the hospital.

Elizabeth Smith, Gloria Olson, Connie Baker, and other direct-entry midwives chose to become midwives to preserve this sense of empowerment for themselves and for other women. They wanted to continue to practice in a unique place, outside society's institutions, which they perceived as restrictive to women, and to

hold onto that change in self-worth that comes through giving birth. Baker identified the relationship between her choosing to become a midwife and her own feelings about being a woman: "I don't know that I had a philosophy of life or birth
that led me to midwifery other than belief that women deserved a fair opportunity
to experience a normal life function without being dissected. However, my becoming a midwife has certainly shaped my life course as a woman and as a mother."
In other words, many direct-entry midwives became midwives because they were
women and mothers themselves. Their own experiences with birth, whether positive or negative, led them to try to make the experience empowering for other
women. As Olson said, midwives are "strongly opinionated and protecting our rights
to be powerful women. Most women don't even think about it. They don't realize
they are not powerful. We are really aware of how painful it is when someone tries
to take our power away from us." To Olson, then, women tend to participate in the
normalization of birth that dictated that birth was too dangerous to take place outside the hospital setting. A midwifery-attended home birth, on the other hand, might
involve, according to Olson, not only physical but emotional labor; therefore, women
needed to birth within the safest psychological environment. During birth a woman
might become more aware of past negative experiences and so reach a new understanding of the gendered nature of those experiences. Olson summarized those impressions in one birth story:

> I was at a birth day before yesterday, and this mother had her first child a
> few years ago, and she had a pretty normal labor, it was a long labor, first
> baby, big baby, but she felt she had a lot of pain about her first birth. They
> took the baby away from her, during her labor she checked out a lot, she
> would just space out, and during her second labor, it was the most interesting
> labor, she would work really hard, hard contractions, close together, then
> all of a sudden she would be hit by a wave of emotion about her first birth—
> about what happened to her and how she felt unsupported and she would
> just sob and weep and her contractions would practically stop for an hour,
> two hours, and she would mourn that past experience . . . I think that women
> have these emotion blocks that come from being second-class citizens in a
> culture. There's no way you can come through it without some emotional
> damage that's going to come up during intimate times and with support it
> [birth] can be a really empowering experience, and generally it is.

Midwives, confirmed Baker, uniquely enable other women to share that experience:
"Midwives are women that other women feel safe with during the vulnerable tran-
sitions of childbearing. I might add that this transition is a normal, non-medical,
non-academic, nonverbal, physiological event, and midwives know that." Therefore, midwives' embodied knowledge, gained through their own birth experiences,
and their experiential knowledge, developed as they attended other women in
women-centered settings, empowered them to offer an alternative experience for
mothers and their families. This experience was discursively defined as an empowering one, and normal home birth awakened or recalled for women that sense
of personal power.

The direct-entry midwives described the experiential knowledge that they regard as authoritative as centered on normal birth. Medical authoritative knowledge extended technological intervention to handle abnormal and pathological conditions. The direct-entry midwives, as characterized by Gloria Olson, taught the "truths" about normal birth:

> I tend to think that traditional midwives will be more and more the teachers in the future of normal birth and living. Normal conception, pregnancy, birth, everything. We will be the small group of keepers of the normal. I read something once . . . that in every generation there is a handful of people who are given the responsibility of holding the truth. And, I always thought that's what traditional midwives are given . . . [the truth] about birth and women.

Moreover, an essential contribution to midwifery experiential knowledge comes from the midwife's efforts to meet the needs of each client, her protocols for handling the specifics of each case. Preserving the laboring mother's choice, then, is essential to direct-entry midwifery care. To Elizabeth Smith, the midwife was "the guardian of certain choices and options," of women's rights. This goal of developing and preserving midwifery experiential knowledge was also reflected during listserv communications at the time of the Minnesota public hearings. For example, for Mary Jane, a participant on the midwifery listserv, the "bottom line" in midwifery care was "letting the woman make her own informed choices. I've just watched too many women be bullied into accepting someone else's decisions over what's right and wrong" (listserv communication, August 30, 1996). For Ellen, a direct-entry midwife and listserv participant who worked with Amish clients in Indiana, choice meant "understanding the mindset" of her clients: "It is not my job to judge a lifestyle that has evolved over several 100s of years" (listserv communication, September 1, 1996). Thus, midwifery experiential knowledge gave the direct-entry midwife the confidence to handle home birth—normal birth in a woman-centered setting—and the means to support her client's own choices for her birth.

The direct-entry midwives then described their midwifery knowledge about birth as a different way of thinking—of seeing and experiencing a different world. Connie Baker described how that thinking affected the Minnesota Midwives' Guild's educational series: "So far it's been totally a women's process—where will people stay if they travel in town and what about their kids is as important as how many questions are on the final exam. So we are really trying to do it in a holistic, loving, and supportive way that makes education a seductive thing, and not a traumatic thing." Baker felt that providing safe child care and comfortable housing to the midwives attending the series was as important as teaching aspects of anatomy and physiology. Thus, as they constructed and disseminated knowledge, midwives and medical caregivers included attitudes about what was normal and comfortable and what was safe or frightening. For example, according to Elizabeth Smith, "Medically trained birth attendants are much more intervention-oriented; they are much more fear-based. They always look at 'what if, what if, what if'; you do have to look at that, but it doesn't have to be the focus."

For some direct-entry midwives, that different way of thinking about birth was discursively constructed in contrast to a patriarchal system. For example, Connie Baker articulated how direct-midwifery knowledge was different from dominant cultural ideas:

> I do think that the dominant culture is this male culture . . . [B]eing a woman puts me in a subculture classification, and that culture was designed by and for men. I think that men have more blinders on—that they are trained to go for what they want, and women are really trained to have a more panoramic view of what's going on, to kind of scope the scene, that we are always looking at dynamics between how we are doing with the kids and [how] the kids [are] doing with each other and [how] our kids [are] doing in the world. I feel that way about birth too—it's hard to look at it in a linear way and say 'if A then B and if B then C.' We do look at it from a lot of different perspectives simultaneously and so it's hard to write this [licensing rules] out and wonder if we will follow it.

Baker described male thinking as linear rather than holistic, as selective rather than inclusive, even as static rather than dynamic.

In line with that view, direct-entry midwives reflected on their gender identities not only within their own discourse community but also within the broader society and culture. These reflections carried over into their attitudes toward and predictions about the licensing and professionalization of midwifery. For example, Connie Baker speculated that, ultimately, in the Minnesota licensing efforts, "midwives will probably not get a fair shake because midwifery is a profession made up of women for the care of other women, and we live in a male-dominant world." In their practices, Baker said, despite the potential empowerment of women through the birth experience, the direct-entry midwives also must acknowledge that they dealt with clients who have inherited and participated in society's messages about gender:

> In staying home with someone with a breech baby or twins . . . there is more emotional work that needs to be done, because women feel that they have been given a very strong surgical message that their body doesn't work and so they have to really hurdle that, determine in the cells of their body that that wasn't the truth and then if it's not a truth they have been truly violated.

Gloria Olson confirmed that the norms of motherhood and birth carried the cultural message that women's embodied and experiential knowledge was inadequate: "We have all been taught that male model [of medicine] and taught that we are inferior and have our prescribed role and told not to overstep it." Moreover, Hope, in her "Epistle to the Midwives" on the midwifery listserv, noted that these messages affected her most basic rights. Without the right to choose where to birth and how to experience one's sexual nature, other choices made no sense, had no impact, according to Hope:

> If I cannot legally make the most elemental choices about my sexual and reproductive life such as choosing where to give birth and who will attend me during this normal physiological process (not to mention the issue of greater safety with midwifery care), then what difference does it make that our democratic institutions "permit" me to vote for the political candidate of my choice? One can not tell the complete story of women's reproductive rights without including its relationship to the criminalization of midwifery and the take-over of the very core of our lives as women by the commercial interests of organized medicine.
>
> (listserv communication, July 25, 1996)

Only in claiming a public space for direct-entry midwifery, in taking the debates over the practice into the public sphere, and in making midwifery visible, even though vulnerable, according to Baker, might more women become empowered through birth, might those patriarchal systems be exposed and challenged:

> I used to feel that we had to keep it [midwifery] underground and protect it and that we were lucky that we found this dark little niche where we could do our women thing. I have evolved to the point where I think that we are entitled to our women culture, to support women in having respectful health care.

Moreover, Rita Ortiz contended that it was time to let go of that oppressed image: "There is a thinking in lay midwifery about really enjoying the underdog status, really enjoying that we are oppressed. Women have been oppressed for a long time, but have actually internalized that oppression and contributed to it. 'You see: we tried [to write licensing rules], and they did us in.'" Thus, Baker, Ortiz, and others not only railed against the system that they believe oppressed them as midwives and as women, the system that limited their choices as to where to birth and how to birth, and the system that they resisted as they wrote the licensing rules for direct-entry midwifery in Minnesota, but they also admitted their own participation in their oppression.

The direct-entry midwives involved in the Minnesota public hearings, along with those who contributed to the midwifery listserv, linked power and gender in describing their own birth experiences and their journeys to midwifery. Working outside what they identified as a system of authoritative knowledge oppressive to women—one that excludes the embodied and experiential knowledge systems they value so highly, the midwives experienced personal freedom and honored the choices of their clients. Birth was both a physical and an emotional event; sexual and reproductive choices were fundamental rights. However, the direct-entry midwives also recognized that only by entering the public sphere would they gain discursive and professional power. These 1990s midwives asked similar questions to those raised throughout the history of midwifery, beginning with Jane Sharp, Elizabeth Cellier, and Elizabeth Nihell in the seventeenth and eighteenth centuries: How can female midwives retain for themselves and their clients the special knowledge midwives bring to birth and also relate to a social and medical system that excludes midwives in essential ways? How can women control their birth experiences and also gain legal access to the scientific tools and procedures that medical professionals claim are strictly within their jurisdiction? How can women feel empowered by birth, a feeling that seems most possible outside the hospital, and still develop discursive and professional power within the public sphere? In Minnesota, at the end of the public hearings that took place between 1991 and 1995, the answer seemed to be that they could not.

The Rhetoric of Midwifery

The Minnesota Midwifery Study Advisory Group and Licensing Rule Writing Group public hearings on direct-entry midwifery represent a local center of the discourse-power-knowledge relationship that Foucault challenges scholars to study. Moreover, the MSAG and LRWG hearings allow us to add gender to the discourse-power-knowledge mix, a factor neglected by Foucault and by scholars such as Abbott and Starr, who have studied the professions. The hearings also add one more chapter to the centuries-old history of midwifery, a story of increasing conflict between medical and state institutions and women's birth knowledge and craft. Finally, a close rhetorical analysis of the hearings adds to our knowledge of distinct persuasive moves within a public sphere, such as boundary spanning. We understand that genre conventions might suppress community voices and that these voices resist the impact of genre conventions on personal ideologies and practices. We see how, through discourse, jurisdictional boundaries are maintained through exclusive claim to scientific knowledge.

The history of midwifery recalls the earliest rhetorical challenges faced by such rhetors as Jane Sharp, who taught her midwives anatomy but also celebrated their distinct knowledge and "touch"; by Elizabeth Cellier, who tried to find a way for midwives to gain professional status and maintain a degree of self-determination; and by Elizabeth Nihell, who defined the jurisdiction of midwifery in contrast to what she considered dangerous and invasive birth instruments. However, to a great extent, with the invention of these instruments, Sharp's, Cellier's, and Nihell's arguments failed. Female midwifery practice was confined to normal birth, however that was defined at given moments in history, but more and more it was narrowly defined to exclude conditions such as breeches and twins. Increasingly, the good midwife must know how to recognize these conditions, how to identify high risk, and how to call for the male physician. At the end of a ninety-year battle for state licensing, British midwives accepted surveillance by the state and supervision by the emerging medical community to gain professional status. In the United States, those who wished to eliminate midwifery care defined birth more and more as a pathology, best handled by a physician in a hospital who would use the event as an opportunity to learn and teach and to develop authoritative medical knowledge about birth. Overturning the Sheppard-Towner Act enabled physicians to handle prenatal care, giving them an important inroad into preventive care for the whole family. The 1970s resistance to physician and hospital care of birth, exemplified by the Santa Cruz Birth Center and the Farm, attempted to turn responsibility and choice back to women and their families; however, government authorities, acting in concert with the medical profession, took steps to reclaim the right to narrowly define the good midwife and the natural process of birth.

This history of midwifery prepares us to understand the MSAG and LRWG hearings, the conversations on the midwifery listserv, and the legal status of midwives in the states that licensed direct-entry midwives in the mid-1990s. Professionalization today for these midwives—much as for Elizabeth Cellier's proposed Midwives' College and for the British midwives celebrating the passage of the 1902 Midwives' Act—means professional status, legal recognition, and a clear sense of jurisdiction. However, professionalization also contributes to the normalization of birth and loss of autonomy and diversity in practice. Thus, as defined in the MSAG hearings, the good midwife not only offers a distinct type of care—one enhanced by a close relationship with the mother, a modern sort of "touch,"—but also knows when to screen out high-risk mothers or to call in the physician. The midwife who attempts to go beyond this definition will encounter opposition from established medicine and even from some members of her own community, as that community attempts to gain professional status and avoid identification as the deviant or other. When the LRWG collaborative method allowed the direct-entry midwives to resist some degree of medical supervision in the licensing rules, to continue to attend breeches and twins at home, and to increase their legal access to medical tools and procedures, medical representatives asserted their authority by successfully lobbying to suspend the licensing rule writing process. Direct-entry midwives, denied use of birth instruments in the seventeenth century, were denied legal access to contemporary birth technologies in the 1990s once again, including drugs such as pitocin and methergine, and forbidden to perform episiotomies and suturing. Midwives who felt confident about handling breeches, twins, and VBACs were not allowed to define safe home birth practice so broadly.

This rhetorical study of midwifery throughout history and in Minnesota in the 1990s increases our understanding of the nature of medical and midwifery knowledge and of the differences between these knowledge systems. It increases our understanding of the role that genre conventions play in suppressing community voices and the attempts of those community members to resist this suppression, the role of science and technology in defending professional jurisdictions, and the relationship between gender and power within discourse.

First, whether set in the seventeenth or the twentieth century, midwifery is a distinct practice offered by and for women. Direct-entry midwifery involves instinct, belief in the natural process of birth, trust in the mother's choice and self-knowledge, and reliance on hands and herbs. Midwives first try non-invasive remedies for unusual conditions, such as breeches and twins, before intervening in the birth process. Even when asking for legal access to scientific tools and techniques, the direct-entry midwife does so only to control emergencies, and some midwives assign the responsibility to make these choices to the mother and her cultural or spiritual support systems. The direct-entry midwife may learn her trade today, as she did yesterday, through apprenticeship and shared birth stories, but she does not dismiss what she can learn about anatomy and physiology through formal educational systems. Those who oppose midwifery or seek to limit its jurisdiction often do so by contrasting the midwife's system of learning to formal education, by contrasting her practice to those professions that lay exclusive claim to scientific knowledge and medical technologies, and by denying that modern medical science can learn anything from midwifery practice. These arguments have been highly successful throughout the history of midwifery and so have driven the practice underground or set strict limits on those direct-entry midwives licensed to practice in the 1990s.

Second, our theories of discourse and knowledge communities must reacknowledge the ability of the rhetor to persuade—by raising her rhetorical status and by challenging the social and professional status assigned to her. The MSAG and LRWG hearings illustrate the rhetor's ability to resist. Within these rhetorical sites, discourse "can be both an instrument and an effect of power, but also a hindrance, a stumbling block, a point of resistance and a starting point for an opposing strategy" (Foucault, *Sexuality* 100–101). Thus, these sites reflect not only the discourse of dominant voices but also the discourse of resistance articulated by the dominated. More specifically, the MSAG and LRWG hearings raise two questions about that resistance. Within the MSAG hearings, Mary Emerson and Rita Ortiz temporarily raised the rhetorical status of direct-entry midwifery by excluding, in essence dominating, another set of voices—the non-guild midwives of Minnesota. Thus, we learn more about to what extent resistance might involve defining and silencing yet another group. We also learn to ask to what extent resistance comes in the form of identifying a new other—or at least making her more uncomfortably visible if she has self-identified as being different, as did Kris House and Karen Mist. Moreover, as witnessed when the Minnesota direct-entry midwives drafted their licensing rules and regulations, persuasive strategies that are effective in public debate might not reflect the diverse ideologies and needs of a community. The direct-entry midwives willing to place breeches and twins on the contraindications list for midwifery care to gain the right to suture, administer pitocin, and perform episiotomies knew that this move did not reflect the abilities and preferences of all midwives. A rhetor who successfully resists the dominant discourse might sacrifice an essential part of her personal or group ideology. This resistance might come in the form of achieving rhetorical status by hiding or discounting some aspect of the special knowledge held by a dominated group.

Third, the MSAG and LRWG public hearings introduce us to a distinct genre: the licensing rules and regulations created by state agencies to regulate a profession. The conventions of this genre define professional jurisdictions and designate hierarchical positions and surveillance strategies. These conventions protect the incumbent profession because that profession is most likely to supervise and limit the newly professionalized field. The genre conventions support the dominant profession's prior standing by excluding or limiting the knowledge systems of the emerging profession. A practice that thrives on autonomy, such as direct-entry midwifery, conflicts with these genre conventions so strongly that practitioners might forgo or never achieve the professionalization they desire. Thus far, our genre theories tend to focus on how genres are created to solve a community problem and to indoctrinate a new member into that community's discourse. We assume that resistance to the conventions of genre indicate important changes within a community or new directions that community decides to take. We do not know fully to what extent a genre silences either those rhetors within the community or those seeking entrance, or to what extent a genre formally assigns dominant roles to community members by these normalizing conventions. This study offers an illustrative case of one discourse community's resistance to a genre and demonstrates how community members' willingness to accept the conventions of that genre might vary greatly.

Fourth, collaborative processes that grant equal rhetorical standing to all voices, such as the equal authority accorded to all participants in the Minnesota hearings, may only work temporarily if the participants have differing professional and social statuses. Given the wide representation on LRWG of physicians, nurses, nurse-midwives, home birth parents, and direct-entry midwives, the process still failed to produce a draft that would survive the scrutiny of those medical organizations and groups that LRWG members represented. Members of LRWG were expected to reach consensus on the licensing rules and employed the shared-document collaborative process to do so. This expectation of consensus seems to mirror the conventions of the licensing genre itself, in which all licensed practitioners must meet the same requirements, all must follow the same protocols, and all must be disciplined for the same transgressions. However, what seems a way to achieve consensus might obscure or postpone inevitable conflict, conflict that might reveal nonnegotiable limits on the product of that collaboration.

Fifth, the study of MSAG and LRWG offers another example of women's complex relationship to the social construction of scientific and technological knowledge systems. The experiential knowledge of the direct-entry midwives, from their confidence and willingness to attend twin and breech births at home and their skill in suturing and performing episiotomies, to their understanding of the fabric of a woman's life, as Connie Baker called it, suggest the uneasy relationship between women's experiential and embodied knowledge and medical knowledge about women's bodies. Legal access to science and technology are claimed by the dominant professional jurisdictions, and, to a great extent, our society has assigned ownership of the science and technology of birth to modern medicine. Midwifery care, as defined over the last two centuries, involves attendance at the normal birth—or, as spelled out in the last draft of the LRWG licensing rules, "without medical care." Direct-entry midwives would prefer to avoid intervening in the natural birth process because, to many home birth mothers and their midwives, intervention through birth instruments and procedures produces iatrogenic problems. However, many of these same direct-entry midwives also seek legal access to scientific and technological tools and procedures when they need them to address emergencies, to screen out high-risk mothers, and to avoid transporting mothers to the hospital for procedures such as suturing. Despite their lack of formal education, many direct-entry midwives have developed skills to attend certain high-risk conditions through direct experience and birth stories, have learned to suture and perform episiotomies from sister midwives, and have acquired drugs such as pitocin from friendly physicians.

Some direct-entry midwives argue that carrying pitocin and suturing are as essential to their practice as wearing latex gloves when examining a mother and delivering an infant—they demand their right to have legal access to such tools. They argue that, without their success in delivering breech babies vaginally, women would have no option other than cesarean section.

Finally, direct-entry midwives describe the personal power, gained through the home birth experience, and they celebrate women's distinct role in procreation. Although, theoretically, we might shy away from so directly linking women's gender identity to their involvement in birth, these midwives do not. We must acknowledge that direct-entry midwives perceive that their and their clients' sense of womanhood and personal power may be best realized through giving birth, through connecting with their bodies through pregnancy. Given this dedication to midwifery and women's empowerment, what choices did the key players in the Minnesota story make at the end of the public hearings in 1995? How were they affected by the outcome?

Having experienced burnout and suffering from decreasing numbers, the guild voted to discontinue much of its political work. Midwives such as Connie Baker, who had long functioned within the guild, became less active and remained unsure of whether licensing was the best solution for Minnesota midwives or whether NARM certification was necessary. Rita Ortiz finished her course in nurse-midwifery and began practice in a local hospital. Mary Emerson left her position as a guild lobbyist to pursue another career. To some extent, the number of guild midwives shrank because uniform protocols and required participation in peer review and reporting statistics seemed a condition of lobbying: "In short, it has been determined that even if we have only a handful of people left—at least that makes the work of lobbying more honest," reported the guild in the July 1997 MANA newsletter (Dixon 13). "How do we justify it otherwise? Very hard stuff, when we all wish we could just sit around sharing birth stories and being a 'sisterhood'"(13). The legal climate seemed particularly threatening at the same time that the guild faced exhaustion. A report in the January 1998 MANA newsletter mentioned that a representative from the Minnesota County Attorney's Association wanted midwives "to be charged with a felony" (Dixon 9). A few months later, the Minnesota Attorney General's office began an investigation of two direct-entry midwives, and the Board of Medical Practice sought legislative relief from its obligation to license the state's direct-entry midwives. Despite these threats to their practice, direct-entry midwives Elizabeth Smith and Julie Dylan became Certified Professional Midwives and were instrumental in creating the Minnesota Council of Certified Professional Midwives. The organization, replacing the Minnesota Midwives' Guild, was created to focus on peer review, educational programs, a midwife defense fund, and political action. However, these Minnesota midwives hoped that they could eventually turn over their legal battle to a consumer organization in the form of the Minnesotans for Midwifery. This organization hosted a picnic for 175 people on May 5, 1998 in the capitol rotunda. Governor Arne Carlson offered his support by signing a proclamation to honor midwives, and at the rally Senator Sandra Pappas read the proclamation and urged political action to preserve midwifery.

Hope for Minnesota direct-entry midwives results from another bill sponsored by state Senator Pappas. Bill SF0383 passed in the Senate on April 15, 1999, by a vote of 61 to 1, and, then passed in the House a few days later. Although Governor Jesse Ventura did not sign the bill, he allowed it to pass into law in January 2000. The law will finally provide a way for the state's direct-entry midwives to become licensed. However, the law will limit direct-entry midwifery to providing care for "those women who are expected to have a normal pregnancy, labor, and delivery,"; normalcy would be determined by a series of screening tests. This screening will be required, and direct-entry midwives will be forbidden to treat any client who refused the tests. Moreover, each licensed midwife will be required to have a written medical consultation plan. Finally, each client must have to sign an informed consent form that specifies the dangers of home birth:

> We realize that there are risks associated with home birth, including the risk of death or disability of either mother or child. We understand that a situation may arise, which requires emergency medical care and that it may not be possible to transport the mother and/or baby to the hospital in time to benefit from such care. We fully accept the outcome and consequences of our decision to have a traditional midwife attend us during pregnancy and at our birth. We realize that our traditional midwife is not licensed to practice medicine. We are not seeking a licensed physician or certified nurse midwife as the primary caregiver for this pregnancy, and we understand that our midwife shall inform us of any observed signs or symptoms of disease, which may require evaluation, care, or treatment by a medical practitioner. We agree that we are totally responsible for obtaining qualified medical assistance for the care of any disease or pathological condition.

Although the law does not allow direct-entry midwives to perform emergency episiotomies, it does allow them to administer oxygen and postpartum antihemorrhagic drugs such as pitocin and to suture first- and second-degree perineal lacerations. Although every three years each licensed midwife must pass thirty hours of continuing education, as approved by the Board of Medical Practice, the law recognizes the NARM exam as an acceptable initial licensing exam. And, although breeches and twins are not mentioned as either sanctioned or contraindicated for home birth, the law refers the reader to the Minnesota Midwives' Guild's *Standards of Care and Certification Guide* for more specific information on normal and abnormal conditions. Finally, a midwifery advisory board, dominated by direct-entry midwives and home birth parents, will distribute information on midwifery practice standards and advise the board on enforcement issues. Thus, the law sponsored by Senator Pappas, herself a home birth parent, will enable those Minnesota direct-entry midwives who pass the NARM exam, and are willing and able to form a relationship with the medical community for screening and backup, to become licensed. Those who reject these restrictions will continue to practice underground.

The margin by which the bill passed the Senate was the result of intense personal lobbying of legislators by the midwives and the Minnesotans for Midwifery organization. When seated across the table from physicians, nurses, and nurse-midwives, during the portion of the story that this book covers, the direct-entry midwives sought professional power to celebrate their knowledge about birth and to expand their practices, and, at least temporarily, gained the rhetorical status to do so within the public hearings. They did so understanding that they must enter a public sphere within a patriarchal system and encounter professionals, whether they be men or women, who have accepted restricted or limited status within that system and may demand that new professionals do so too. Many of the direct-entry midwives involved in the Minnesota hearings perceived a highly gendered system of the professions. We must acknowledge that, because of that perception, the efforts of direct-entry midwives and their home birth clients to legitimize midwifery within the system of the professions will continue to be fraught with the challenges and complexities of the centuries-old rhetorical struggle over gender and power and the validity of differing knowledge systems.

APPENDIX A

Additional Notes on Methodology and Sources

The Genesis of this Project

I came to this project by accident—a lucky one, that is. I showed up early to meet a friend for dinner who was attending a set of public hearings on midwifery. And so, I sat in on Rachel Waters's testimony on the Minnesota Obstetrics Management Initiative and the first part of Rita Ortiz's story of how she came to midwifery. I had just joined the Department of Rhetoric and become an affiliate of the Center for Advanced Feminist Studies at the University of Minnesota. I was eager to find a research study that would build upon my dual interest in the rhetoric of science and technology and feminist studies. The hearings would provide a chance to do a rhetorical study of the debates surrounding the highly gendered community of direct-entry midwives. Also, I had access to a wealth of information—the hearings were open to the public, and the Board of Medical Practice recorded the testimony and was quite willing to loan audiotapes to me, which I then transcribed.

Two colleagues joined me in the first part of this project as we analyzed the testimony offered during the Midwifery Study Advisory Group hearings. That joint effort resulted in a 1996 *Quarterly Journal of Speech* article. When I learned that the proposed legislation based on the first set of recommendations had failed, I decided to go on with the project, this time alone, and not only transcribed the tapes of the Licensing Rule Writing Group but also attended each hearing to understand better the major players and their interactions. Thus, I started my own apprenticeship in midwifery.

As I had not had a child myself, let alone delivered one, I had to learn a whole new culture, including the terms, the ideologies, the history, and the current challenges in order to appreciate the hearings. For example, I had to learn how an episiotomy might be avoided, the differences between degrees of perineal tearing, the risks of vaginal birth after cesarean section (VBAC), and the uses of pitocin, from the points of view of two discourse communities, the medical community and the direct-entry midwifery community, who had different authoritative knowledge systems about birth. However these two knowledge systems were defined publicly, I realized that I also had to avoid essentializing these communities, as it was clear that individual physicians and midwives often held different opinions on such matters.

Until the Board of Medical Practice suspended the hearings for the first time in August of 1994, I sat in the back of the hearings and wrote verbatim what seemed essential testimony, as at times the audio recordings were muffled, and took notes to help me identify voices on the recordings. I became a familiar figure to a few hearing participants, particularly the ones who had attended my early public presentation of the *QJS* article at the Humphrey Institute at the University of Minnesota, and to the Board of Medical Practice staff members who loaned me the audiotapes and kindly ensured that I got copies of all licensing rule drafts. For the majority of participants, I had developed no ethos, no credibility, but when it became clear that events outside of the hearings had led to their August 1994 suspension, I needed to consult with participants on a face-to-face basis. I asked similar questions of each rhetor; for example, I asked each midwife how she came to midwifery, and I asked each person whether she would support licensing of traditional midwifery, given the latest licensing rule draft. However, I hesitate to call these consultations interviews. Their purpose was not to gather and compare data or to trace trends; instead, they were to help me understand the nature of the conversations and decisions that took place outside the public hearings or to learn the motivation and rhetorical strategies of statements made in the public hearings. Although at times I add a clarifying statement from these information conversations, my analysis focuses on the public testimony and the documents generated by that testimony. All members with whom I consulted kindly helped me understand, from their points of view, the events and conflicts outside the hearings that manifested themselves within the public discussions. As I was now a familiar addition to the hearings when they reconvened several months later, the members of the Minnesota Midwives' Guild invited me to attend a strategy meeting and a peer review session. Such opportunities allowed me to more fully understand this community, which up to this point, had chosen to remain underground. It also became quite clear to me that the rhetorical strategies used by guild representatives in the public hearings were often carefully selected and practiced in these private guild meetings. Even though the Minnesota hearings were open to the public and all testimony became a matter of public record, I have used pseudonyms for all hearing participants because some direct-entry midwives continue to practice underground. This strategy encompasses not only the public testimony but also the consultations I had with key rhetors at the public hearings and the letters and other written statements I received to help me understand the philosophies and motivations of those who testified. Whenever I decided to quote directly from these conversations outside the public hearings, I requested the permission of the speaker and allowed her to review those quoted statements and, in a few cases, alter specific words in order to clarify her thinking or mask her identity. However, in some cases, I have had to include certain identifying features, such as country of origin, professional affiliation, and source of the testimony. Although I am sure that the Minnesota home birth community and the specific medical organizations may recognize their colleagues, their identities will not be known to the larger reading public. I have retained the real names of midwives and other key figures who published their thoughts in more formal sources, such as *MANA News,* so that the reader who wishes might find her way back to these documents.

During both the Minnesota hearings, the midwives often referred to activities in other states to support their arguments that midwives should be entitled to access to drugs or granted permission to perform certain procedures or they warned that particular restrictions had not worked well in other states. To understand their arguments, I joined the Midwives' Association of North America (MANA) and began receiving such publications as the *MANA News* and *Midwifery Today,* which placed these arguments within a broader context. Also, I obtained the licensing rules of all states in which midwifery is legally permitted and a sampling of those states in which it is outlawed. Finally, as it became clear that it was essential to place the Minnesota story into a national context—that the same conversations were occurring elsewhere and therefore my findings could be generalized, I become a lurker on the Midwifery listserv at midwife@fensende.com. At the time of my study, the listserv was maintained by Sabrina, a childbirth educator in Palo Alto, California, and major domo, an automated listserver. A lurker, of course, does not contribute to or affect the conversation. However, at one point, I needed clarification about midwifery laws in other states and so I posted a request that was answered by a member of MANA. My posting made clear to the listserv participants that a researcher was reading their postings; no participant protested. However, the listserv participants were well aware that the listserv had attracted lurkers and worried that some might trace postings in order to pursue legal action against midwives operating illegally in some states. To preserve the anonymity of the listserv participants, I have given them all pseudonyms (even though they themselves might already be using pseudonyms) and noted just the date when they posted their message, and, in some cases, their affiliation to midwifery (for example, "a CNM who does home births in the state of Indiana"); I include no last names or e-mail addresses. I use the postings as texts to confirm or generalize about the practices and philosophies of midwives rather than observing the behavior of subjects using the particular communication medium of the listserv (see the fair practice and privacy guidelines I followed as noted in Gurak 138–139). Finally, in quoting from this listserv, to preserve the tone of the discussions, I seldom corrected spelling, grammar, or punctuation errors; I inserted a [sic] only for the most glaring errors. In some cases, I placed in square brackets a definition of an abbreviation or medical term within the message.

Finally, I want to remark on the interdisciplinary nature of this project and explain my choices in presenting the findings. My initial intention was to study what Michel Foucault called a local center of a power-knowledge relationship (*Sexuality* 52), as I mention in chapter 1, and to inform Foucault's theories by studying a gendered discourse community. I also had read Andrew Abbott's fine book on the system of the professions but had noticed that gender, and certainly women's experiential knowledge, did not figure into his theories or cases. To understand fully the Minnesota hearings and texts, I gained additional expertise in current rhetorical theory, such as genre studies; to appreciate the history of the midwifery community, I recovered some primary historical documents and read thoroughly the many excellent secondary sources on this history; to analyze the ideologies in current home birth and midwifery communities, I studied the recent tensions among feminist theorists and postmodernists about the nature of experience and the social construction of woman; to understand the opposition to midwifery among medical practitioners, I explored the research on professionalism and the nature of expertise and authoritative knowledge; and to understand the significance of science and technology within the Minnesota hearings, I probed the recent research in both rhetorical theory and feminist theory on the social construction of science. Thus, the analysis contained within this book is highly interdisciplinary.

Finally, I debated as to whether to present my findings as an argument or as a narrative. In the end, I decided that the story was of such significance, that the ways in which the Minnesota hearings progressed were so important, and that the personal voices of the rhetors were so vivid, that, to a great extent, the narrative must carry the argument, rather than simply presenting the narrative as evidence to support conclusions. The home birth and midwifery community has been little understood by scholars who have not read the secondary material and has been invisible to the majority of the general public. When I shared the subject of this project with my family and both my academic and social communities, they would usually respond with surprise that midwives still existed, that home birth was not illegal, and that women might choose to birth in a setting where prescription pain medications and sophisticated monitoring technologies were not readily and immediately available. So I wanted to avoid letting my scholarly analysis overshadow the voices and stories coming from one of the few public conversations between midwives and medical practitioners. However, this project is a case study, with all the richness of detail usually present in this method of gathering and analyzing data. So for those readers interested in the specifics of my information sources, I provide the final section of this appendix.

Sources of Information

- Legislative rules and actions that preceded and followed the public hearings, in particular Minnesota statute 148.30-32, Minnesota Board of Medical policy 5600.2000, and the legislation presented by Minnesota State Senators Sandra Pappas and Carol Flynn and House Representative Kay Brown.
- Transcriptions of Midwifery Study Advisory Group hearings in which the regulatory options for direct-entry midwives in Minnesota were discussed (October 23, 1991; November 7, 1991; November 22, 1991; December 3, 1991; January 8, 1991; April 29, 1992; and May 11, 1992). My observational notes of the November 7, 1991 public hearing.
- The final report of the Advisory Group, written by the Minnesota Department of Health, Health Occupations Program, and presented to the Minnesota Board of Medical Practice on June 1, 1992.
- Informal conversations with the chair of the public hearings and with the executive director of the Board of Medical Practice, the past president of the

Minnesota Midwives' Guild, and the lobbyist for the Guild after an early analysis of the public hearings. A conversation with the executive director of the Board of Medical Practice before the final public hearing (1 June 15, 1995).

- Observational notes on and transcriptions of all public hearings that pertained specifically to the licensing rules as convened by the Board of Medical Practice (December 1, 1993; January 13, 1994; February 15, 1994; April 21, 1994; June 21, 1994; July 28, 1994; August 30, 1994; March 28, 1995; and June 15, 1995). Observational notes and minutes from the Minnesota Board of Medical Practice meeting on November 23, 1996, at which the Minnesota Midwives' Guild defended the NARM exam.

- Text of the five drafts of the licensing rules that emerged during the discussions of the rule writing group. Text of other licensing rules and regulations produced by the Board of Medical Practice, whose boilerplate language appeared in the midwifery rules drafts.

- An in-depth consultation with the Board of Medical Practice staff member who drafted the five versions of the licensing rules. Notes of this staff member's phone conversations and letters that preceded the controversial August 10, 1994, meeting of the rule writing group, when the group was suspended for six months.

- Twelve in-depth consultations (eleven face-to-face and one long distance) between September 1994 and January 1995 with key members of the rule writing group: five members of the Minnesota Midwives' Guild; two non-Guild midwives; the lobbyist for the Guild; two nurses; one nurse-midwife; and one physician. These members represented various organizations, such as the Minnesota chapter of the American College of Nurse-Midwifery, the Minnesota Medical Association (Ob/Gyn), the Minnesota Midwives' Guild, and the Minnesota Nursing Association. The Minnesota Midwives' Guild also invited me to attend a strategy meeting and a peer review session.

- Text of the rules of all other states that license, certify, or register direct-entry midwives in the United States and a sampling of the states that outlaw direct-entry midwifery.

- Texts from the public, nonmoderated, noncopyrighted listserv of direct-entry and certified nurse-midwives, midwife@fensende. com, in the summer and fall of 1996, and documents offered on individual midwives' World Wide Web home pages. In May 1996, there were 168 direct-entry midwives, CNMs, physicians, home birth parents, and others who were members of midwife@fensende.com. They were located throughout the United States as well as in Canada, New Zealand, England, Germany, and Australia. Organizations such as MANA and journals such as *Midwifery Today* had representatives who contributed to this public listserv.

Glossary of Birth Terms

This appendix defines the birth terms essential to understanding the Minnesota midwifery public hearings, the legal statutes, and the listserv communications included in this study. It is not meant to be inclusive of all birth conditions or as detailed as a medical dictionary or birth manual. Instead, it should give the reader an understanding of the conditions of pregnancy, labor, and birth that concerned participants in the midwifery hearings and some of the possible medical and midwifery ways to respond to those conditions.

Asphyxia   Decrease in the amount of oxygen and increase in the amount of carbon dioxide in the body as caused by interference with respiration. The baby suffering asphyxia would need to be resuscitated.

Bi-manual compression   Used to control bleeding by placing one hand externally on top of the uterus and inserting one hand into the vagina and up against the uterus and then pressing the two hands together.

Breech birth   The biggest risk with breech birth occurs when the baby's body is born and its head is too large to deliver. In **frank breech** births, the baby emerges bottom first with the legs extended upwards over the chest. In **complete breech** births, the legs are up and crossed. A mother may be successful in helping her baby turn to **vertex** with postural tilting or lying with her hips elevated. An experienced midwife may try to turn the baby who persisted in the breech position by external version. However, as Elizabeth Davis comments, external version "requires great expertise in fetal palpation and a highly refined sense of touch" (67). Although physicians also attempt external version, an alternative to assisting a mother whose baby is known to be in a breech position would be cesarean section. In the home birth setting, midwives must be prepared to handle the occasional surprise breech or transport quickly to the hospital.

Contracted pelvis   A shortened pelvis that impedes delivery of the baby.

Cord prolapse The umbilical cord may become compressed by the baby's head as the baby descends. Cord prolapse affects the flow of blood to the baby, and fetal heart tones often indicate that the baby is suffering this problem. Repositioning the mother and administering oxygen might correct the problem at home or the mother might need to be transported to the hospital immediately.

Deelee (or DeLee) suction The DeLee trap is a suction device used to remove mucus or meconium from the newborn's mouth. The trap consists of a piece of tube that is inserted into the baby's mouth and that leads into a container or trap; the caregiver sucks on a second piece of tube and that also leads into the container.

Effacement The shortening and softening of the cervix as the baby descends and puts pressure on the lower uterine tissues. An indication that the woman is in labor.

Episiotomy Incision of the perineum during labor to avoid tearing of the perineum or to aid in the immediate delivery of a baby in distress.

Eye prophylaxis A newborn's eyes are usually treated with antibacterial drops, such as erythromycin, penicillin, or silver nitrate, a few hours after birth.

Fetal heart tones (FHT) Normally a baby's heart beats from 120 to 160 beats per minute. The caregiver might use a Doppler, fetal monitor, or sonogram to track the baby's heartbeat during pregnancy and delivery.

Fibroma A fibroid tumor in the uterus.

Fillet A birth instrument invented about the same time as the forceps. The fillet consisted of a strip of silk or leather which would be looped over the fetal head and secured at each end of a handle to form a noose to pull the child out.

Forceps A birth instrument invented by the Chamberlen family of England in the early 1700s. The two blades of the forceps were used to grasp the baby's head and pull it out. Similar birth instruments included the **vectis**, which had a single blade; the **fillet**, which had a loop to fit over the fetal head; blunt **hooks** to bring down the child's thighs in a breech delivery; **crotchets and knives** to puncture the dead child's head; and the **speculum matricis** to dilate the vagina so that the surgeon or male midwife could cut out obstructions (Wilson 65; Wertz and Wertz 34).

Hemorrhage Can be **intrapartum** (during labor) or **postpartum** (after delivery). Intrapartum bleeding is often caused by placenta praevia and placental abruption. After the birth of the baby and before the delivery of the placenta, hemorrhage might be caused by partial placental separation, cervical lacerations, and vaginal tears (Davis 141). After the delivery of the placenta, hemorrhage might be caused by the uterus lacking tone (uterine atony), retained placental fragments, or sequestered clots (Davis 143–144). Various measures to address hemorrhage include nipple stimulation to cause the uterus to contract; administration of pitocin, tincture of angelica, or methergine; bi-manual compression; or manual removal of the placenta.

Hep lock   Heparin is an anticoagulant produced by the liver. A "lock" or "block" would help control bleeding during delivery.

Iatrogenic   Referring to problems caused by a caregiver's words or actions.

Incompetent cervix   A cervix that opens during the second trimester of pregnancy and allows the premature baby to be born. Caused by trauma to the cervix and often treated by sewing the cervix closed until labor begins.

Inversion of the uterus   Turning the uterus inside out by pulling on the umbilical cord in an attempt to deliver the placenta. Such action can lead to the death of the mother.

Malpresentation   A general term that includes breech births in which the baby emerges bottom first with the legs extended upwards over the chest (frank breech) or the legs up and crossed (complete breech), **footlings** in which the baby's legs emerge first, **transverse lie** in which the baby lies horizontally to the birth canal, and shoulder dystocia when the baby's head has emerged but its shoulder becomes stuck behind the mother's pubic bone. Even though one twin might be in the easy vertex position, the second may be malpresented. Turning a baby by repositioning the mother and by manual manipulation by the caregiver is called **version**.

Meconium   The baby's first bowel movement. If aspirated by the baby during delivery, meconium can cause respiratory problems.

Methergine   A drug used to stop postpartum hemorrhage, and, during the Minnesota midwifery hearings, considered more effective but more risky than pitocin.

Multiple gestation   More than one baby in the womb. During the midwifery hearings in Minnesota, much debate centered around direct-midwives' ability and home birth parents' desire to deliver "breeches and twins" at home. The risks involve **cord prolapse**, particularly if one of the babies is in the breech position, **placental abruption**, and **postpartum hemorrhage**.

Ophthalmia neonatorum   Severe conjunctivitis in a newborn.

Perineal tears (degrees)   Tearing of the mass of tissue, muscle, and skin between the vagina and rectum. Tearing can be measured in degrees—with first degree the least severe and fourth degree the most severe; in fourth-degree tears, not only the skin but also the muscles tear all the way to the anal sphincter. (Some caregivers rate tears from first- to third-degree only). Slight tearing (first degree) may heal without suturing, but severe tearing (second through fourth) requires repair. Midwives often try to help the mother avoid tearing by lubricating the perineum and gradually stretching the tissue through massage.

Pitocin   A synthetic form of **oxytocin**, which is the hormone in women that causes uterine contractions at the onset of labor. Pitocin may be administered in a hospital setting to start or speed up labor. Also, pitocin may be used in hospital or home births (where permitted) to control extreme postpartum hemorrhage, particularly due to lack of tone and contraction in the uterus, as the woman recovers from labor.

Placental abruption   Premature separation of the placenta, caused by cord entanglement, preeclampsia, or other physical trauma. If the abruption occurs late in pregnancy or early in delivery, it can be fatal to the mother and baby. If it occurs just before delivery, the mother and baby can often survive.

Placenta praevia   The placenta is implanted low in the uterus. The first symptom of placenta praevia might be bleeding, as small portions of the placenta detach and are shed. If the placenta totally or partially covers the cervical area, then a cesarean section is required. Vaginal delivery might still be possible if the placenta lies close to the cervical area but does not cover it, although the mother must be watched for excessive bleeding.

Preeclampsia (and eclampsia)   Preeclampsia causes high blood pressure, protein in the urine, and other symptoms in pregnant women. If left untreated, preeclampsia can evolve into eclampsia, which causes convulsions and coma and can cause death. Women who have experienced preeclampsia in previous pregnancies have a 25 to 50 percent chance of developing the condition again (Carlson, Eisenstat, and Ziporyn 498). Women with this condition are carefully monitored, and their labor is often induced as soon as the fetus is viable.

Prolonged rupture of the membranes (PROM)   When more than twenty-four hours pass between the time the mother's "water breaks" and the onset of labor and delivery of her baby, risk of infection increases so dramatically that labor is often induced.

Puerperium   Period following the third stage of labor until the pelvic organs return to normal (three to six weeks).

RhoGam   The anti-antigen administered to a mother whose Rh factor is negative and her baby's is positive. RhoGam prevents isoimmunization, a condition produced when the mother manufactures antibodies against the baby's positive cells and causes anemia in the infant.

Shoulder dystocia   This birth complication occurs when the baby's head has been birthed, but the baby's anterior shoulder is stuck behind the mother's public bone. The baby's chest may become compressed, so that the baby suffers brain damage or death. A midwife who feels comfortable continuing to assist in the delivery of the baby may ask the mother to change her position to loosen the pelvis and may try to maneuver the baby with her hands and fingers or dislodge the shoulder by exerting pressure from behind the baby's shoulder.

Suturing   Perineal tears and episiotomies may be sutured rather than allowed to heal on their own. Midwives such as Ina May Gaskin assume that experienced midwives are able to repair first- and second-degree tears (*Spiritual Midwifery* 377). Suturing involves stitching the wound closely with or without the administration of local anesthetic.

Twilight sleep   A condition induced by a combination of morphine and scopolamine, introduced in 1914 to give laboring women relief from pain and block the memory of giving birth (Rooks 22).

Vacuum extractor   A device that uses a suction cup attached to the fetus's head to add traction during delivery.

Vaginal birth after cesarean section (VBAC)   Mothers frequently were told in the past that once they had a cesarean section, they must deliver all subsequent babies through this surgery, because the conditions that prevented vaginal delivery, such as "failure to progress" or small pelvic structures, would persist. Classical or vertical incisions, which were common in the past, were inclined to rupture during subsequent labors and deliveries. However, bikini-line or horizontal incisions, which are now the norm, are unlikely to rupture, and many midwives are willing to work with the mother to overcome some of the conditions that led to the initial cesarean.

Vectis   A birth instrument invented about the same time as the forceps. The vectis consisted of a single blade curved to fit around and rotate the fetus's head.

Version   Turning the fetus into the head down or vertex position by manually manipulating it through the mother's abdominal wall. Instruments such as the forceps also provide the needed traction to turn the child to the feet or to perform **podalic version**.

Rhetors Involved in the Minnesota Hearings and Chronology of the Hearings

Because the Minnesota hearings are complicated not only by the number of participants, representing a variety of discourse communities, but also by the different drafts and documents that emerged, this appendix offers a list of those participants and a brief chronology of the Midwifery Study Advisory Group (MSAG) and Licensing Rule Writing Group (LRWG) hearings. All participants have been assigned pseudonyms except for the representatives from the Department of Health, Tom Hiendlmayr, and the executive director for the Board of Medical Practice, Leonard Boche. Because his name appears on official documents, I also did not assign a pseudonym to Phillip McAfee, the policy analyst who worked with LRWG in the first hearings; the board staff member who assumed McAfee's responsibility consented to a face-to-face consultation and therefore I have given her the pseudonym of Jessica Ramsey.

Rhetors within the Direct-Entry Midwifery Community Who Participated in Minnesota Hearings

Mary Emerson, who was president of the International Cesarean Awareness Network/Cesarean Prevention Movement of Southwest Minnesota, a home birth parent, and lobbyist for the guild, gave the opening testimony in the MSAG hearings. Emerson used the rhetorical strategy of boundary spanning to establish a positive image of midwifery knowledge and the guild midwife. During the LRWG hearings in the summer of 1994, Emerson saw that, although it might be difficult for the direct-entry midwives to hear, the licensing rules and regulations process was not working, as the medical community lobbied for its suspension.

GUILD MEMBERS

Rita Ortiz was a key rhetor during the MSAG and LRWG hearings. She gave testimony for the guild during the November 7, and 22, 1991, MSAG hearings. Ortiz learned midwifery during the 1970s birth movement and helped found the Minnesota Midwives' Guild. Ortiz expressed political awareness of how direct-entry midwives would have to accept normalization of their practices with professionalization.

Gloria Olson was a guild midwife who was uncertain of the rhetorical strategies used by Emerson and Ortiz before MSAG and argued to include breeches and twins in the licensing rules and regulations produced by LRWG.

Connie Baker had experience with midwifery in other countries, such as South America, and worried about the loss of diversity that she feared would accompany professionalization of direct-entry midwifery. Baker offered an extensive sewing metaphor to distinguish between midwifery and medical care. Baker herself gave birth at the Farm and learned much about midwifery practice there.

Julia Dylan began in the guild as an apprentice midwife and eventually moved into a leadership position. Dylan was a strong supporter of licensing but also requested that standards of practice include the ability to carry pitocin, perform episiotomies, and other such controversial procedures as a tradeoff for giving up the ability to deliver twins and breeches at home. Dylan also had substantial knowledge of the licensing rules and regulations in other states and how these rules affected the actual practices of direct-entry midwives.

Elizabeth Smith served her apprenticeship with the guild and, along with Julia Dylan, was a strong supporter of licensing. During LRWG, she and Dylan requested that the direct-entry midwives be given legal sanction to carry pitocin, perform episiotomies, and suture.

NON-GUILD MEMBERS

Karen Mist and Kris House often worked together to support home birth parents within their Christian fellowship community. They testified before the December 3, 1991, MSAG hearing, and House was an active participant in the LRWG hearings.

Greta Godwin fought before LRWG to include breeches and twins in the scope of practice of direct-entry midwifery. Godwin did not function in the Christian fellowship community, as did Mist and House, but also did not favor licensing or state surveillance of direct-entry midwifery.

Rhetors within the Medical Community Who Participated in Minnesota Hearings

Rachel Waters, a pathologist in the Department of Laboratory Medicine, Pathology, and Ob/Gyn at the University of Minnesota, testified about the Minnesota Obstetrics Management Initiative or MOMI project on November 7, 1991, before the MSAG group. The MOMI project identified and ranked twenty-five thousand risk factors in pregnancy.

Judy Miller, a physician, played a major role in the LRWG hearings. She represented the American College of Obstetrics and Gynecology and the Minnesota Ob/Gyn Society and often referred to the opinions of these organizations when she spoke before LRWG.

Emma Davidson, a nurse, represented the Minnesota Nurses' Association and cautioned the LRWG participants several times that the medical community would be uncomfortable with the scope of practice of direct-entry midwifery as defined in the emerging licensing rules and regulations.

Henrietta Kramer, a nurse-midwife, in the April 21, 1994, LRWG meeting, presented an extensive list of contraindications for home birth, including breeches and twins. Kramer represented the Twin Cities chapter of the American College of Nurse Midwives and kept in frequent touch with Emma Davidson during the LRWG hearings.

Elaine English, a nurse, representing the Board of Nursing, infrequently attended LRWG meetings until the summer of 1994 when she publicly warned the direct-entry midwives that their request for legal access to birth technologies would jeopardize their licensing efforts.

Rhetors Representing State Agencies during the Minnesota Hearings

DEPARTMENT OF HEALTH

Tom Hiendlmayr participated in the MSAG hearings and wrote the final report on behalf of MSAG.

BOARD OF MEDICAL PRACTICE

Leonard Boche, executive director of the Board of Medical Practice, attended the initial meetings of MSAG and LRWG and suspended the LRWG hearings on August 30, 1994, and June 5, 1995.

Joan Montgomery, a former citizen member of the board, chaired the MSAG discussions and the majority of LRWG hearings. Montgomery led the LRWG participants in the August 30, 1994, meeting to recognize that the rule writing process had met too much opposition from the medical community to survive.

Phillip McAfee, a policy analyst with the board, responded to the letter from the assistant Steele Country attorney who challenged the board to regulate the direct-entry midwives in weighing the board's options. At his urging, the Board created the LRWG. He was replaced very early during the LRWG hearings by Jessica Ramsey.

Jessica Ramsey, a board staff member, has a nursing degree and is also a lawyer. She drafted all but the first of the licensing rules and regulations drafts for LRWG, served as an informal co-chair at several hearings, interpreted the conventions of the genre for LRWG participants, received reactions from various participants who preferred to express their concerns outside the hearings, fielded reactions from the Minnesota Medical Association, and eventually agreed with other Board members that the rule writing process was not working.

Chronology of the Minnesota Hearings

Midwifery Study Advisory Group (MSAG)
October 23, 1991—organizational meeting of the MSAG group

November 7, 1991—testimony of Rachel Waters and Rita Ortiz

November 22, 1991—continued testimony of Rita Ortiz

December 3, 1991—testimony of Kris House and Karen Mist

January 8, 1991—continued conversations and drafting of the MSAG recommendations

April 29, 1992—continued conversations and drafting of the MSAG recommendations

May 11, 1992—continued conversations and drafting of the MSAG recommendations

LICENSING RULE WRITING GROUP (LRWG)

December 1, 1993—Jessica Ramsey provides the hearing participants with the first draft of the direct-entry midwifery licensing rules and regulations (dated November 30, 1993). The draft, which includes thirteen conditions that would be "unsafe" for home birth, gives the LRWG participants a detailed introduction to the conventions of the licensing rules and regulations genre.

January 13, 1994—Three groups offer drafts of the scope of practice section of the direct-entry midwifery licensing rules and regulations. The Minnesota Midwives' Guild's draft is extensive and based on the guild's *Standards of Care and Certification Guide*. Two physicians submitted drafts—one independently and one representing the American College of Obstetrics and Gynecology and the Minnesota Ob/Gyn Society. Both focus on definitions of normal birth; however, the latter assumes that some published document would contain more specific conditions and contraindications.

February 15, 1994—The second draft is presented to the LRWG participants containing privacy issues that seem to negate birth stories and peer review within the direct-entry midwifery community. The direct-entry midwives resist the "hard line" taken on conduct with clients that seems to negate their close relationships with generations of home birth clients and request that their practice be described in positive terms, resisting the conventions of the genre that focused on disciplinary action and prohibited conduct. Direct-entry midwives participating in the licensing rule writing process wish to foreground the benefits of the midwife forming a relationship with her home birth parents rather than the aspects of practice that would be prohibited by the state and overseen by medical care givers.

April 21, 1994—LRWG again uses the shared-document collaborative writing process to draft a list of contraindications for home birth. The guild members had previously agreed among themselves that they would no longer deliver breeches and twins at home if, by this compromise, they could gain legal access to certain drugs and permission to carry out certain procedures. However, this rhetorical strategy fails, as the direct-entry midwifery community, publicly divided on the issue of breeches and twins and the collaborative process used by LRWG had permitted the conditions to be left within the scope of practice for direct-entry midwifery. The meeting ends with Judy Miller's warning that the licensing process would fail unless breeches and twins were contraindicated for home birth.

June 21, 1994—Minnesota Midwives' Guild members protest the notion of required medical consultation. They propose instead individual midwifery protocols and informed consent agreements between the direct-entry midwife and her client substitute for required medical consultation. The LRWG examines two examples of informed consent—one used by physicians in the hospital setting and one proposed by direct-entry midwives as more reflective of their ideologies and practices. During this meeting, discussion over legal access to birth technologies begins.

July 28, 1994—The meeting of LRWG focuses the direct-entry midwives' legal access to obtain and administer pitocin, a drug effective in stopping postpartum hemorrhage, to perform emergency episiotomies at home, and to suture first- and second-degree perineal tears at home.

August 30, 1994—Given the number of complaints received by the Board of Medical Practice about the content of the emerging licensing rules and regulations, the Board decides to suspend the hearings. In particular, the direct-entry midwives' requests for legal access to the technologies of birth, exclusively claimed by the medical community, so alienated the medical community in Minnesota that the board felt that, based on the August 30, 1994 draft of the rules and regulations, the process would fail. The rules and regulations appearing in the fourth draft produced by LRWG would invite too many objections and not survive the scrutiny of an administrative law judge.

March 28, 1995—The Board of Medical Practice reconvenes LRWG and presents a fifth draft of the licensing rules and regulations. This draft, however, does not contain the special services section that grants midwives the legal right to carry pitocin and oxygen, suture, and perform episiotomies.

June 15, 1995—The Board of Medical Practices suspends LRWG once more when it discovers that licensing fees would far exceed the midwives' ability to pay.

NOTES

CHAPTER 1   *The Current Debate over Direct-Entry Midwifery in the United States*

1. Rita Ortiz offered this testimony to the Midwifery Study Advisory Group, which met in St. Paul, Minnesota, on November 7, 1991. All testimony quoted in this chapter came from that November 1991 hearing, unless otherwise noted. In the past, Rita Ortiz would have been called a traditional or lay midwife, to distinguish her philosophy and practice from that of nurse-midwives. In fact, some of the documents that come out of the Minnesota public hearings and those in other states still use the term traditional midwives. However, Ortiz and her sister midwives usually prefer the term direct entry—indicating that they enter directly into midwifery education and practice, rather than through the discipline of nursing. Although this testimony and that of others is a matter of public record, having been offered during public hearings and recorded for review by the Minnesota Board of Medical Practice and Department of Health, and although the midwifery listserv, which I monitored for several months, is a nonmoderated, public one, I have used pseudonyms throughout this book. See appendix A for a fuller description of my rationale for these choices.
2. Although certain information was communicated to me by key rhetors in the Minnesota debates, again I have preserved the anonymity of these rhetors, including those who participated in the computer listserv.
3. This physician, called Judy Miller in this study, shared this impression with me in personal correspondence on November 17, 1994.
4. Although the terms *midwifery knowledge* and *medical knowledge* might not capture the complexity of these two knowledge systems, they help me avoid overly packed sentences throughout this book. I thank Robbie Davis-Floyd for helping me sort through these complexities and selecting the vocabulary to express them.

CHAPTER 2   *Rhetorical Analysis and the Midwifery Debates*

1. A *metaphor* implies a comparison between two seemingly unlike objects to reveal similarities; an *analogy* also compares items that appear to be quite different in order to develop a sustained thought, such as making the unfamiliar seem familiar, arguing a point, or changing feelings on a subject; an *enthymeme* leaves out the major premise of the traditional syllogism, often to convince readers or listeners that the premise is common

knowledge or an accepted standard; a *definition* places a word or concepts in a general category and then distinguishes that word or concept from others in the same category.

2. See also Winsor, "Constructing" 127; Swales, *Genre;* Latour and Woolgar 55.
3. This comment appeared on a midwifery listserv located at midwife@fensende.com. This listserv provided a means of contextualizing the Minnesota hearings. All listserv communications noted throughout this book originated at this e-mail address. In general, I have not edited these comments for correct spelling and grammatical form but instead have preserved the exact language used in the original message.
4. Olson shared this sense of empowerment with me during a personal consultation outside the public hearings on January 21, 1995.
5. See also Swales 58 and Miller 37.
6. See Treichler 123 for further distinctions between meaning and definition.
7. Freedman and Medway 11; Devitt 613.
8. Testimony offered to the Midwifery Study Advisory Group, November 7, 1991, St. Paul, Minnesota.
9. Threads are strings of messages on one topic, and a flame is a blunt or insulting message that may anger, intimidate, or silence a participant (see, for example, Anderson).
10. A great many scholars have speculated about how women gain or are denied access to computers, express their liking or fear of them, learn how to program or use them, and apply this knowledge to selected activities (see, for example, Davidson, Savenye, and Orr; Durndell; Durndell, Siann, and Glissov; Hall and Cooper; Hawkins; Jessup; Kiesler, Sproull, and Eccles; Kramer and Lehman; Ogletree and Williams; Turkle; Turkle and Papert). Now scholars have begun to focus on how communication on the Internet might be affected by gender. Some speculate that gender, race, and class become invisible, while others conclude that gender bias still exists on the Internet. For example, Dale Spender concludes, "The discourse is male; the style is adversarial" (198), and Nancy Kaplan and Eva Farrell note that ". . . women frequently feel ignored, silenced, even abused in electronic conversations" (np). More specifically, Spender proposes that "males who in real life probably wouldn't dream of butting in on a group of women, appear to have no compunction about posting messages to women-only groups on the net. A significant number of these postings are sexually explicit and abusive" (196).

    When a participant's spouse tried unsuccessfully to "unsubscribe" from the midwifery listserv and inadvertently sent a message to the entire list, under the heading "bumbling idiots," another thread about flaming started. In this thread, one of the male participants, George, speculates that the flamer feels freer to scold females and would not dare do so with a discussion group of men or in a face-to-face setting:

    > WOA . . . Hold on a second, I'm not okay with your communications with this list. Now, I'm not going to call you a so-and-so or insult you either on the list or in email. Basically, anything I say now, or from here on are things I'd say if you were standing infront of me . . .
    >
    > I'm not okay with you abusing people on this list nor am I okay with you telling people, in effect, "Don't post what I sent you" when you have done just that.
    >
    > Let this issue die. You don't need to prove your manhood. (That's not a flame or a swipe at you. You know that status of your manhood, just like you know what your personality and character are, what anyone else may say or think about it doesn't matter because they can't change what it is no matter what they say.)
    >
    > Stop ripping on the midwives on this list.
    >
    > I feel angry and upset that you're abusing the people on this list, specifically you've directed your posts at the women on this list, knock it off, this is not the place for it.

If you have any comments you want to make to me, tell me in email. P.S. If we were a group of men or you were speaking to us face to face I wonder if you'd speak to us the way you've chosen to on-line. (listserv communion, September 14, 1996)

CHAPTER 3   *The Rhetorical History of Midwifery*

1. Historical studies of traditional midwifery include Borst; DeVries; Donegan; Donnison; Kitzinger; Leavitt; Litoff, *Midwife Debate*; Litoff, *American Midwives*; Wertz and Wertz; and Wilson. Other works on the history of medical care and technology often focus or touch on traditional midwifery and include Arms; Arney; Corea; Davis-Floyd; Gross; Martin (*Woman in the Body*); Mitford; Oakley, *Captured*; Romalis; Rothman, *In Labor*; Rothman, *Recreating*; Rowland; and Starr.
2. See also Kramer and Sprenger; Barstow.
3. See, for example, Donegan 25; Donnison 2.
4. Also available to English midwives was a general text in the vernacular, Eucharius Roesslin's *Der Swangern Frawen und Hebammen Rosengarten*, which was translated by Richard Jonas and printed by Thomas Raynalde in 1540 as *The Byrth of Mankynde, Otherwise Named the Womans Booke*.
5. Medical men, such as Percivall Willughby (1596–1685), who criticized female midwives for being illiterate and motivated by money rather than knowledge, also reflect such a combination of beliefs. For example, Willughby's remedy for "flooding" or hemorrhage was a drink made of hog's dung and ashes of toad (Donnison 16).
6. Cellier had earlier entered into public debate by attesting to the harm that war brought to midwives and their clients. Women whose husbands were engaged in Civil War missed "necessary comfort and benevolence," best witnessed by the midwives who attended them. The midwives themselves were "also undone, for as women are helpers unto men, so are we unto women in all their extreamities, for which we were formerly well paid, and highly respected in our parishes for our great skill and mid-night industry, but now our Art doth fail us" ("Just Petition" 1–2).
7. See also Sablosky.
8. See also Smellie, *Treatise* 442.
9. See also Dewees; Millikin.
10. According to Josephine Baker's 1912 report, thirteen states had regulatory laws for midwives; only Utah and Ohio had schools for midwives (see Baker, table 1). Van Blarcom reported in 1914 that American midwives practiced without restriction in thirteen states and that they had no laws about their training in fourteen other states. According to Van Blarcom, midwives in twelve states and the District of Columbia had to pass an examination to receive a license, in six they were restricted to "normal" births, and in seven the "existing state provisions for their regulation are so inadequate as to be practically without effect" (quoted in Litoff, *Midwife Debate* 170). Finally, in New York and Pennsylvania, 1913 legislatures enacted laws that made possible the "adoption of satisfactory systems of licensure, registration and control in these states" (170). In 1912, New York City issued licenses to 1,395 midwives. In a 1923 issue of *JAMA*, Anna Rule offered a more comprehensive breakdown by state of midwifery regulation. She reported that at that time Massachusetts was the one state in which midwives had no legal status. In the other states, physicians were always required to attend abnormal births, but lack of funding generally made control and supervision of the midwife difficult. Rule reported the following about specific states:

- Arizona midwives "shall not give drugs, give injection into birth canal or make internal examinations; shall secure physician for abnormal cases."
- California: "shall not give drugs, use instruments, make internal examinations or give injection into birth canal; shall attend normal cases only; must have specified equipment."
- Alabama required of its midwives "[k]nowledge of midwifery; freedom from communicable disease; moral character."
- Maryland required the "[a]bility to read and write; certificate of physician showing attendance at 5 cases; 3 certificates of character."
- Minnesota required a diploma from school of midwifery or successful completion of an examination.
- New Jersey required graduation from a "common school; certificate or diploma from school of midwifery or maternity hospital having 1,800 hours' instruction, and examination" (988–989).

Rule also reported that "the state health authorities are somewhat perplexed in their effort to find practical means of handling the midwife situation. However, eighteen progressive health departments have already decided that trained, licensed and supervised midwives should be provided at least for rural communities" (990). Rule reminds her readers that regardless of their attitude toward urban midwives, in rural communities in which physicians were scarce, families must depend on traditional midwives.

11. See also Grace Abbott.
12. The Frontier Graduate School of Midwifery was established in 1939 to educate nurse midwives; the American College of Nurse Midwives was founded in 1955.
13. Several studies demonstrated that there was no difference in mortality between hospital and home births and that, indeed, more birth injuries occurred in the hospital; see, for example, Mehl et al.; Sagov and Brodsky.
14. See also Gilgoff for additional birth stories and Davis for similar midwifery techniques.
15. See also Annas 51, 59.

CHAPTER 4   *The Minnesota Midwifery Study Advisory Group:*
Professional Jurisdictions and Boundary Spanning

1. Rita Ortiz shared this statement with me in a consultation outside the Minnesota public hearings on 23 November 1994.
2. Again, I have used pseudonyms for the majority of rhetors quoted in this chapter. However, I have retained the real names of the executive director of the Board of Medical Practice, Leonard Boche, and the representative from the Department of Health, Tom Hiendlmayr. Although the voice of Elizabeth Smith does not appear in this chapter, in the chapters that follow, she plays a key role.
3. A version of this chapter appeared as "The Rhetoric of Midwifery: Conflicts and Conversations in the Minnesota Home Birth Community in the 1990s," written with Billie Wahlstrom and Carol Brown and published in the *Quarterly Journal of Speech* 82 (November 1996): 383–401. Smith shared this comment in a consultation with me outside the Minnesota public hearings on January 13, 1995.
4. All quotations in this section are taken from the October 23, 1991 MSAG hearing, unless otherwise noted.
5. Mary Emerson shared this impression with me in a consulation outside the Minnesota public hearings on November 14, 1994.
6. The theories of Michel Foucault provide an additional framework and vocabulary for

interpreting the rhetorical challenge Mary Emerson undertook. For example, Foucault believed that knowledge and truth about any subject could be negotiated through discourse because power is not located primarily within groups or individuals in opposition to each other, not owned, but instead exercised through relationships. If power is not the privilege of the dominant class, but, as Foucault says, "the overall effect of its strategic positions," then any group challenging the status of another must take into account their own current and potential relationship with the group—"an effect that is manifested and sometimes extended by the position of those who are dominated," as Foucault said (*Discipline* 26–27).

7. See also Smith, *Everyday*; Smith, *Conceptual*; Longino, "In Search"; Longino, "Subjects."

8. In many states, cultural history or economic factors influence the legal status of direct-entry midwifery. Arkansas' General Assembly found that "adequate maternal care is not readily available in some parts of the state resulting in undue hardship to poor expectant mothers" (Arkansas Pt. 100.101). Also, Florida's legislature noted that "access to prenatal care and delivery services is limited by the inadequate number of providers of such services and that the regulated practice of midwifery may help reduce this shortage" (Florida Pt. 467.002). On the other hand, New Mexico and Texas have a long history of direct-entry midwifery within their Hispanic communities. Overall, even in states where direct-entry midwives are legally licensed and home birth encouraged, the number of home births remains quite small. For example, Arkansas reported in July 1995 that the total number of births attended by licensed midwives since 1986 was 1,123, with 130 maternal transports and 22 infant transports (Penn).

9. All quotations in this section are taken from the November 7, 1991 MSAG hearing, unless otherwise noted.

10. All quotations from Ortiz in this section, unless otherwise noted, are taken from the November 7, 1991, and from the November 22, 1991, MSAG hearings.

11. Rita Ortiz shared these comments with me in a consultation outside the Minnesota public hearings on November 23, 1994.

12. See also Nancy Fraser, "False" 71.

13. Feminist scholars have debated to what extent Foucauldian theory is useful in investigating gendered communities and effecting change in patriarchal societies and institutions. (Some of the leading voices in the debate are found in Ramazanoglu's and Diamond and Quinby's collections as well as individual articles and monographs such as Hartsock; Bell; McNay, *Foucault and Feminism*; Benhabib; Sawicki.) For some feminist scholars, because Foucault fails to focus on the disadvantages to women as a gender in societies and institutions, his theories cannot inform feminists' desire to change those societies and institutions. For other feminist scholars, Foucault's focus on the discourse of sexuality connects with feminist concerns with the female body as a site of repression or potential power. And, for other feminist scholars, Foucault's study of how social labels of "normal" and "abnormal" influence groups or individuals to cooperate or resist is useful—a scholarly "camp" in which this book finds a home.

14. All quotations in this section are taken from the December 3, 1991, MSAG hearing, unless otherwise noted.

15. House further explained her journey to midwifery in a consultation with me outside the Minnesota public hearings on January 7, 1995.

16. House offered this definition of screening in a consultation with me outside the Minnesota public hearings on January 7, 1995.

17. Gloria Olson offered these observations in a consultation that took place on January 13, 1995.

18. Greta Godwin offered these observations in a consultation that took place on January 7, 1995.

CHAPTER 5   *Licensing Rules and Regulations:*
Normalizing the Practice of Midwifery

1. Julia Dylan offered this comment in a consultation with me outside the Minnesota public hearings on January 6, 1995. Elizabeth Smith shared this impression in a consultation on January 13, 1995.
2. See also Bazerman and Paradis.
3. See also Berkenkotter and Huckin 29; Swales, "Discourse Analysis"; Swales, "Discourse Communities"; Swales, *Genre.*
4. See also Wiener; Bruffee, "Liberal Education"; Farkas; Bruffee, *Short Course.*
5. For more information on conflict and collaboration, see Burnett and Ewald, Karis; Trimbur; Burnett; Janis; Putnam.
6. Statements taken from the Licensing Rule Writing Group hearings are noted by the date of the hearing or by explanatory footnotes. Statements such as this one by Julia Dylan (January 6, 1995) and the following one by Gloria Olson (January 21, 1995) were offered in consultative sessions outside the public hearings.
7. This comment was offered in a consultation outside the Minnesota public hearings on January 13, 1995.
8. This comment was offered in a consultation outside the Minnesota public hearings on January 7, 1995.
9. This comment was offered in a consultation outside the Minnesota public hearings on January 7, 1995.
10. This comment was offered in a consultation outside the Minnesota public hearings on January 13, 1995.
11. This comment was offered in a consultation outside the Minnesota public hearings on January 13, 1995.
12. This comment was offered in a consultation outside the Minnesota public hearings on January 13, 1995.
13. This comment was offered in a consultation outside the Minnesota public hearings on January 7, 1995.
14. See also Sullivan and Weitz for a survey of Arizona midwives in the early 1980s; Baldwin; Janssen, Holt, and Myers; and Myers et al. for information on midwives in Washington state; Schramm, Barnes, and Bakewell for Missouri midwives.
15. All references in this section pertain to this first draft of the licensing rules unless otherwise noted.
16. The gender and status of the participants might affect their desire to collaborate in the first place and their interpretations of conflict, whether they perceive it as substantive, procedural, or interpersonal. Carol Gilligan notes that some women may seek collaboration or connection with others and base their decisions on an ethic of care, an emphasis on interpersonal harmony. This connection might seem uncomfortable to male participants who have accepted individualism and competition as essential to their gender roles (see also Chodorow and Belenky et al. for more explanation of this possible difference). Female participants might more readily define substantive conflict as interpersonal conflict or feel uncomfortable when the debate becomes volatile (Lay 20–23). Regardless of gender, low-status individuals may be more likely to avoid con-

flict or interpret conflict as interpersonal, while high-status individuals consider the same conflict substantive.

17. All references in this section pertain to the draft dated February 15, 1994, unless otherwise noted.

18. All references in this section are from the February 15, 1994, LRWG hearing unless otherwise noted.

19. All references in this section are from the June 21, 1994, LRWG hearing unless otherwise noted.

20. California midwives had the same problem in establishing a relationship with physicians; see, for example, Bennett 11.

21. In states where direct-entry midwives are legal by statute but licensure is not available, midwives often encounter hostility from physicians. For example, a home birth midwife working in Athens, Georgia, relates the following story on the midwifery listserv:

> A few years ago (on New Year's Eve) I was working with a wonderful Korean couple with their first pregnancy. The mother spoke no English and the father's was poor. The mother and I did real well with the communication of touch. I ended up having to transport her. When we got to the ER I went in with her and was told to sit in the waiting room and that the "hospital administrator would deal with me!" They then seperated [sic] the father from the mother (of course, just to do the paper work, they said) and I could hear this poor woman crying all over the ER. The OB came out to talk to me and in front of the ER patients told me I had no right to "dump my problems on her, especially on New Years Eve and that I would be hearing from her attorney." This OB has the highest C/S rate in the state of Georgia, and of course, my client had one . . . Luckily, out of my 500 some odd births I haven't transported that many, but when I have I always come home and wonder why I continue. Not only is it a disruption of care to my clients but it really knocks me back. The hospital and physician never consider her excellent pre-natal care or comprehensive lab work or any other positives I give. It's only that I am not MD (or at least an CNM) and I don't work there. It's hard enough to just leave a home birth even when the reason is totally justified but to be met at the hospital with such anger and hostility, it's bad. (listserv communication, 30 August 1996)

22. The following is a portion of one CNM's informed consent form for VBAC:

> Consent for Vaginal Birth After Cesarean Section At Home
>
> 1. I have had one or more previous cesarean sections (C/S), have records documenting a lower uterine segment incision, and desire a vaginal birth after C/S at home with my current pregnancy . . .
>
> 3. My midwife has informed me regarding:
>   A) The relative risks of VBAC:
>   - Complete rupture of the uterus: occurs in less than 1% of women having a VBAC; can lead to severe internal hemorrhage of the mother and death of the baby; this risk does not appear to be greater for women with a previous uterine incision than for women who have a normal uterus;
>   - Incomplete rupture of the uterus: occurs about 1% of the time; no symptoms and usually does not require any additional care;
>   B) The relative benefits of VBAC:
>   - Prevention of death and potential complications of surgery (blood loss, infection, injury to bowel urinary tract, etc., blood clots in the legs), a Public Citizen Report places maternal death rate at 18.4 per 100,000 women with elective C/S and less than half that for a vaginal birth;

- Faster recovery time after birth
- Easier time with breastfeeding without abdominal incision
- Less than half the cost of a C/S
- Decreased death and injury in baby resulting from surgical delivery
- Resultant positive emotional state from successful vaginal birth

I understand that, in the case of a complete uterine rupture, adverse consequences can be catastrophic in a matter of minutes. By choosing to have a VBAC outside of the hospital setting, I realize that I may not be diagnosed as quickly as having a potential rupture and that I may not receive emergency treatment and/or surgery as quickly as I would if I were having my baby inside of the hospital. It is possible that loss of time in transfer could be harmful or even fatal to myself and/or my baby.

4. After considering the above information, I believe that the benefits of VBAC at home outweigh the risks in my situation, and I choose to seek care with Grace _____ and pursue a VBAC at home rather than in the hospital.

(Grace, listserv communication, August 8, 1996)

Grace's form ensures that the midwife-client relationship includes a discussion of both risks and benefits.

23. This comment was offered by Emma Davidson in a consultation outside the Minnesota public hearings on November 23, 1994.

24. All references in this section are from the January 13, 1994, LRWG hearing unless otherwise noted.

25. Because this book focuses on the legal status of direct-entry midwives in the United States, readers who wish current information on midwives in other countries should refer to Orzack and Calogero; Weitz; Ratcliff; Malin and Hemminki; Tyson; Kaufman; Treffers et al.; Sparks; Benoit; and the "International Midwife Features" in *Midwifery Today.*

26. This comment was offered by Henrietta Kramer in a consultation outside the Minnesota public hearings on 9 November 9, 1994.

27. This comment was offered by Emma Davidson in a consultation outside the Minnesota public hearings on November 23, 1994.

28. This comment was offered in a consultation outside the Minnesota public hearings on November 23, 1994.

29. This comment was offered in a consultation outside the Minnesota public hearings on January 21, 1995.

30. This comment was offered in a consultation outside the Minnesota public hearings on January 7, 1995.

31. This comment was offered in a consultation outside the Minnesota public hearings on January 13, 1995.

32. This comment was offered in a consultation outside the Minnesota public hearings on January 21, 1995.

CHAPTER 6   *Jurisdictional Boundaries: Claiming Authority*
over Scientific Discourse and Knowledge

1. Dylan shared this impression with me in a consultation outside the hearings on January 6, 1995, and Miller shared hers through personal correspondence on November 17, 1994.

2. See also Rothschild, *Machina Ex Dea*; Rothschild, *Women*; Rossiter.

3. See appendix B for further definitions of these techniques; see also Davis; Gaskin, *Spiritual Midwifery*.

4. See, for example, Birke 171; Keller, *Secrets* 20–24.

5. See Oakley, *Wisewoman* 57; Mies 37; see also Rowland.

6. See Wajcman 13; see also Martin; Stanley; Cowan.

7. See also Grint and Gill; Wilson and Laennec.

8. See also Harding, *Whose Science?* 47.

9. Connie Baker shared this impression with me during a consultation outside the Minnesota midwifery hearings on January 13, 1995.

10. Rita Ortiz's remark offered in this section comes from an outside consultation on November 23, 1994.

11. Davidson offered this comment in a consultation outside the LRWG hearings on November 23, 1994.

12. All references in this section are to the April 14, 1994, LRWG hearing, unless otherwise noted.

13. Although I have given informal definitions of the less commonly known birth terms in the text of this chapter, for a more thorough description turn to appendix B.

14. Olson offered this comment in a consultation outside the LRWG hearings on January 21, 1995.

15. Although I have generally quoted testimony offered during the LRWG hearings in the order in which it was given, in this case I have included a statement made by Godwin in a later hearing (July 28, 1994).

16. See, for example, Rooks 144–145; 376.

17. This comment came from personal correspondence with Miller on November 17, 1994.

18. The direct-entry midwives' comments, analyzed in this section of the chapter, were taken from consultations outside the LRWG hearings between November 1994 and January 1995. At this point, the midwives were looking back not only at their failure to reach consensus but also at the first breakdown of the rule writing process. Connie Baker and Elizabeth Smith shared their comments on January 13, 1995, Kris House on January 7, 1995, and Gloria Olson on January 21, 1995.

19. At this point in the Minnesota story, the reader might need to consult appendix C, which gives a list of the MSAG and LRWG hearings and the specific decisions made during each hearing.

20. All references in this section are to the June 21, 1994, and July 28, 1994, LRWG hearings, unless otherwise noted.

21. Julia Dylan shared this impression with me during a consultation outside the Minnesota midwifery hearings on January 6, 1995. Elizabeth Smith shared the statement that follows on January 19, 1995 and Gloria Olson offered hers on January 21, 1995.

22. See also Torstendahl 3; Gross 72–73; Rubin 36–37.

23. Olson's statement was offered in a consultation outside the Minnesota midwifery hearings on January 21, 1995.

24. Ortiz's statement was offered in a consultation outside the Minnesota midwifery hearings on November 11, 1994.

25. Jessica Ramsey shared this information with me in a consultation outside the LRWG hearings on September 19, 1994.

26. Kramer shared this assessment with me in a consultation outside the hearings on November 9, 1994.

27. English shared this assessment with me in a consultation outside the hearings on November 18, 1994.

28. Miller shared these impressions with me in personal correspondence on November 17, 1994.

29. Dylan shared this concern with me in a consultation outside the hearings on January 6, 1995.

30. Emerson shared this concern with me in a consultation outside the hearings on November 14, 1994.

31. All references in this section are from the August 30, 1994, LRWG hearing, unless otherwise noted.

32. The August 1994 LRWG hearing proved not to be the last public discussion of licensing Minnesota's direct-entry midwives. Seven months later, the board was challenged again by state officials to proceed in good faith to fulfill its statutory requirements to license the direct-entry midwives or to move to repeal the statute that demanded it license this group. Thus, it recalled LRWG to respond to a very different set of licensing rules. The board had spent the last seven months working with an expert in test development at the University of Minnesota and with NARM representatives to establish the validity of the latest version of the NARM exam. By the time LRWG reconvened in March 1995, a fifth draft of the rules had been written by Jessica Ramsey and other board staffers. This draft reflected "some administrative changes" that the board felt necessary to "make it possible to administer the rules." The special services section of the draft—the section that granted direct-entry midwives the right to administer pitocin and oxygen, suture, and perform emergency episiotomies—had been removed. Also, the contraindications for home birth section had been deleted, as the board intended to use the final results of Rachel Waters's risk assessment MOMI study to redraft this section. The MOMI study would have certainly listed breeches and twins as contraindicated for home birth. However, by June 15, 1995, the board announced that it had encountered yet another obstacle to licensing Minnesota direct-entry midwives. According to Minnesota statute 215, each regulated profession must carry the cost of the regulation. The licensing fees for direct-entry midwives would be too much for them to bear. The fees would have to recover all of the board's investments, the stipends of the Midwifery Advisory Board members, and the unpredictable costs of any disciplinary actions against licensed midwives. Rather than a $95 licensing fee, as noted in the fifth draft, the board anticipated a fee of $1,000 to $1,400 per year, a tenth of some midwives' incomes. Therefore, the Minnesota Board of Medical Practice suspended the Licensing Rule Writing Group and again declared the licensing effort a failure.

CHAPTER 7   *Issues of Gender and Power: The Rhetoric of Direct-Entry Midwifery*

1. The comment from Henrietta Kramer came from an outside consultation on November 9, 1994. Gloria Olson shared her comment in an outside consultation on January 21, 1995. Unless otherwise noted, in this chapter all of Kramer's and Olson's comments came from these consultations.

2. Hawkesworth has reviewed the many different ways that scholars have used gender—for example, as an attribute of individuals, an interpersonal relation, and a mode of social organization; as a reflection of status, sex roles, and sexual stereotypes; as a structure of consciousness, psyche, and "internalized" ideology; as a result of attribution, socialization, disciplinary practice, and "accustomed stance"; as an effect of language; as a feature of power and a "mode of perception"; as "relations of power manifested in domination and subordination"; and as a liberating or as an imprisoning attribute (650–651).

3. Using Foucault to analyze gender and power is, of course, problematic. Foucault generally conceives of gender as a given—not a point of resistance and not as an aspect of

one group holding power over another. Nancy Hartsock and other feminist scholars propose that these gender relations are neglected in Foucault's studies and need to be addressed in future studies: "[B]ecause power relations are less visible to those who are in a position to dominate others, systematically unequal relations of power ultimately vanish from Foucault's account of power" (Hartsock 165). Foucault's focus on individuals makes it difficult, according to Hartsock, "to locate domination, including domination in gender relations. He has on the one hand claimed that individuals are constituted by power relations, but he has argued against their constitution by relations such as the domination of one group by another" (169; see also McNay, *Feminism* 38). To overcome these limitations in Foucault's theories of discourse and power, to extend an analysis of resistance, we need then to capture the voices and experiences of those groups who are dominated and who resist that domination. As Hartsock says, "We need to develop our understanding of difference by creating a situation in which hitherto marginalized groups can name themselves, speak for themselves, and participate in defining the terms of interaction, a situation in which we can construct an understanding of the world that is sensitive to difference" (158). To do this, we must treat these dominated voices and perspectives not as subjugated but as "primary and constitutive of a different world" (Hartsock 171). We need to understand the knowledge systems of such a world as direct-entry midwifery and how these systems are affected by the lives of those within them, their experiential and embodied knowledge. We need to understand how these knowledge systems constitute resistance to the dominant knowledge about women and their bodies. Therefore, to understand the Minnesota direct-entry midwifery hearings, to place them within a national and historical context, we must listen to the voices of the midwives themselves, to appreciate their perceptions of how their voices had been suppressed or supported because of their place as women and as bearers of children.

4. Unless otherwise noted, in this chapter all of Elizabeth Smith's comments were taken from a consultation outside the Minnesota hearings on January 13, 1995.

5. Unless otherwise noted, in this chapter all of Mary Emerson's comments were taken from a consultation outside the Minnesota hearings on November 14, 1994.

6. Unless otherwise noted, Connie Baker's comments in this chapter were taken from a consultation outside the Minnesota hearings on January 13, 1995.

BIBLIOGRAPHY

Abbott, Andrew. *The System of Professions: An Essay on the Division of Expert Labor.* Chicago: University of Chicago Press, 1988.

Abbott, Carrie. "Regional Reports. Region 5, West." *MANA News* (Midwives' Alliance of North America, Newton, Kan.) (May 1995): 10.

Abbott, Grace. "Administration of the Sheppard-Towner Act, Plans for Maternal Care." *Transaction of the American Child Hygiene Association* 13 (1922): 194–201.

Alaska Department of Commerce and Economic Development. Division of Occupational Licensing. Statutes and Regulations for Certified Direct-Entry Midwives. (A. S. && 08.65.190 [1994]).

Anderson, Judy "yduJ." "Not for the Faint of Heart: Contemplations on Usenet." *Wired Women: Gender and New Realities in Cyberspace.* Ed. Lynn Cherny and Elizabeth Reba Weise. Seattle, Wash.: Seal Press, 1996, 126–138.

Annas, George. "Legal Aspects of Home Birth." *Home Birth: A Practitioner's Guide to Birth Outside the Hospital.* Ed. Stanley E. Sagov, Richard I. Feinbloom, and Peggy Spindel with Archie Brodsky. Rockville, Md.: Aspen Systems Corp, 1984, 51–63.

"Are Our Obstetrical Principles Unscientific?" *JAMA* 7 (August 7, 1886): 155–157. Editor's reply.

Aristotle. *Rhetoric, Book I. The Rhetorical Tradition: Readings from Classical Times to the Present.* Ed. Patricia Bizzell and Bruce Herzberg. Boston: Bedford Books, 1990.

Arkansas Department of Health. *Regulations Governing the Practice of Lay Midwifery* (Ark. Code Ann && 17–85–101, 20–7–109 [1992]).

Arms, Suzanne. *Immaculate Deception: A New Look at Women and Childbirth in America.* Boston: Houghton Mifflin, 1975.

Arney, William Ray. *Power and the Profession of Obstetrics.* Chicago: University of Chicago Press, 1982.

Baker, S. Josephine. "Schools for Midwives." *American Journal of Obstetrics and the Diseases of Women and Children* 65 (1912): 256–270. Reprinted in Judy Barrett Litoff, ed. *The American Midwife Debate: A Sourcebook on Its Modern Origins.* New York: Greenwood Press, 1986, 153–166.

Baldwin, Rahima. "A Call for Unity and Support." *Special Delivery* 3.2 (1980): 3.

Balsamo, Anne. *Technologies of the Gendered Body: Reading Cyborg Women.* Durham, N.C.: Duke University Press, 1997.

Barnes, Diana. "From the President." *MANA News* (Midwives' Alliance of North America, Newton, Kan.) (November 1994): 3, 16.

————. "From the President." *MANA News* (Midwives' Alliance of North America, Newton, Kan.) (July 1995): 3, 11.

Barstow, Anne Llewellyn. *Witchcraze: A New History of the European Witch Hunt*. San Francisco: Pandora, 1994.

Bazerman, Charles. *Shaping Written Knowledge: The Genre and Activity of the Experimental Article in Science*. Madison: University of Wisconsin Press, 1988.

————, and James Paradis. "Introduction." *Textual Dynamics of the Professions: Historical and Contemporary Studies of Writing in Professional Communities*. Ed. Charles Bazerman and James Paradis. Madison: University of Wisconsin Press, 1991, 3–10.

Becker, Ellie, Meria Long, Vicki Stamler, and Pacia Sallomi. *Midwifery and the Law. A Mothering Special Edition*. Sante Fe, N.M.: Mothering Magazine, *1990*.

Belenky, Mary Field, Blythe McVicker Clinchy, Nancy Rule Goldberger, and Jill Mattuck Tarule. *Women's Ways of Knowing: The Development of Self, Voice, and Mind*. New York: Basic Books, 1986.

Bell, Vikki. *Interrogating Incest: Feminism, Foucault, and the Law*. London: Routledge, 1993.

Benhabib, Seyla. "Feminism and Postmodernism." *Feminist Contentions: A Philosophical Exchange*. Ed. Seyla Benhabib, Judith Butler, Drucilla Cornell, and Nancy Fraser. New York: Routledge, 1995, 17–34.

Bennett, Maggie. "Regional Reports. Region 6, Pacific." *MANA News* (Midwives' Alliance of North America, Newton, Kan.) (May 1995): 10–12.

Benoit, Cecilia. "The Professional Socialisation of Midwives: Balancing Art and Science." *Sociology of Health & Illness* 11.2 (1989): 160–180.

Benson, Ralph C. *Handbook of Obstetrics and Gynecology*. Los Altos, Calif.: Lange Medical Publications, xxx.

Berkenkotter, Carol, and Thomas N. Huckin. *Genre Knowledge in Disciplinary Communication: Cognition/Culture/Power*. Hillsdale, N.J.: Lawrence Erlbaum Associates, 1995.

Birke, Linda. *Women, Feminism, and Biology. The Feminist Challenge*. New York: Methuen, 1986.

Bitzer, Lloyd. "The Rhetorical Situation." *Philosophy and Rhetoric* 1 (1968): 1–14.

Blair, Carole, and Martha Cooper. "The Humanist Turn in Foucault's Rhetoric of Inquiry." *Quarterly Journal of Speech* 73 (1987): 151–171.

Bordo, Susan. *Unbearable Weight: Feminism, Western Culture, and the Body*. Berkeley: University of California Press, 1993.

Borst, Charlotte G. *Catching Babies: The Professionalization of Childbirth, 1870–1920*. Cambridge, Mass.: Harvard University Press 1995.

The Boston Women's Health Book Collective. *Our Bodies, Ourselves*. New York: Simon and Schuster, 1971.

Bowland et al. v Municipal Court for Santa Cruz City, etc., 1 Civil 35739, 134 Cal Rptr. 630. California Supreme Court Decision, December 6, 1976.

"British Midwifery Law." *The Law Reports: The Public General Statutes, Passed in the Second Year of the Reign of His Majesty King Edward the Seventh*. Vol. XL. London: Eyre & Spottiswoode. July 31, 1902.

Browner, Carole H., and Nancy Press. "The Production of Authoritative Knowledge in American Prenatal Care." *Childbirth and Authoritative Knowledge: Cross-Cultural Perspectives*. Ed. Robbie E. Davis-Floyd and Carolyn F. Sargent. Berkeley: University of California Press, 1997, 113–131.

Bruffee, Kenneth A. "Liberal Education and the Social Justification of Belief." *Liberal Education* 68 (1982): 95–114.

————. *A Short Course in Writing: Practical Rhetoric for Teaching Composition through Collaborative Learning.* 3rd ed. Boston: Little, Brown, 1985.

Burnett, Rebecca E. "Conflict in Collaborative Decision-Making." *Professional Communication: The Social Perspective.* Ed. Nancy Roundy Blyler and Charlotte Thralls. Newbury Park, Calif.: Sage, 1992, 144–162.

Burnett, Rebecca E., and Helen Rothschild Ewald. "Rabbit Trails, Ephemera, and Other Stories: Feminist Methodology and Collaborative Research." *Journal of Advanced Composition* 14.1 (winter 1994): 21–51.

Carlson, Karen J., Stephanie A. Eisenstat, and Terra Ziporyn. *The Harvard Guide to Women's Health.* Cambridge, Mass.: Harvard University Press, 1996.

Cellier, Elizabeth. "To Dr. . . . : An Answer to His Queries Concerning the Colledg of Midwives." London, 1687.

————. "The Midwives just Petition or, A complaint of divers good Gentlewomen of that faculty. Shewing to the whole Christian world their just case of their sufferings to these distracted Times, for their want of Trading. Which said complaint they tendered to the House on Monday last, being the 23 of Jan. 1643." London: 1643.

————. "A Scheme for the Foundation of a Royal Hospital, and Raising a Revenue of Five or Sex-thousand Pounds a Year, by, and for the Maintenance of a Corporation of skilful Midwives, and such Foundlings, or exposed Children, as shall be admitted therein. As it was proposed and addressed to his Majesty King James II." Independently published in June 1687. London: Harlein Miscellany, 1745, vol. 4.

Chamberlen, Hugh. "Translator to the Reader." In Mauriceau, François. *The Diseases of Women with Child, and in Child-bed.* 2nd ed. Trans. Hugh Chamberlen. London: John Darby, 1683.

Chamberlen, Paul (?). *Dr. Chamberlain's Midwives Practice: or a Guide for Women in the High Concern of Conception, Breeding, and Nursing Children.* London: Thomas Books, 1665.

Chapman, Edmund. *Treatise on the Improvement of Midwifery.* 3rd ed. London: L. David and C. Reymers, 1759.

Chodorow, Nancy. *The Reproduction of Mothering: Psychoanalysis and the Sociology of Gender.* Berkeley: University of California Press, 1978.

Coe, H. C. "The Immediate Application of the Forceps to the After-coming Head in Cases of Version with the Partial Dilation of the Os." *JAMA* 12 (January 19, 1889): 101.

Colorado. State Legislature. *Rules and Regulations for Approval of Direct-Entry Midwifery: General Authority C.R.S. 12–37–106, Section 12–37–103,* July 1, 1993.

"Complete Dilation of the Cervix Uteri, an Essential Condition to the Typical Forceps Operation." *JAMA* 5 (August 29, 1885): 238–240.

Condit, Celeste. *Decoding Abortion Rhetoric: Communicating Social Change.* Urbana: University of Illinois Press, 1990.

Corea, Gena. *The Machine: Reproductive Technologies from Artificial Insemination to Artificial Wombs.* London: The Women's Press, 1985.

Corson, Hiram. "On the Statistics of 3,036 Cases of Labor," *JAMA* 7 (July 31, 1886): 138–139.

Costigan, James T. "Introduction: Forests, Trees, and Internet Research." *Doing Internet Research: Critical Issues and Methods for Examining the Net.* Ed. Steve Jones. Thousand Oaks, Calif.: Sage, 1999, xvii–xxiv.

Cowan, Ruth Swartz. *More Work for Mother: The Ironies of Household Technology from the Open Hearth to the Microwave.* New York: Basic Books, 1983.

Crowell, R. Elisabeth. "The Midwives of New York." *Charities and the Commons* 17 (January 1907): 667–677. Reprinted in Litoff, Judy Barrett, ed. *The American Midwife Debate: A Sourcebook on Its Modern Origins.* New York: Greenwood Press, 1986, 36–49.

Culpepper, Nicholas. *A Directory for Midwives: Or, A Guide for Women, In their Conception, Bearing, and Suckling their Children. . . .* London: Norris, Bettlesworth, Ballard and Batley, 1724.

Cutter, Irving S., and Henry R. Viets. *A Short History of Midwifery.* 1st ed. London: W. B. Saunders Co., 1964.

Davidson, Gayle V., Wilhelmina C. Savenye, and Kay B. Orr. "How Do Learning Styles Relate to Performance in a Computer Applications Course?" *Journal of Research on Computing in Education* 24.2 (1992): 348–358.

Davis, Elizabeth. *Heart & Hands: A Midwife's Guide to Pregnancy & Birth.* 2nd ed. Berkeley, Calif.: Celestial Arts, 1987.

Davis-Floyd, Robbie E. *Birth as an American Rite of Passage.* Berkeley: University of California Press, 1992.

———. "Birth of a Dream, Death of a Dream: The Development of Direct-Entry Midwifery in New York." Paper presented at the Joint Meetings of the Society for Applied Anthropology and the Society for Medical Anthropology, Seattle, Wash., March 1997.

———. "The Development of Direct-Entry Midwifery in North America: Implications for Health Care Policy." Paper presented at the American Anthropological Association, San Francisco, 1996.

Davis-Floyd, Robbie, and Elizabeth Davis. "Intuition as Authoritative Knowledge in Midwifery and Home Birth." *Childbirth and Authoritative Knowledge: Cross-Cultural Perspectives.* Ed. Robbie E. Davis-Floyd and Carolyn F. Sargent. Berkeley: University of California Press, 1997, 315–349.

Dawkes, Thomas. *The Midwife Rightly Instructed.* London: J. Oswald, 1736.

De Lee, Joseph B. "Progress Toward Ideal Obstetrics." *Transactions of the American Association for the Study and Prevention of Infant Mortality* 6 (1915): 114–123. Reprinted in Litoff, Judy Barrett, ed. *The American Midwife Debate: A Sourcebook on Its Modern Origins.* New York: Greenwood Press, 1986, 102–109.

Devitt, Amy J. "Genre, Genres, and the Teaching of Genre." *College Composition and Communication* 47 (1996): 605–615.

DeVries, Raymond G. *Regulating Birth: Midwives, Medicine, & the Law.* Philadelphia: Temple University Press, 1985.

Dewees, William B. "New Axis-Traction Obstetric Forceps," *JAMA* 19 (July 9, 1892): 32–33.

Diamond, Irene, and Lee Quinby, eds. *Feminism & Foucault: Reflections on Resistance.* Boston: Northeastern University Press, 1988.

Dixon, Kerry. "Regional Reports. Region 4, Midwest—Minnesota." *MANA News* (Midwives' Alliance of North America, Newton, Kan.) (May 1997): 6.

———. "Regional Reports. Region 4, Midwest—Minnesota." *MANA News* (Midwives' Alliance of North America, Newton, Kan.) (July 1997): 12–13.

———. "Regional Reports. Region 4, Midwest—Minnesota." *MANA News* (Midwives' Alliance of North America, Newton, Kan.) (January 1998): 8–9.

———. "Regional Reports. Region 4, Midwest—Minnesota." *MANA News* (Midwives' Alliance of North America, Newton, Kan.) (September 1998): 9.

Doheny-Farina, Stephen. *The Wired Neighborhood.* New Haven, Conn.: Yale University Press, 1996.

Donegan, Jane. *Women & Men Midwives: Medicine, Morality, and Misogyny in Early America.* Westport, Conn.: Greenwood Press, 1978.

Donnison, Jean. *Midwives and Medical Men: A History of Inter-Professional Rivalries and Women's Rights.* New York: Schocken Books, 1977.

Durand, Mark A. "The Safety of Home Birth: The Farm Study." *American Journal of Public Health* 82.3 (March 1992): 450–453.

Durndell, Alan. "Why Do Female Students Tend to Avoid Computer Studies?" *Research in Science & Technological Education* 8.2 (1990): 163–170.

Durndell, Alan, Gerda Siann, and Peter Glissov. "Gender Differences and Computing in Course Choice at Entry into Higher Education." *British Educational Research Journal* 16.2(1990): 149–162.

Edgar, J. Clifton. "The Education, Licensing and Supervision of the Midwife." *American Journal of Obstetrics and the Diseases of Women and Children* 73 (March 1916): 385–398. Reprinted in Litoff, Judy Barrett, ed. *The American Midwife Debate: A Sourcebook on Its Modern Origins.* New York: Greenwood Press, 1986, 129–143.

El Halta, Valerie. "Normalizing the Breech Delivery." *Midwifery Today* 38 (summer 1996): 22–24, 41.

Emmons, Authur Brewster, and James Lincoln Huntington. "The Midwife: Her Future in the United States." *American Journal of Obstetrics and the Diseases of Women and Children* 65 (March 1912): 383–404. Reprinted in Litoff, Judy Barrett, ed. *The American Midwife Debate: A Sourcebook on Its Modern Origins.* New York: Greenwood Press, 1986, 115–126.

Farkas, David K. "Collaborative Writing, Software Development, and the Universe of Collaborative Activity." *Collaborative Writing in Industry: Investigations in Theory and Practice.* Ed. Mary M. Lay and William M. Karis. Amityville, N.Y.: Baywood, 1991, 13–30.

Fernback, Jan. "There Is a There There: Notes Toward a Definition of Cybercommunity." Doing Internet Research: Critical Issues and Methods for Examining the Net. Ed. Steve Jones. Thousand Oaks, Calif.: Sage, 1999, 203–220.

Florida Agency for Health Care Administration, Division of Medical Quality Assurance, Council of Licensed Midwifery, Tallahassee, Chapter 467 and Rule 59 DD, F. A. C. January 1995.

Foucault, Michel. *The Birth of the Clinic: An Archaeology of Medical Perception.* Trans. A. M. Sheridan Smith. New York: Vintage, 1975.

———. *Discipline and Punish: The Birth of the Prison.* Trans. Alan Sheridan. New York: Vintage, 1979.

———. *The History of Sexuality. Volume I: An Introduction.* Trans. Robert Hurley. New York: Vintage Books, 1990.

———. *Power/Knowledge: Selected Interviews and Other Writings 1972–1977.* Ed. Colin Gordon. Trans. Colin Gordon, Leo Marshall, John Mepham, and Kate Soper. New York: Pantheon, 1980.

———. "The Subject and Power." Afterword. *Michel Foucault: Beyond Structuralism and Hermeneutics.* Ed. Hubert L. Dreyfus and Paul Rabinow. 2nd ed. Chicago: University of Chicago Press, 1983, 208–226.

Frankenberg, Scott. "Report to the Birth Seminar, March 25, 1972." In Raven Lang. *Birth Book.* Felton, Calif.: Genesis Press, 1972.

Fraser, Nancy. "False Antitheses: A Response to Seyla Benhabib and Judith Butler." *Feminist Contentions: A Philosophical Exchange.* Ed. Seyla Benhabib, Judith Butler, Drucilla Cornell, and Nancy Fraser. New York: Routledge, 1995, 59–74.

———. "Rethinking the Public Sphere: A Contribution to the Critique of Actually Existing

Democracy." *Habermas and the Public Sphere*. Ed. Craig Calhoun. Cambridge, Mass.: MIT Press, 1992, 107–142.

Freedman, Aviva, and Peter Medway. "Locating Genre Studies: Antecedents and Prospects." *Genre and the New Rhetoric*. Ed. Aviva Freedman and Peter Medway. London: Taylor and Francis, 1994, 1–20.

Fry, Henry D. "The Application of Forceps to Transverse and Oblique Positions of the Head. Description of a New Forceps." *JAMA* 13 (November 9, 1889): 651–657.

Gaskin, Ina May. "Regional Reports. Region 3, South." *MANA News* (Midwives' Alliance of North America, Newton, Kan.) (May 1995): 6.

———. *Spiritual Midwifery*. 3rd. ed. Summertown, Tenn.: The Book Publishing Company, 1990.

Gieryn, Thomas F. "Boundary-Work and the Demarcation of Science from Non-Science: Strains and Interests in Professional Ideologies of Scientists." *American Sociological Review* 48 (1983): 781–795.

Giffard, William. *Cases in Midwifery*. London: B. Motte, T. Wotton, & L. Guilliver, 1734.

Gilgoff, Alice. *Home Birth*. New York: Coward, McCann & Geoghegan, Inc., 1978.

Gilligan, Carol. *In a Different Voice: Psychological Theory and Women's Development*. Cambridge, Mass.: Harvard University Press, 1982.

Goodnight, G. Thomas. "The Personal, Technical, and Public Spheres of Argument: A Speculative Inquiry into the Art of Public Discourse." *Journal of the American Forensic Association* 18 (spring 1982): 214–227.

Grint, Keith, and Rosalind Gill. *The Gender-Technology Relation: Contemporary Theory and Research*. London: Taylor & Francis, 1995.

Gross, Stanley J. *Of Foxes and Hen Houses: Licensing and the Health Professions*. Westport, Conn.: Quorum Books, 1984.

Grosz, Elizabeth. *Volatile Bodies: Toward a Corporeal Feminism*. Bloomington: Indiana University Press, 1994.

Gurak, Laura. *Persuasion and Privacy in Cyberspace: The Online Protests over Lotus Marketplace and the Clipper Chip*. New Haven, Conn.: Yale University Press, 1997.

Hall, Joan, and Joel Cooper. "Gender, Experience and Attributions to the Computer." *Journal of Educational Computing Research* 7.1 (1990): 51–60.

Haraway, Donna J. *Simians, Cyborgs, and Women: The Reinvention of Nature*. New York: Routledge, 1991.

Harding, Sandra. "Rethinking Standpoint Epistemology: What Is 'Strong Objectivity'?" *Feminist Epistemologies*. Ed. Linda Alcoff and Elizabeth Potter. New York: Routledge, 1993, 49–82.

———. *The Science Question in Feminism*. Ithaca, N.Y.: Cornell University Press, 1986.

———. *Whose Science? Whose Knowledge? Thinking from Women's Lives*. Ithaca, N.Y.: Cornell University Press, 1991.

Hartley, E. C., and Ruth E. Boynton. "A Survey of the Midwife Situation in Minnesota." *Minnesota Medicine* 7 (1924): 439–446.

Hartsock, Nancy. "Foucault on Power: A Theory for Women?" *Feminism/Postmodernism*. Ed. Linda J. Nicholson. New York: Routledge, 1990, 157–175.

Hawkesworth, Mary. "Confounding Gender." *Signs* 22.3 (1997): 649–685.

Hawkins, Jan. "Computers and Girls: Rethinking the Issues." *Sex Roles* 13.3/4 (1985): 165–180.

Hazell, Lester Dessez. "A Study of 300 Elective Home Births," *Birth and the Family Journal* 2.1 (1975): 11–18.

Huntington, James Lincoln. "The Midwife in Massachusetts: Her Anomalous Position." *Boston Medical and Surgical Journal* 168 (March 1913): 418–421. Reprinted in Litoff, Judy Barrett, Ed. *The American Midwife Debate: A Sourcebook on Its Modern Origins.* New York: Greenwood Press, 1986, 110–116.

Illg, Susan. "A Recommendation Regarding the Legal and Regulatory Status of Traditional Midwives in Minnesota." Unpublished master's thesis, University of Minnesota, Public Affairs, June 1991.

"International Midwifery Features." *Midwifery Today* 40 (winter 1996): 41–61.

Jacobi, Abraham. "The Best Means of Combatting Infant Mortality." *Journal of the American Medical Association* 58 (June 1912): 1735–1744. Reprinted in Litoff, Judy Barrett, Ed. *The American Midwife Debate: A Sourcebook on Its Modern Origins.* New York: Greenwood Press, 1986, 177–199.

Jacobus, Mary, Evelyn Fox Keller, and Sally Shuttleworth. "Introduction." *Body/Politics: Women and the Discourses of Science.* Ed. Mary Jacobus, Evelyn Fox Keller, and Sally Shuttleworth. New York: Routledge, 1990, 1–10.

Janis, I. L. *Victims of Groupthink: A Psychological Study of Foreign Policy Decisions and Fiascoes.* 2nd ed. Boston: Houghton Mifflin 1982.

Janssen, Patricia A., Victoria Holt, and Susan J. Myers. "Licensed Midwife-Attended, Out-of-Hospital Births in Washington State: Are They Safe?" *Birth* 21.3 (September 1994): 141–148.

Jessup, Emily. "Feminism and Computers in Composition Instruction." *Evolving Perspectives on Computers and Composition Studies: Questions for the 1990s.* Ed. Gail E. Hawisher and Cynthia L. Selfe. Urbana, Ill.: National Council of Teachers of English, 1991, 336–355.

Jordan, Brigitte. "Authoritative Knowledge and Its Construction." *Childbirth and Authoritative Knowledge: Cross-Cultural Perspectives.* Ed. Robbie E. Davis-Floyd and Carolyn F. Sargent. Berkeley: University of California Press, 1997, 55–79.

Kaplan, Nancy, and Eva Farrell. "Weavers of Webs: A Portrait of Young Women on the Net." *Arachnet Electronic Journal on Virtual Culture* 2.3 (July 1994): np.

Karis, Bill. "Conflict in Collaboration: A Burkean Perspective." *Rhetoric Review* 8 (1989): 113–126.

Kaufman, Karyn J. "The Introduction of Midwifery in Ontario, Canada." *Birth* 18.2 (June 1991): 100–103.

Keller, Evelyn Fox. *A Feeling for the Organism: The Life and Work of Barbara McClintock.* New York: W. H. Freeman, 1983.

———. *Secrets of Life/Secrets of Death: Essays on Language, Gender and Science.* New York: Routledge, 1992.

Kiesler, Sara, Lee Sproull, and Jacquelynne S. Eccles. "Pool Halls, Chips, and War Games: Women in the Culture of Computing." *Psychology of Women Quarterly* 9 (1985): 451–462.

Kitzinger, Sheila. *The Midwife Challenge.* London: Pandora, 1988.

Kobrin, Frances E. "The American Midwife Controversy: A Crisis in Professionalization." *Bulletin of the History of Medicine* 40 (1966): 350–363.

Korte, Diana. "Midwives on Trial." *Mothering* 76 (fall 1995): 53–57.

Kramer, Heinrich, and James Sprenger. *The Malleus Maleficarum.* Trans. Montague Summers. 1486. reprt. New York: Dover, 1971.

Kramer, Pamela E., and Sheila Lehman. "Mismeasuring Women: A Critique of Research on Computer Ability and Avoidance." *Signs* 16.1 (1990): 158–172.

Lang, Raven. *Birth Book.* Felton, Calif.: Genesis Press, 1972.

Latour, Bruno, and Steve Woolgar. *Laboratory Life: The Construction of Scientific Fact.* Princeton, N.J.: Princeton University Press, 1986.

Lay, Mary M. "Interpersonal Conflict in Collaborative Writing: What We Can Learn from Gender Studies." *Journal of Business and Technical Communication* 3.2 (1989): 5–28.

———, Billie J. Wahlstrom, and Carol Brown. "The Rhetoric of Midwifery: Conflicts and Conversations in the Minnesota Home Birth Community in the 1990s." *Quarterly Journal of Speech* 82 (1996): 383–401.

Leavitt, Judith Walzer. *Brought to Bed: Childbearing in American 1750–1950.* New York: Oxford University Press, 1986.

Litoff, Judy Barrett, ed. *The American Midwife Debate: A Sourcebook on Its Modern Origins.* New York: Greenwood Press, 1986.

———. *American Midwives: 1860 to the Present.* Westport, Conn.: Greenwood Press, 1978.

Logue, Cal M., and Eugene F. Miller. "Rhetorical Status: A Study of its Origins, Functions, and Consequences." *Quarterly Journal of Speech* 81 (1995): 20–47.

Longino, Helen. "In Search of Feminist Epistemology." *The Monist* 77 (1994): 472–485.

———. "Subjects, Power and Knowledge: Description and Prescription in Feminist Philosophies of Science." *Feminist Epistemologies.* Ed. Linda Alcoff and Elizabeth Potter. New York: Routledge, 1993, 101–120.

Louisiana. "Midwife Practitioners Act." Revised Statutes 37:3240–37.3257, 1988.

McAfee, Phillip. Memo to H. Leonard Boche on "Midwife Regulation" August 5, 1993.

McCloskey, Donald N. *The Rhetoric of Economics.* Madison: University of Wisconsin Press, 1985.

McKerrow, Raymie E. "Critical Rhetoric: Theory and Praxis." *Communication Monographs* 56 (1989): 91–111.

———. "Critical Rhetoric and the Possibility of the Subject." *The Critical Turn: Rhetoric and Philosophy in Postmodern Discourse.* Ed. Ian Angus and Lenore Langsdorf. Carbondale: Southern Illinois University Press, 1993, 51–67.

McNay, Lois. *Foucault: A Critical Introduction.* New York: Continuum, 1994.

———. *Foucault and Feminism: Power, Gender and the Self.* Cambridge, Mass.: Polity Press, 1992.

Malin, Maili, and Elina Hemminki. "Midwives as Providers of Prenatal Care in Finland—Past and Present." *Women & Health* 18.4 (1992): 17–34.

MANA Core Compentencies. Revised October 1994. *MANA News* (Midwives' Alliance of North America, Newton, Kan.) (November 1994): 31–33.

MANA News (Midwives' Alliance of North America, Newton, Kan.) (July 1995): 3.

Marschall, Marlene E., commissioner of health. Letter to H. Leonard Boche, executive director, Minnesota Board of Medical Practice, accompanying Minnesota Department of Health, "Regulation of Traditional Midwifery in Minnesota: Considerations and Recommendations," June 1, 1992.

Martin, Emily. *Flexible Bodies: The Role of Immunity in American Culture from the Days of Polio to the Age of AIDS.* Boston: Beacon, 1994.

———. *The Woman in the Body: A Cultural Analysis of Reproduction.* Boston: Beacon, 1992.

Maubray, John. *The Female Physician.* London: James Holland, 1724.

Mead, E. S. "Discussion." *JAMA* 23 (August 18, 1894): 277.

The Medical Repository, n.s. 8 (1823–1824): 224–225.

Mehl, L., L. A. Leavitt, G. H. Peterson, and D. C. Creevy. "Home Birth versus Hospital Birth: Comparisons of Outcomes of Matched Populations." Paper presented at the meetings of the American Public Health Association, Miami, 1977.

Memmi, Albert. *The Colonizer and the Colonized.* Boston: Beacon Press, 1967.

Midwifery Licensing Series. Minnesota Midwives' Guild. Handout to Rule Writing Group, August 30, 1994.

Mies, Maria. "Why Do We Need All This? A Call Against Genetic Engineering and Reproductive Technology." *Made To Order: The Myth of Reproductive and Genetic Progress.* Ed. Patricia Spallone and Deborah Lynn Steinberg. Oxford, N.Y.: Pergamon Press, 1987.

Miller, Carolyn R. "Genre as Social Action." *Quarterly Journal of Speech* 70 (1984): 151–167. Also, reprinted and revised in *Genre and the New Rhetoric.* Ed. Aviva Freedman and Peter Medway. London: Taylor and Francis, 1994, 23–42.

————, and S. Michael Halloran. "Reading Darwin, Reading Nature; Or, on the Ethos of Historical Science." *Understanding Scientific Prose.* Ed. Jack Selzer. Madison: University of Wisconsin Press, 1993, 106–126.

Millikin, Dan. "Report of a Case in which the Child's Arm Became Engaged in the Fenestrum of the Obstetric Forceps," *JAMA* 16 (June 27, 1891): 906–908.

Minnesota Board of Medical Examiners. "Physician Assistant Rules and Related Acts," November 1990.

Minnesota Board of Medical Practice. Minutes of the Board Meeting, September 14, 1996.

Minnesota Board of Medical Practice. "Proposed Rules for Midwifery Licensure and Registration." Drafts November 30, 1993; February 14, 1994; July 26, 1994; August 30, 1994; March 20, 1995.

Minnesota Board of Medical Practice. Public Policy Committee. "Home Births and Midwifery Policy Memo," September 1993.

Minnesota Department of Health. "Adopted Permanent Rules Relating to the Registration of Respiratory Care Practitioners," August 28, 1991.

Minnesota Department of Health. *Regulation of Traditional Midwifery in Minnesota: Considerations & Recommendations. A Report to the Minnesota Board of Medical Practice.* Minneapolis: Health Occupations Program, June 1, 1992.

Minnesota Medical Association. Personal correspondence to Minnesota Board of Medical Practice. July 26, 1994.

Minnesota Midwives' Guild. *Standards of Care and Certification Guide.* 1989. Revised 1995.

Minnesota State Legislature. *Midwifery.* Rules Pt. 5600.2000.

Minnesota State Senate SF 1409. Proposed coding for new law in Minnesota Statutes, Chapter 148, Section 148.491, March 22, 1993.

Minnesota Statutes, Chapter 148 (Proposed as SF 1409 and HF 1677), March 22, 1993. Sponsored by Senators Pappas and Flynn; Representative Brown.

Mitford, Jessica. *The American Way of Birth.* New York: Dutton, 1992.

Montana. Department of Commerce. "Direct-Entry Midwifery." *Professions and Occupations: Administrative Rules,* Chapter 27, March 31, 1994.

Mosher, George C. "The Management of Lingering Labor," *JAMA* 19 (July 9, 1892): 33–36.

Myers, Susan J., Patricia A. St. Clair, Stephen S. Gloyd, Philip Salzberg, and Joanne Myers-Ciecko. "Unlicensed Midwifery Practice in Washington State." *American Journal of Public Health* 80.6 (June 1990): 726–728.

Nelson, John S., Allan Megill, and Donald N. McCloskey. "Rhetoric of Inquiry." *The Rhetoric of the Human Sciences: Language and Argument in Scholarship and Public Affairs.* Madison: University of Wisconsin Press, 1987, 3–18.

New Hampshire. "Regulations Governing Lay Midwives." Chapter He-P 3100.

New Mexico Department of Health. "Regulations Governing the Practice of Licensed Midwifery." DOH 93–9. July 9, 1993.

New Mexico Midwives Association. *Policies and Procedures.* nd.

Nihell, Elizabeth. *A Treatise on the Art of Midwifery. Setting Forth Various Abuses therein, especially as to the Practice with Instruments: The Whole Serving to put all Rational Inquirers in a fair Way of very safely forming their own Judgement upon the Question; Which it is best to employ, In Cases of Pregnancy and Lying-in, A Man-Midwive; or, a Midwife.* London: A. Morley, 1760.

Oakley, Ann. *The Captured Womb: A History of the Medical Care of Pregnant Women.* Oxford, U.K.: Basil Blackwell, 1986.

———. "Wisewoman and Medicine Man: Changes in the Management of Childbirth." *The Rights and Wrongs of Women.* Ed. J. Mitchell and Ann Oakley. Harmondsworth, U.K.: Penguin, 1976.

Ogletree, Shirley M., and Sue W. Williams. "Sex and Sex-Typing Effects on Computer Attitudes and Aptitude." *Sex Roles* 23.11/12 (1990): 703–712.

Oregon. Administrative Rules, Board of Direct Entry Midwifery, Chapter 332, Divisions 1–30. July 1994.

Orzack, Louis H., and Caroline Calogero. "Midwives, Societal Variation, and Diplomatic Discourse in the European Community." *Current Research on Occupations and Professions* 5 (1990): 43–69.

Pall Mall Gazette, September 9, 1880, 11.

Parker, Jennifer D. "Ethnic Differences in Midwife-Attended US Births." *American Journal of Public Health* 84.7 (July 1994): 1139–1141

Penn, MariMikel. "Regional Reports. Region 9, South Central." *MANA News* (Midwives' Alliance of North America, Newton, Kan.) (November 1994): 14–15.

———. "Regional Reports. Region 9, South Central." *MANA News* (Midwives' Alliance of North American, Newton, Kan.) (July 1995): 10.

Public Policy Committee. Memo to Minnesota Board of Medical Practice on "Home Births and Midwifery Policy," September 1993. Adopted by the Board of Medical Practice September 11, 1993.

Pugh, Benjamin. *A Treatise of Midwifery, Chiefly with Regard to the Operation, with Several Instruments in that ART . . .* London: J. Buckland, 1754.

Pulley, Debby. "Legislative Committee Report." *MANA News* (Midwives' Alliance of North America, Newton, Kan.) (November 1994): 21.

Putnam, Linda L. "Conflict in Group Decision-Making." *Communication and Group Decision-Making.* Ed. R.Y. Hirokawa and M. S. Poole. Beverly Hills: Sage, 1986, 175–196.

Ramazanoglu, Caroline, ed. *Up Against Foucault: Explorations of Some Tensions between Foucault and Feminism.* London: Routledge, 1993.

Ratcliff, Kathryn Strother. "Midwifery in East London: Responding to the Challenges." *Women & Health* 22.1 (1994): 49–78.

Reagan, Leslie J. *When Abortion Was a Crime: Women, Medicine, and Law in the United States, 1867–1973.* Berkeley: University of California Press, 1997.

Roesslin, Eucharius. *Der Swangern Frawen und Hebammen Rosengarten.* Trans. Richard Jonas. *The Byrth of Mankynde, Otherwise Named the Womans Booke.* London: Thomas Rayhalde, 1540.

Romalis, Shelly, ed. *Childbirth: Alternatives to Medical Control.* Austin: University of Texas Press, 1981.

Rooks, Judith Pence. *Midwifery and Childbirth in America.* Philadelphia: Temple University Press, 1997.

Rothman, Barbara Katz. *In Labor: Women and Power in the Birthplace.* New York: London, 1982.

————. *Recreating Motherhood: Ideology and Technology in a Patriarchal Society*. New York: Norton, 1989.

Rothschild, Joan. *Machina Ex Dea: Feminist Perspectives on Technology*. New York: Pergamon, 1984.

————. *Women, Technology and Innovation*. Oxford, U.K.: Pergamon, 1982.

Rowland, Robyn. *Living Laboratories: Women and Reproductive Technologies*. Bloomington: Indiana University Press, 1992.

Rubin, Stephen. "The Legal Web of Professional Regulation." *Regulating the Professions: A Public-Policy Symposium*. Ed. Roger D. Blair and Stephen Rubin. Lexington, Mass.: Lexington Books/Heath, 1980, 29–60.

Rule, Anna R. "The Midwife Problem in the United States." *JAMA* 81 (September 22, 1923): 989–992.

Sablosky, Ann H. "The Power of the Forceps: A Comparative Analysis of the Midwife—Historically and Today." *Women and Health* 1 (January/February 1976): 10–13.

Sagov, Stanley E., and Archie Brodsky. "The Issue of Safety." *Home Birth: A Practitioner's Guide to Birth Outside the Hospital*. Ed. Stanley E. Sagov, Richard I. Feinbloom, and Peggy Spindel, with Archie Brodsky. Rockville, Md.: Aspen Systems Corporation, 1984, 17–49.

Said, Edward. *Orientalism*. New York: Vintage, 1978.

Sauer, Beverly A. "Sense and Sensibility in Technical Documentation: How Feminist Interpretation Strategies Can Save Lives in the Nation's Mines." *Journal of Business and Technical Communication* 7.1 (1993): 63–83.

Sawicki, Jana. *Disciplining Foucault: Feminism, Power, and the Body*. New York: Routledge, 1991.

Sawyer, Peggy. "Letter to the Editor." *MANA News* (Midwives' Alliance of North America, Newton, Kan.) (October 1995): 916–917.

Schiebinger, Londa. *Nature's Body: Gender in the Making of Modern Science*. Boston: Beacon, 1993.

Schlinger, Hilary. "New York State: Witch-hunt or Political Strategy?" *MANA News* (Midwives' Alliance of North America, Newton, Kan.) (January 1996): 1, 24–25.

Schramm, Wayne R., Diane E. Barnes, and Janice M. Bakewell. "Neonatal Mortality in Missouri Home Births, 1978–84." *American Journal of Public Health* 77.8 (August 1987): 930–935.

Scott, Joan W. "Gender: A Useful Category of Historical Analysis." *American Historical Review* 91.5 (December 1986): 1053–1075.

Seaman, Valentine. *The Midwives Monitor and Mother's Mirror*. New York: Isaac Collins, 1800.

"Setting the Standards for Midwifery: The NARM Certified Professional Midwife." *MANA News* (Midwives' Alliance of North America, Newton, Kan.) (July 1995): 1, 17.

Sharp, Jane. *The Midwives Book or the whole Art of Midwifery Discovered Directing Childbearing Women how to behave themselves in their Conception, Breeding, Bearing, and Nursing of Children*. Orig. London: S. Miller, 1671; reprinted New York: Garland, 1985.

Smart, Carol. *Feminism and the Power of Law*. London: Routledge, 1989.

Smart, Graham. "Genre as Community Invention: A Central Bank's Response to Its Executives' Expectations as Readers." *Writing in the Workplace: New Research Perspectives*. Ed. Rachel Spilka. Carbondale: Southern Illinois Press, 1993. 124–140.

Smellie, William. *A Collection of Cases and Observations in Midwifery to Illustrate His Former Treatise, or First Volume on that Subject*. London: D. Wilson and T. Durham, 1754.

————. *A Collection of Preternatural Cases and Observations in Midwifery*, 2nd ed. London: D. Wilson and T. Durham, 1766.

————. *A Treatise on the Theory and Practice of Midwifery*, 3rd. ed. London: D. Wilson & T. Durham, 1756.

Smith, Dorothy. *The Everyday World as Problematic: A Feminist Sociology*. Boston, Mass.: Northeastern University Press, 1987.

————. *The Conceptual Practices of Power: A Feminist Sociology of Knowledge*. Boston, Mass.: Northeastern University Press, 1990.

Smith-Rosenberg, Carroll. *Disorderly Conduct: Visions of Gender in Victorian America*. New York: Knopf, 1985.

Sonnenstuhl, Pat. "Midwifery in the United States." Communication submitted to midwife@fensende.com. Copies sent to sci.med.midwifery and sci.med.nursing. May 24, 1996.

South Carolina Department of Health and Environmental Contro, Chapter 61. "Standards for Licensing Midwives." Regulation 61–24, July 23, 1993.

Sparks, Barbara Taylor. "A Descriptive Study of the Changing Roles and Practices of Traditional Birth Attendants in Zimbabwe." *Journal of Nurse-Midwifery* 35.3 (May/June 1990): 150–161.

Spender, Dale. *Nattering on the Net: Women, Power and Cyberspace*. North Melbourne, Victoria, Australia: Spinfex, 1995.

Stanley, Autumn. *Mothers and Daughters of Invention: Notes for a Revised History of Technology*. Metuchen, N.J.: Scarecrow Press, 1993.

Starr, Paul. *The Social Transformation of American Medicine*. New York: Basic Books, 1982.

Stewart, William S. "When Should the Obstetric Forceps Be Used? And What Form of Instrument Is Required?" *JAMA* 13 (November 30, 1889): 770–771.

Stone, Sarah. *A Complete Practice of Midwifery*. London: T. Cooper, 1737.

Sullivan, Deborah A., and Rose Weitz. *Labor Pains: Modern Midwives and Home Birth*. New Haven, Conn.: Yale University Press, 1988.

Sullivan, Mary Ellen. "Development of the North American Registry Exam for Midwives." Testing Consultant to the Midwives' Alliance of North America. Initial Report, March 1992.

Swales, John. "Discourse Analysis in Professional Contexts." *Annual Review of Applied Linguistics* 11 (1990): 103–114.

————. "Discourse Communities, Genres, and English as an International Language." *World English* 7 (1988): 211–220.

————. *Genre Analysis: English in Academic and Research Settings*. Cambridge, U.K.: Cambridge University Press, 1990.

Texas. "Midwifery Act." Statute 4512i. Amended by Chapter 337. 1993.

Torstendahl, Rolf. "Introduction: Promotion and Strategies of Knowledge-Based Groups." *The Formation of Professions: Knowledge, State and Strategy*. Ed. Rolf Torstendahl and Michael Burrage. London: Sage, 1990, 1–10.

Treffers, Pieter, Martine Easkes, Gunilla Kleiverda, and Dik van Alten. "Home Births and Minimal Medical Interventions." *JAMA* 264.17 (November 7, 1990): 2203, 2207–2208.

Treichler, Paula. "Feminism, Medicine, and the Meaning of Childbirth." *Body/Politics: Women and the Discourses of Science*. Ed. Mary Jacobus, Evelyn Fox Keller, and Sally Shuttleworth. New York: Routledge, 1990, 113–138.

Trimbur, John. "Consensus and Difference in Collaborative Learning." *College English* 51 (1989): 602–616.

Tulip, Rosalyn. "Regional Reports. Region 4, Midwest." *MANA News* (Midwives' Alliance of North America, Newton, Kan.) (November 1994): 7–10.

Turkle, Sherry. "Computational Reticence: Why Women Fear the Intimate Machine." *Technology and Women's Voices: Keeping in Touch*. Ed. Cheris Kramarae. New York: Routledge and Kegan Paul, 1988, 41–61.

———. *Life on the Screen: Identity in the Age of the Internet*. New York: Simon and Schuster, 1995.

Turkle, Sherry, and Seymour Papert. "Epistemological Pluralism: Styles and Voices within the Computer Culture." *Signs* 16.1 (1990): 128–157.

Tyson, Holliday. "Outcomes of 1001 Midwife-Attended Home Births in Toronto, 1983–1988." *Birth* 18.1 (March 1991): 14–19.

Van Blarcom, Carolyn Conant. "Midwives in America." *American Journal of Public Health* 4 (March 1914): 197–207. Reprinted in Litoff, Judy Barrett, ed. *The American Midwife Debate: A Sourcebook on Its Modern Origins*. New York: Greenwood Press, 1986, 117–176.

Van Pelt, William, and Alice Gillam. "Peer Collaboration and the Computer-Assisted Classroom: Bridging the Gap between Academia and the Workplace." *Collaborative Writing in Industry: Investigations in Theory and Practice*. Ed. Mary M. Lay and William M. Karis. Amityville, N.Y.: Baywood, 1991, 170–205.

Varney, Helen. *Nurse Midwifery* 2nd ed. Oxford, U.K.: Blackwell Scientific, 1987.

Wajcman, Judy. *Feminism Confronts Technology*. University Park: Pennsylvania State University Press, 1991.

Washington Department of Health. "The Laws Relating to Midwifery." Chapter 18.50 RCW, July 1992.

Weitz, Rose. "English Midwives and the Association of Radical Midwives." *Women & Health* 12.1 (1987): 79–89.

Wertz, Richard W., and Dorothy C. Wertz. *Lying-In: A History of Childbirth in America*. New York: The Free Press, 1977.

Wiener, Harvey S. "Collaborative Learning in the Classroom: A Guide to Evaluation." *College English* 48.1 (1986): 52–61.

Willughby, Percival. *Observations in Midwifery. As Also the countrey Midwifes Opusculum or Vade Mecum*. Ed. H. Blenkinsop. Warwick, U.K.: H. T. Cooke and Son, 1863.

Wilson, Adrian. *The Making of Man-Midwifery: Childbirth in England, 1660–1770*. Cambridge, Mass.: Harvard University Press, 1995.

Wilson, Deborah S., and Christine Moneera Laennec. *Bodily Discursions: Genders, Representations, Technologies*. Albany, N.Y.: SUNY Press, 1997.

Winsor, Dorothy. "Constructing Scientific Knowledge in Gould and Lewontin's 'The Spandrels of San Marco.'" *Understanding Scientific Prose*. Ed. Jack Selzer. Madison: University of Wisconsin Press, 1993, 127–143.

———. *Writing Like an Engineer: A Rhetorical Education*. Mahwah, N.J.: Lawrence Erlbaum, 1996.

"Women's Health Care Initiative: The ACNM Commitment to Excellence." *MANA News* (Midwives' Alliance of North America, Newton, Kan.) (July 1995): 1, 17.

Wyoming Board of Medicine. Phone Interview, May 25, 1995.

Ziegler, Charles Edward "The Elimination of the Midwife." *JAMA* 60 (January 4, 1913): 32–38.

INDEX

Abbott, Andrew, 28, 102, 130, 151, 191
abortion, 23
American College of Nurse-Midwives
(ACNM), 7; Certification Council and
Division of Accreditation, 8; and the
Certified Midwife, 8, 27; representative
to Minnesota midwifery hearings, ix, 8,
10, 149
American College of Obstetrics and
Gynecology, 67, 127; California
Chapter, 73; Minnesota Chapter, 11,
124; representative to Minnesota
midwifery hearings, 11, 139
American Medical Association, attitude
toward midwifery in 1912, 64;
California Chapter, 72; involvement in
repeal of Sheppard-Towner Act, 65–66.
See also Minnesota Medical Association
Aristotle, 20, 22, 46
Arms, Suzanne, 67
asphyxia, 195
athletic trainers, in Minnesota, 114–115
Aveling, J. J., 58

"Baker, Connie," 109, 110, 135, 143, 163,
176, 177, 178, 179, 185, 202
Baker, S. Josephine, 62, 209 n. 10
Balsamo, Anne, 20, 22, 171
Bell, Vicki, 88
bifurcated consciousness, 85
bi-manual compression, 195
biopower, 173
birth: abnormalcy, 11, 22; high-risk, 11;
normalcy of, 5, 10, 18, 22, 23, 44, 64,

90, 92. *See also* normalization, of birth;
technologies, of birth
birth stories, 68–69, 70–71, 76, 118, 170.
See also knowledge, through birth
stories; midwifery practice, modern
direct-entry, and birth stories
body as boundary concept, 171; as cyborg,
23, 172; as machine, 24, 134; social
perceptions of, 23; theories of, 22–25
Boche, Leonard, 80, 114, 163, 164, 203
Borst, Charlotte, 27
boundary-spanning, techniques of, 18, 78,
79–80, 81–87, 92, 101
Bowland et al. v. Municipal Court, 72,
121
Bradley, Robert, 67
breech births, definition, 185. *See also*
midwifery practice, modern direct-entry,
and breech birth; midwifery practice,
pre-twentieth-century, and breech birth
British midwives, licensing of, 44, 58–61,
75, 181
British Nurses' Association, 60
Brown, Jerry (governor of California), 72
Browner, Carole, 31

California Association of Midwives, 73, 74
Carlson, Arne (governor of Minnesota),
185
Cellier, Elizabeth, 19, 44, 49–50, 62, 75,
108, 115, 170, 180, 181, 209 n. 6
Central Midwives' Board, 60
Certified Nurse-Midwife (CNM). *See*
nurse-midwife